Human *in Vitro* Fertilization and Embryo Transfer

Human *in Vitro* Fertilization and Embryo Transfer

Edited by
Don P. Wolf
and
Martin M. Quigley
University of Texas Health Science Center
Houston, Texas

Plenum Press • New York and London

Library of Congress Cataloging in Publication Data

Main entry under title:

Human in vitro fertilization and embryo transfer.

Includes bibliographical references and index.
1. Fertilization in vitro, Human 2. Embryo transplantation. I. Wolf, Don P. II. Quigley, Martin M. [DNLM: 1. Fertilization in vitro. 3. Embryo transfer, WQ 205 H9174]
RG135.H86 1984 618.1′78 83-27133

ISBN-13: 978-1-4684-4714-9 e-ISBN-13: 978-1-4684-4712-5
DOI: 10.1007/978-1-4684-4712-5

Softcover reprint of the hardcover 1st edition 1984

A Division of Plenum Publishing Corporation
233 Spring Street, New York, N.Y. 10013

FOREWORD

The births of more than 100 apparently normal infants at term following pregnancies initiated by *in vitro* fertilization and embryo transfer testifies to the successful clinical application of insights obtained from studies in reproductive biology over the last 20 years. In women, these studies have included: 1) characterization of the changes in blood hormone profiles throughout ovulatory menstrual cycles; 2) documentation of the hormonal composition of antral fluid in developing and degenerating preovulatory follicles; 3) correlation of these observations with the state of oocyte maturation and the fertilizability of the oocyte; 4) application of pharmacologic agents for perturbing the normal hormone profiles to regulate the number of preovulatory follicles developing and the time of ovulation; and 5) development of non-invasive methods for monitoring follicular development.

Optimizing methods for maturing and fertilizing eggs, for monitoring normal development *in vitro*, and for transferring and achieving implantation of embryos are continuing concerns of physicians and scientists responsible for extant programs. In addition, all serious students of reproductive biology should critically examine every facet of the processes which must concatenate to assure birth of normal infants following pregnancies achieved by these methods.

However, the literature which contains the informational substrate is dispersed widely in a plethora of journals not always readily accessible. Bringing the essentials together facilitates both rapid retrieval of data and access to relevant literature.

In producing such a resource, Wolf and Quigley have relied not only on their own experience in establishing a successful program but also on the skills of colleagues in reproductive biology to produce a review of the state of the art. The results of their efforts should be of particular interest to persons planning to provide *in vitro* fertilization and embryo transfer as therapy for infertility not otherwise treatable.

Finally, while addressing scientific issues, Wolf and Quigley have not ignored the ethical and legal problems arising from *in vitro* fertilization and embryo transfer. Attention to these problems should assist physicians and reproductive scientists in acquiring and maintaining public support for these procedures and the research opportunities they provide.

Griff T. Ross

ACKNOWLEDGMENTS

The development of a program in *in vitro* fertilization and embryo transfer, encompassing both a clinical service for the treatment of infertile couples and a research effort in basic reproductive biology, could not have been accomplished without the assistance and expertise of many devoted individuals, not the least of which are the patients, who by their participation expressed confidence not only in *in vitro* fertilization and embryo transfer as a viable treatment modality, but also in our ability to provide this service.

Obviously, most of the authors of this text have been and are continuing to be active members in this program. On behalf of these authors and ourselves, we wish to acknowledge those who have played a role in this program.

This endeavor was undertaken with the full support and encouragement of Dr. Berel Held, the former Chairman of the Department of Obstetrics and Gynecology at The University of Texas Health Science Center at Houston. Dr. Held graciously provided the departmental resources necessary for personnel recruitment and equipment purchases, and met the laboratory space needs of this program.

We wish to thank Dr. Alex Lopata of the University of Melbourne who visited this Institution in 1981 and provided helpful suggestions prior to our first treatment cycles. Additionally, we wish to thank Dr. Roger Pepperill, Chairman of the Department of Obstetrics and Gynecology at the University of Melbourne, who made possible a visit by one of us (MMQ) to Australia, as well as to Drs. Ian Johnston and Alan Trounson who generously shared their time, knowledge and expertise during that visit.

The assistance provided by the Committee for the Protection of Human Subjects of The University of Texas Health Science Center is also acknowledged, especially that of Drs. William Fields and Samuel Dreizen, as well as Mrs. Paula Knudson.

We have been fortunate over the past several years to have had an outstanding group of professionals associated with our IVF-ET program. The enthusiastic support and expertise shared by Griff T. Ross, M.D., Ph.D. is gratefully acknowledged. In the outpatient facilities and in the operating room these individuals include: Terri Benter, R.N., Sue Chambers, R.N., Tressie Dunlap, L.V.N., Sandy Hardwick, R.N., Kathleen Karlman, R.N., Barbara Miller, Marilyn Siebel, L.V.N., Margaret Sissons, L.V.N., Roxanne Watkins, R.N., Taryn Wilbur, R.N. and Shelly Willis, R.N.

The Endocrine Laboratory, now directed by Albert Berkowitz, Ph.D., has had excellent technical assistance by Stephanie Gilbert, Nancy Shih, Kari Tate, Susan Wilbourne, and Che-Sen Wan. In the Embryo Culture Laboratory, a special note of appreciation is expressed to Pramila Dandekar. Pramila, who is now involved in the IVF-ET program at the University of California in San Francisco, was instrumental in establishing our initial laboratory protocols and in applying the preimplantation mouse embryo bioassay to the assessment of culture conditions. More recently, both Denise Ochs, Ph.D., and Eve Shen have made contributions to the staffing of the embryo culture facilities. Appreciation is also expressed to Ruby Shorter who has responded promptly and appropriately to our requirements for glassware processing and in maintaining sterile inventories of our specialized supplies.

We wish to acknowledge the contribution of Herbert Fritche, Ph.D. of The University of Texas M.D. Anderson Tumor Institute, who has provided sensitive assays for hCG and to Sidney Bottoms, M.D. and Glen Tse who provided statistical expertise. Jane Barnett and Susan Ward have consistently, cheerfully and resourcefully dealt with our often unusual and more often "emergency" purchasing needs. Gail Coppersmith and Robin Judy in the Ultrasound Division of the Department of Radiology are also recognized for their role in providing daily ultrasonograms, as is Rose Griswold, who filled a dual role as patient financial counselor as well as organizer of treatment records.

Special thanks belong to Charlie Anderson for his advice concerning the computer applications. Charlie is responsible for designing the first set of computer data forms used in our record keeping.

Appreciation is expressed to Mrs. Pierre Soupart who graciously donated to this Department all of her late husband's photomicrographs, several of which are published for the first time in Chapter 12. Many companies have donated or loaned equipment during the initial phase of our program while others have custom designed or custom modified the specialized instrumentation necessary in this new enterprise. Among companies deserving of mention are Forma Scientific (micro-processor gas mixing incubator, oxygen monitor), Monoject Division of Sherwood Medical (Tomcat catheters), MicroPro (InfoStar), Olympus of America (loan of laparoscopic video equipment). In addition, William Merz, President of American V. Mueller, has been most helpful with the custom design and fabrication of embryo transfer catheter guides and aspiration needle cannulas. Russell Pelham, Ph.D., and Benjamin Duce of Serono Laboratories have been helpful in securing the IND documentation necessary for the use of Serophene and Pergonal in our research protocols.

The Office of Public Affairs of The University of Texas Health Science Center, particularly Ina Fried and Joe Sigler, has been helpful in all our media relations. The Media Production Department and UTHSC-TV have been impressive in their production of top quality work.

Appreciation is also expressed to the secretarial staff, Beth Johnson, Sandra League, Nancy Mann, Anna Miller, and Wanda Smith, not only for assistance in the production of this text but also in the preparation of innumerable letters, notes, abstracts and manuscripts emanating from this IVF-ET program. Last but by no means least, a special acknowledgement goes to Gail Alexander and Marjorie Stringer. These capable ladies have not only done more than their share of secretarial work, but their efforts have been critical to the production of this text. In addition, Marjorie somehow finds the time to be a constant source of information and support to those patients involved in our program.

Finally, a note of deep appreciation goes to our families for their tolerance and understanding, for inevitably, an undertaking of the present magnitude impacts on family life.

Don P. Wolf
Martin M. Quigley
October, 1983

CONTENTS

1

HISTORICAL BACKGROUND AND ESSENTIALS FOR A PROGRAM IN *IN VITRO* FERTILIZATION AND EMBRYO TRANSFER

Don P. Wolf and Martin M. Quigley

In the last 18 months, explosive growth has occurred around the world in the establishment of programs offering *in vitro* fertilization-embryo transfer (IVF-ET) as a treatment modality for certain types of human infertility. One of the characteristics of a rapid growth phase in the application of a relatively sophisticated new technology is a lack of standardization in approaches as well as a predominence of ancedotal accounts of results. Only now, after several years, are we beginning to see the establishment of a suitable reference base. This includes the excellent general work by R. G. Edwards entitled "Conception in the Human Female" which provides an extensive description of the endocrinology, physiology and morphology of reproductive events in the human (Edwards, 1980). Additionally, several symposia proceedings are now available (Edwards and Purdy, 1982; Beier and Lindner, 1983; Crosgnani and Rubin, 1983) which provide a great deal of useful information relating specifically to aspects of IVF-ET as conducted by individual programs. To date, however, there is not yet available a reference with sufficient detailed information from any one program to be suitable for those groups planning or establishing IVF-ET programs. The present effort was undertaken with two objectives foremost. Firstly, the provision of a current review or summary of those areas of human reproductive physiology most relevant to IVF-ET. This objective is represented by chapters on the hypothalamic control of the menstrual cycle (Chapter 4), maturation of the follicular microenvironment (Chapter 5), sperm capacitation (Chapter 11), oogenesis, fertilization and development (Chapter 12) and implantation (Chapter 16). These chapters are also designed to provide sufficient understanding of "normal" events in human reproductive physiology to appreciate the extent of disruption inherent in IVF-ET. Extensive bibliographic citations have been encouraged to give credit to the large number of individuals who have made significant contributions and to encourage the reader to explore these subjects further. Secondly, the most immediate purpose of this text was to provide a complete description of all areas of a single IVF-ET program. A practical manual, if you will, which describes all areas of an IVF-ET program including patient selection and screening (Chapter 3), the use of clomiphene citrate (Chapter 6) and menopausal gondotrophins (Chapter 7) in follicular recruitment, the monitoring of follicular recruitment by ultrasonography (Chapter 8) and by peripheral estrogen determination (Chapter 9), laparoscopic follicular aspiration (Chapter 10), laboratory details (Chapter 13), techniques in embryo transfer (Chapter 15), program coordination (Chapter 18) and data processing (Chapter 19). Our intentions, in addition to providing a reference source for groups involved in IVF-ET, is to encourage the detailed accounting of IVF-ET programs such that we can move towards a standardization of procedures. We have also included chapters on the legal and ethical considerations of IVF-ET and related technologies. Appendicies have been used to incorporate a complete listing of the items of equipment, supplies and chemicals utilized by our program as well as specific addresses of our suppliers and ordering information. Most of the authors contributing to this text have purposefully been chosen from individuals directly involved in the in vitro fertilization and embryo transfer program of the Department of Obstetrics and Gynecology of The University of Texas Medical School at Houston. This decision was predicated on the desire to provide a unified, comprehensive description of all aspects of one program.

HISTORICAL BACKGROUND

As a prerequisite to successful IVF-ET, it was, of course, necessary to develop, in the laboratory, conditions supportive of preimplantational development. While this subject will not be treated in detail here, it is appropriate to at least direct the reader to reviews of the subject. Extensive experimentation in the mouse and rabbit, primarily, has led to an appreciation of the role of a number of parameters in preimplantation embryonic growth including, pH, osmolarity, gas atmosphere, metabolic and ion requirements, and macromolecular components (Brinster and Troike, 1979; Biggers, 1979; Brackett, 1981).

The in vitro fertilization of mammalian ova enjoys a surprisingly long history. The earliest attempts summarized by

Thibault (1969), date back to 1878 (Shenk, 1878), and include experiments in both the rabbit, most notably by Pincus and co-workers, and the human, by Rock and Menkin. However, the first confirmed success was not recorded until 1959 when M.C. Chang reported his work in the rabbit. Chang utilized genetic markers to provide irrefutable proof that mother and offspring were different, the latter the product of IVF-ET (Table 1). It is appropriate that the first confirmed in vitro fertilization and embryo transfer be attributed to M.C. Chang, for his pioneering studies in the laboratory of Gregory Pincus set the stage for much that has followed. For instance, the technique of mounting a group of intact eggs on a slide for subsequent scoring was reported by Chang in 1952, as was a technique for spreading the whole blastocyst for the examination of histological details (Chang, 1952 and 1954). Another factor which almost certainly contributed to the success of in vitro fertilization of mammalian eggs was the observation that sperm require pretreatment, normally in the female genital tract, before they are capable of fertilizing an egg. This process, termed capacitation, was discovered simultaneously by Chang and Austin in 1951. While an awareness of the phenomenon of capacitation was critical to the success of early attempts at in vitro fertilization, our understanding of the molecular-level events associated with capacitation is still very limited. What we do know is discussed in detail in Chapter 11. The next species to succumb to the new developing technology was the hamster. Successful in vitro fertilization was reported in 1964, again eminating from M.C. Chang's laboratory in collaboration with Yanagimachi (1964), followed successively by the mouse in 1968; and then, perhaps somewhat surprisingly, by the in vitro fertilization of human oocytes (Edwards et al., 1969). It is interesting to note that the development of non-human primate models has lagged far behind the work occurring in humans. The first reported success with non-human primates was with the squirrel monkey in 1973 followed only very recently by the baboon, the chimpanzee, the cynomolgus and the rhesus monkey. While it may appear at first glance that the human served as a model for the non-human primate, it is hoped that these sub-human primate model systems will be highly valuable to the further improvement of protocols in human IVF-ET.

HUMAN IVF-ET

Ovarian oocytes of most mammals, at birth, are arrested in the prophase of meiosis-I (dictytate or germinal vesicle stage). In the hours between the LH surge and ovulation the first meiotic division is resumed and completed, and the second meiotic division is initiated. This resumption of meiosis is termed preovulatory

Table 1. Chronology of mammalian *in vitro* fertilization

Year	Species	Reference
1878–1958	Unconfirmed attempts at IVF	Summarized by Thibault, 1969
1959	Rabbit	Chang, 1959
1964	Hamster	Yanagimachi and Chang, 1964
1968	Mouse	Whittingham, 1968
1969	Human	Edwards et al., 1969
1970	Cat	Hamner et al., 1970
1972	Guinea Pig	Yanagimachi, 1972
1973	Rat	Miyamoto and Chang, 1973
1973	Squirrel Monkey	Gould et al., 1973
1977	Cow	Iritani and Niwa, 1977
1978	Pig	Iritani et al., 1978
1979	Baboon	Gould, 1979
1982	Cynomolgus Monkey	Kreitmann et al., 1982
1983	Rhesus Monkey	Bavister et al., 1983
1983	Chimpanzee	Gould, 1983

maturation and requires approximately 24 to 36 hours in the human (Edwards, 1975; Chapter 12). A second meiotic arrest occurs prior to ovulation in most mammals at metaphase II. Normally, completion of meiosis is dependent upon sperm-egg fusion at fertilization. It has been known for many years that, when oocytes are removed from the follicular environment (regardless of the state of the development of the follicle) they will spontaneously mature to metaphase II *in vitro* (Pincus and Saunders, 1939). Beginning in the mid 1960's, several investigators, most prominently Edwards, used this knowledge and attempted the *in vitro* fertilization of human oocytes which had been recovered from excised ovaries and matured *in vitro* (Edwards et al., 1969). While Edwards' efforts met with success, the percentage of fertilization was very low and there was a correspondingly high rate of abnormal fertilizations. At approximately this time, Steptoe was pioneering the use of the laparoscope in gynecology. The application of the laparoscope to oocyte retrieval allowed the collection of human oocytes which had been matured *in vivo*. Insemination of these oocytes resulted in a much higher fertilization rate (Edwards et al., 1970). From 1970 through 1975 Steptoe and Edwards attempted *in vitro* fertilization using a variety of ovulation inducing drugs to time follicular development and to increase the number of recoverable oocytes. However, their only clinical success was a tubal ectopic pregnancy

(Steptoe and Edwards, 1976). By the mid-seventies, they were proceeding on the assumption that the use of ovulation inducing drugs so distorted the hormonal environment that the establishment of a pregnancy following in vitro fertilization and embryo transfer was impossible. Accordingly, they switched to detecting the onset of the LH surge in a spontaneous menstrual cycle by measurements of urinary LH at three hour intervals. By scheduling a laparoscopic aspiration at 24 to 28 hours after the onset of the spontaneous LH surge, they achieved four pregnancies, the most notable resulting in the birth of the baby Louise Brown on July 25, 1978 (Edwards et al., 1980).

In 1979, a team in Melbourne, Australia formed from both the University of Melbourne and Monash University duplicated Steptoe's and Edwards' success (Lopata et al., 1980). In the next year, the two Melbourne teams, now working independently, established that the clomiphene citrate-stimulated ovulatory cycle (with or without hCG) was compatible with the establishment of pregnancies and in fact they demonstrated that the use of clomiphene resulted in a higher percentage of patients undergoing embryo transfer and hence an increased pregnancy rate overall (Trounson et al., 1981; Johnston et al., 1981). This work contributed substantially to the development of IVF-ET as clomiphene stimulation supports the development of several preovulatory follicles and an increase in the total number of oocytes recovered per patient.

In this country, Howard and Georgianna Jones started a program of IVF-ET in 1980. This program pioneered the exclusive use of hMG in follicular recruitment and served to introduce the developing technology to the American public.

At this writing, there are a multitude of groups around the world involved in IVF-ET with live births resulting from at least five programs in the U.S.A. and others in Australia, France, West Germany, England, and Austria. The vast majority of these successful pregnancies have resulted from oocyte retrieval performed during the course of a stimulated ovulatory cycle.

ESSENTIALS OF A PROGRAM FOR IVF-ET

Treatment of human infertility by IVF-ET requires a unique cooperation of both basic scientists and clinicians. At the present time, the success rate for IVF-ET is relatively low and there are marked differences among established groups in the treatment protocols utilized. As experience is gained around the world, however, it is expected that there will be additional changes and refinements of treatment protocols and a continued increase in the clinical pregnancy rate. At the present time, IVF-ET is still investigational and repeated success requires the integrated cooperation of a large team representing many different disciplines.

During the course of a treatment cycle, an IVF-ET program must function seven days a week. Accordingly, it is necessary that there be at least two, if not three, individuals fully capable of performing each of the functions involved in the treatment program. First, there must be a trained reproductive endocrinologist able to supervise the management and monitoring of follicular development. Second, there must be an experienced laparoscopist, able to perform both oocyte recoveries and embryo transfers. There must be surgical facilities with anesthesia coverage for oocyte retrieval seven days per week. The embryo laboratory should be supervised by an individual with advanced knowledge of and experience in mammalian reproductive physiology. Obviously all technicians involved in media preparation, gamete and embryo handling must be appropriately trained. As part of the monitoring of follicular development, there must be available the capabilities for daily follicular ultrasonographic measurements and radioimmunoassays for luteinizing hormone and estradiol. Finally, a clinical coordinator is highly desirable if not absolutely essential to an IVF-ET program.

In our view, the above constitutes the minimum requirements for an active IVF-ET program designed primarily to provide a service to the infertile couple. In an academic setting, of course, additional requirements would be tailored to the specific needs and research interests of the team.

SUMMARY AND CONCLUSIONS

Treatment of human infertility by in vitro fertilization and embryo transfer is still in its developmental stages. Successful application of these techniques requires a multidisciplinary team approach with integration of basic science and clinical experience. As these technologies are rapidly developing, the team should have the experience and capability necessary to evaluate and change the treatment protocols as needed. This text is intended as a reference source to provide both a comprehensive summary of the physiologic processes involved in follicular growth, oocyte maturation, capacitation, and fertilization, as well as a practical description of the clinical and laboratory aspects of a functioning IVF-ET program.

REFERENCES

Austin, C.R., 1951, Observations on the penetration of the sperm into the mammalian egg, Aust. J. Sci. Res. Ser. B, 4:581.

Bavister, B.D., Boatman, D.E., Leibfried, L., Loose, M., and Vernon, M.W., 1983, Fertilization and cleavage of rhesus monkey oocytes in vitro, Biol. Reprod., 28:983.

Beier, H.M., Lindner, H.R., eds., 1983, "Fertilization of the Human Egg In Vitro: Biologic Basis and Clinical Application," Berlin, Springer-Verlag.

Biggers, J.D., 1979, Fertilization and blastocyst formation, in: "Animal Models for Research on Contraception and Fertility," N.J. Alexander, ed., Harper & Row, New York.

Brackett, B.G., 1981, Applications of in vitro fertilization, in: "New Technologies in Animal Breeding," B.G. Brackett, G.E. Seidel, Jr., and S.M. Seidel, eds., Academic Press, New York.

Brinster, R.L., and Troike, D.E., 1979, Requirements for blastocyst development in vitro, J. Anim. Sci., 49:308

Chang, M.C., 1951, Fertilizing capacity of spermatozoa deposited into the fallopian tubes, Nature, (London), 168:697.

Chang, M.C., 1952, Fertilizability of rabbit ova and effects of temperature in vitro on their subsequent fertilization and activation in vitro, J. Exp. Zool., 121:351.

Chang, M.C., 1954, Development of parthenogenetic rabbit blastocysts induced by low temperature storage of unfertilized ova, J. Exp. Zool., 125:127.

Chang, M.C., 1959, Fertilization of rabbit ova in vitro, Nature, (London) 184:466.

Crosignani, P.G., and Rubin, B.L., eds., 1983, "In Vitro Fertilization and Embryo Transfer," Academic Press, London.

Edwards, R.G., 1975, Physiological aspects of human embryo transfer, in: "Progress in Infertility," S.J. Behrman and R.W. Kistner, eds., Boston, Little, Brown.

Edwards, R.G., and Purdy, J.M., eds., 1982, "Human Conception In Vitro," London, Academic Press.

Edwards, R.C., 1980, "Conception in the Human Female," Academic Press, New York.

Edwards, R.G., Bavister, B.D., and Steptoe, P.C., 1969, Early stages of fertilization in vitro of human oocytes matured in vitro, Nature (London), 221:632.

Edwards, R.G., Steptoe, P.C., and Purdy, J.M., 1970, Fertilization and cleavage in vitro of preovulator human oocytes, Nature, (London)227:1307.

Edwards, R.G., Steptoe, P.C., and Purdy, J.M., 1980, Establishing full-term human pregnancies using cleaving embryos grown in vitro, Brit. J. Obstet. Gynaecol., 87:737.

Gould, K.G., Cline, E.M. and Williams, W.L., 1973, Observations on the induction of ovulation and fertilization in vitro in the squirrel monkey (Saimiri sciureus), Fertil. Steril., 24:260.

Gould, K.G., 1979, Fertilization in vitro of non-human primate ova: present status and rational for further development of the technique, in: "Report to the Ethics Advisory Board, Appendix: HEW Support of Research Involving Human In Vitro Fertilization Embryo Transfer," U.S. Gov. Printing Off., Washington, D.C..

Gould, K.G., 1983, Ovum recovery and in vitro fertilization in the chimpanzee, Fertil. Steril., 40:378.

Hamner, C.E., Jennings, L.L. and Sojka, N.J., 1970, Cat (felis katus) spermatozoa require capacitation, J. Reprod. Fertil., 23:477.

Iritani, A., and Niwa, K., 1977, Capacitation of bull spermatozoa and fertilization in vitro of cattle follicular oocytes matured in culture, J. Reprod. Fertil., 50:119.

Iritani, A., Niwa, K., Imai, H., 1978, Sperm penetration in vitro of pig follicular oocytes matured in culture, J. Reprod. Fertil., 54:379.

Johnston, I., Lopata, A., Speirs, A., Hoult, I., Kellow, G., and DuPlessis, Y., 1981, In vitro fertilization: The challenge of the eighties, Fertil. Steril., 36:699.

Kreitmann, O., Lynch, A., Nixon, W.E. and Hodgen, G.D., 1982, Ovum collection, induced luteal dysfunction, in vitro fertilization, embryo development and low tubal ovum transfer in primates, in: "In Vitro Fertilization and Embryo Transfer," E.S.E. Hafez and K. Semm, eds., MTP Press Ltd., Lancaster.

Lopata, A., Johnston, I.W.H., Hoult, I.J., Speirs, A.I., 1980, Pregnancy following intrauterine implantation of an embryo obtained by in vitro fertilization of a preovulatory egg, Fertil. Steril., 33:117.

Miyamoto, H., and Chang, M.C., 1973, Fertilization of rat eggs in vitro, Biol. Reprod., 9:384.

Pincus, G., and Saunders, B., 1939, The comparative behavior of mammalian eggs in vivo and in vitro VI. The maturation of human ovarian ova, Anat. Rec., 75:537.

Shenk, S.L., 1878, Das Saugetierdi Kunstlich befruchtet ausserhalb der Muttertieres, Mitt. Embryol. Inst. Univ. Wien, 1877.

Steptoe, P.C., and Edwards, R.G., 1976, Reimplantation of a human embryo with subsequent tubal pregnancy, Lancet, 7:880.

Thibault, C., 1969, Fertilization of the mammalian egg, in: "Fertilization," Vol. 2, C.B. Metz and A. Monroy, eds., Academic Press, New York.

Trounson, A.O., Leeton, J.F., Wood, C., Webb, J. and Wood, J., 1981, Pregnancies in humans by fertilization in vitro and embryo transfer in the controlled ovulatory cycle, Science, 212:681.

Whittingham, D.G., 1968, Fertilization of mouse eggs in vitro, Nature (London), 220:592.

Yanagimachi, R., and Chang, M.C., 1964, In vitro fertilization of hamster ova, J. Exp. Zool., 156:361.
Yanagimachi, R., 1972, Fertilization of guinea pig eggs in vitro, Anat. Rec., 174:9.

2

LEGAL ISSUES RAISED BY IN VITRO FERTILIZATION AND EMBRYO TRANSFER

Lori B. Andrews

The successful clinical application of in vitro fertilization has given rise to a brave new legal field. As more actors have become involved in the drama of reproduction, various legal precedents have been consulted to sort out the rights and responsibilities of the doctors, gamete donors, and couples participating in the process, as well as the rights of the children created by this technique. Alternatives to in vitro fertilization (such as in vivo fertilization with embryo transfer) and research applications of in vitro fertilization raise additional legal issues.

There are numerous statutes and regulations that can affect in vitro fertilization: laws governing fetal research, the protection of human subjects, artificial insemination, paternity, and adoption. In addition, some states have adopted specific in vitro fertilization laws. Yet the process raises far more sophisticated legal issues than these laws are able to handle. In particular, many of these statutes may violate the constitutional rights of privacy of the couples seeking to conceive through in vitro fertilization.

CONSTITUTIONAL BASIS OF THE RIGHT TO PROCREATE

The Constitution of the United States gives strong protection to people's procreation decisions. The U.S. Supreme Court has said that both married and single individuals have a right of privacy to be free from governmental intrusion into their decision whether to bear a child.[1]

In a series of cases, the U.S. Supreme Court has struck down state laws that interfered with that decision. The Court struck down an Oklahoma law that required forced sterilization of habitual criminals because the law was an unjust interference with the right to procreate.[2] The Court also struck down state laws that limited access to contraceptives[3] and abortion,[4] on the grounds that such laws interfered with the right to privacy to make procreation decisions.

All of these cases dealt with the right to decide whether or when to bear children. The open question with the new reproductive technologies is: Does the right to privacy also cover a couple's decision how to get pregnant? That is, does an infertile couple have a fundamental privacy right to use in vitro fertilization, either with their own gametes, with those of donors, or with gestation by a surrogate carrier?

A strong privacy argument can be made for these infertility treatments. In most instances, they represent the final step in a couple's lengthy quest for a child that is biologically theirs. Along the way they probably tried surgery and other treatments that were unsuccessful. Thus, a law denying that couple IVF-ET as a treatment would cut off their ability to have a child just as the sterilization proposed in the Oklahoma case would have irrevocably ended the criminal's procreative capabilities.

If a fundamental right to an infertility treatment to start a pregnancy does exist (like the right to an abortion to end one), a state law restricting in vitro fertilization in any manner will be upheld only if the state can prove the law furthers a compelling need in the narrowest way possible. For example, the state might be able to prove that there are compelling reasons to have a law preventing a fertile woman from using in vitro fertilization - for example, where the woman wants to avoid the burden of pregnancy by having her fertilized egg implanted in a paid surrogate. But even if the state had a compelling reason to prevent that type of in vitro fertilization-surrogate carrier arrangement, it could not constitutionally forbid all types of in vitro fertilization, but rather could only prohibit the particular troublesome arrangement.

The general rule is that when a state adopts a law that impinges on reproduction, that law must be a narrow one so that it does not improperly interfere with the couple's right to privacy. However, the constitutional right of privacy does not require that the government fund the medical service that people need to fulfill their procreative choice. For example, even though the constitutional right of privacy prohibits the government from forbidding abortions during the first two trimesters, the government is not constitutionally required to pay for abortions for indigent women.[5] Thus, even if the constitutional right of privacy requires the government to allow in vitro fertilization to take place, it would not require the government to pay for the procedure for poor couples.

LAWS REGARDING WHETHER IVF MAY TAKE PLACE

When abortion was legalized in the mid-1970's, legislators felt that in order for people to maintain respect for human dignity, it was necessary to pass laws restricting experimentation on abortuses or on pregnant women who intended to abort. In 1975, the National Commission for the Protection of Human Subjects of Biomedical and Behavioral Research published recommendations governing research with fetuses.[6] The Commission concluded that fetal research was ethically acceptable only if appropriate prior research with animals and nonpregnant humans had been undertaken, the knowledge sought by the research was important and unobtainable by alternative means, the risks and benefits to the mother and fetus of the research had been analyzed and described, proper informed consent was obtained and the subjects of the research were equitably selected. The Commission's report led to the adoption of federal regulations covering federally funded fetal experimentation;[7] however, these regulations do not extend to in vitro fertilization because they define a "fetus" as beginning with implantation.[8]

In the wake of the Roe v. Wade abortion decision[4] and the Commission's report, 23 states have adopted laws governing fetal research.[9] Rather than taking the Commission's approach of spelling out the circumstances in which fetal research may take place, most of these state laws delineate broad prohibitions against fetal research. In addition, unlike the federal regulations, many of the state laws potentially cover in vitro fertilization. Fifteen states explicitly extend their coverage to research on embryos.[10] In eight other states, the term "fetus" is not defined sufficiently to determine whether or not the law applies to the preimplantation embryo.[11]

Of the 23 states with fetal research laws, 11 cover such research only where it is done at a time when abortion is anticipated or subsequent to an abortion.[12] Others cover only research with a fetus that exhibits a heartbeat, spontaneous respiratory activity, spontaneous voluntary muscle movement or pulsation of the umbilical cord.[13] Laws of these two types would not extend their reach to in vitro fertilization since the procedure does not involve an abortion and, by the time the fetus exhibits the capabilities mentioned, it is no longer part of ex utero research but rather is developing in utero in the course of a normal pregnancy.

Laws that ban research on fetuses in a more general manner, however, might preclude the practice of in vitro fertilization. In Michigan, for example, there can be no research on a live human embryo if its life or health may be jeopardized.[14] The Minnesota law forbids experimenting on a living human conceptus, including one conceived outside the body, unless the experiment protects the conceptus' health or life, or scientific evidence has shown that sort of experimentation to be harmless.[15] In Rhode Island, there can be no experimentation on a live human embryo before or after expulsion from the mother's womb.[16]

The laws restricting fetal research present an even greater potential barrier to an alternative to in vitro fertilization, in vivo fertilization followed by embryo transfer. The latter technique may be requested by a woman who is infertile because she has no ovaries, no ova, inaccessible ovaries, or a genetic defect she does not wish to pass on. Her husband's sperm can be used to inseminate another woman who will carry the embryo for five days. At the end of that period of time, the embryo will be flushed out of the woman's uterus and then implanted in the uterus of the previously infertile woman. There have already been two reported pregnancies through the use of this technique.[17]

Embryo transfer after in vivo fertilization is within the reach of the fetal research statutes in a number of states. Louisiana law, for example. prohibits the "conduct on a human embryo or fetus in utero, of any experiment or study except to preserve the life or improve the health of said human embryo or fetus."[18]

In at least 17 other states, the statutes regulating fetal research might also prohibit the practice of embryo transfer after in vivo fertilization.[19] A greater number of statutes would extend regulation to this procedure rather than to in vitro fertilization because, under many of these laws, the definition of abortion would seem to encompass the flushing technique used in embryo transfer. Hence, where in vitro fertilization is untouched by statutes that limit their scope to research on the fetus aborted or intended to be aborted, in vivo fertilization and embryo transfer appears to qualify in some states as experimentation or research in connection with an abortion.

Intuitively it may seem that embryo transfer should not fall within these statutes. Indeed, the federal guidelines for federally-funded fetal research do not cover the practice since abortion is defined as the termination of pregnancy, and pregnancy is understood as beginning at implantation. If the state statutes followed these provisions, the flushing of a fertilized ovum before implantation would not be considered an abortion, and embryo transfer, like in vitro fertilization, would not be covered by the statutes regulating research in connection with an abortion. However, some state laws (as well as some cases) define pregnancy as starting with fertilization and abortion as the extraction or expulsion of the product of conception.[20] For example, in Oklahoma, an abortion includes the administration of any substance intended to cause expulsion of a conceptus, zygote, morula, blastocyst, or embryo.[21] Similarly, in Wyoming, the definition of abortion covers any procedure administered to a woman carrying an embryo or fetus with the intent of producing the premature expulsion, removal or termination of that embryo or fetus.[22] Statutes with definitions such as these would cover the technique of embryo transfer, as would more general statutes prohibiting experimenting on embryos.

The fetal research laws are also broad enough in some states to put restraints on the women whose ovum are fertilized and transferred. If such women are paid a certain fee per cycle to participate in the research, they might be affected by the laws of two states prohibiting a woman from selling a fetus for experimentation.[23] The laws of an additional eight states reach even women who merely give away[24] or permit[25] someone to use a fetus.

While the fetal research statutes were enacted without recognition of the potential of in vitro or in vivo fertilization and embryo transfer, more recent state laws specifically single out in vitro fertilization. An in vitro fertilization law was enacted in Pennsylvania to monitor the procedure.[26] The law provides that anyone conducting in vitro fertilization must file quarterly reports with the Department of Health describing the names of everyone conducting or assisting in the process, the locations where the fertilization takes place, names and addresses of the individuals or institutions sponsoring the procedures, the number of eggs fertilized, the number of embryos destroyed or discarded and the number of women implanted with embryos. However, the names of the donors or recipients of the gametes are not required.

In Illinois, the legislature adopted a statute that restricts in vitro fertilization in an unusual way.[27] It makes a physician who fertilizes a women's egg outside of her body the custodian of the offspring for purposes of an 1877 child abuse act. The physician is criminally liable if he endangers the life or health of the embryo. Thus, the law doesn't prohibit in vitro fertilization directly, but raises so many concerns in the minds of Illinois physicians that few are willing to undertake the procedure at this point.

It seems incongruous to deal with the modern issue of in vitro fertilization by referring to an 1877 law. When lawmakers in the late 1800's designed that particular child protection law, they expected it to mean that a parent or guardian would provide sufficient food, clothing, and shelter so that a child would remain healthy. But physicians have no idea how prosecutors or judges will interpret this law to cover *in vitro* fertilization. What must a physician do to provide adequate care to a two-cell, four-cell, or eight-cell embryo? Can a physician be prosecuted for child abuse if the district attorney believes the physician should have provided different nutrients in the embryo's medium or should have stored the petri dish with the embryo at a different temperature? Will the physician commit a crime if he discards an embryo that is not dividing properly?

The Illinois law also makes it a crime for the physician to permit anyone else to endanger the individual created by *in vitro* fertilization. It is hard to determine what that means. Must the physician police the conduct of the pregnant woman carrying the fertilized eggs? Must he see to it that she does not drink excessively, smoke, or ride on airplanes? Under the Illinois law, the physician's duties are unclear. He may be susceptible to widespread liability with respect to the actions he takes that affect the embryo.

Several additional laws have been proposed that would also affect *in vitro* or *in vivo* fertilization. The proposed federal Human Life Bill would give all the legal rights of personhood to an embryo from the moment of conception. This would put a clinician offering *in vitro* or *in vivo* fertilization in an uncomfortable position. If anything happened to the embryo, the physician could be charged with murder. Perhaps the physician would be prohibited from undertaking the two procedures altogether since, once the embryo was given the full rights of a human being, its consent to the procedure would be necessary, yet legally impossible to obtain. Although parents often give proxy consent for children, the potential parents of an *in vitro* embryo may be disqualified from consenting on its behalf if they are viewed as having too great a conflict of interest regarding whether the embryo will be conceived.

Another law that has been proposed is one that would provide that *in vitro* fertilization may be performed only if the physician intends to implant all the embryos produced back into the woman. This proposed law may seem infinitely preferable to the law currently in force in Illinois, which subjects the physician to unclear duties with respect to the embryo. But the proposed law imposes undue limitations upon the physician's discretion, since he may feel obligated to evidence his intention by implanting an embryo that is not dividing properly and will not survive (even though such a useless procedure will waste the time of the couple, the physician and his staff, will unnecessarily tie up the operating room and a hospital bed, increase the financial burden on the couple, and carries a small risk that the woman will contract an infection because of the insertion process).

A law requiring the intent to implant all embryos would also serve to stifle in vitro fertilization technology, rather than allowing it to develop in ways to increase a couple's options. Soon, it might be possible for genetic diseases to be detected in an embryo while it is in vitro. Tests could be performed on one cell of the in vitro embryo to determine if it would suffer from particular hereditary diseases or if it had a significant chromosomal abnormality such as Down's Syndrome. If the child did have such a defect, the couple might wish not to have it reimplanted. They should have such a right--after all, they would have a right to abort that same fetus if they learned of the defect five months later through amniocentesis. But a law with an intent requirement might not allow the physician to provide them with that option. The physician might be guilty of a felony if he performed genetic screening on an embryo since those tests could be used as proof that he didn't really intend to implant all embryos created by the procedure.

Likewise, a law with an intent requirement might prevent physicians from offering another option - the freezing of embryos. For years, sperm banks have offered frozen sperm. In this way, a man who is about to start taking drugs that might affect his fertility or a man who works in an environment that might be hazardous to spermatogenesis can have his healthy sperm frozen and later have a physician use them to inseminate the man's wife. But human embryo freezing may run afoul of the proposed law which might require that the physician intend to implant all embryos at the same time, immediately after fertilization.

CHALLENGES TO THE LAW

If a state law appears to impede a new reproductive technology, that does not mean that physicians and couples in that state will have to forego the particular infertility treatment. If the state law is ambiguous or was adopted without specific reference to in vitro or in vivo fertilization, the physician can ask the State Attorney General or State District Attorney for an opinion to learn whether it actually proscribes the procedure. In Massachusetts in May 1983, the District Attorney for the Boston area rendered an opinion that in vitro fertilization would not violate the Massachusetts fetal research statute if all the fertilized eggs used were implanted in the woman.[28] In addition, an argument could be made that *in vitro* fertilization should not be covered by the fetal experimentation statutes at all on the grounds that it is no longer experimental. The Board of Directors of the American Fertility Society at its March 1982 Annual Meeting adopted a resolution endorsing *in vitro* fertilization as "the acceptable treatment for achieving pregnancy for couples whose wives have absent or irreparably damaged fallopian tubes." But even though its therapeutic value is recognized, the process of *in vitro* fertilization is constantly being refined and thus would probably still be viewed as experimental. Newer variations such as embryo freezing or *in vivo* fertilization and embryo transfer would definitely be considered experimental at this point.

If the proposed infertility treatment is definitely prohibited, the physician and the couple who want the treatment could join together in a lawsuit against the state to have the law declared unconstitutional on the grounds that it violates the couple's constitutional right to privacy to decide to bear a child. Such a lawsuit has been instituted to challenge the Illinois *in vitro* law.[29] A couple, Mary and John Smith, and their physician brought suit against the Illinois Attorney General and the prosecuting attorney to prevent them from enforcing the Illinois *in vitro* fertilization law.

"While the legislature apparently views *in vitro* fertilization as a crime," argued the attorneys for the couple, "to many childless couples it is seen as a possible miracle." The attorneys (including this author) asserted that "The *in vitro* provision implicates and eviscerates both marital privacy and the individual privacy right to make and effectuate childbearing decisions. Procreation is universally recognized by every culture and religion as a fundamental element of the institution of marriage. For many married couples it is the essence of family. The desire to produce one's own offspring is, for most couples, as primary as the need to eat or sleep." Because of the constitutional protection given the extremely important childbearing decision, the lawsuit contended that the Illinois law interfering with that decision should be declared unconstitutional.

In response to the suit, the State's Attorney and the Illinois Attorney General rendered an opinion that the physician's actions would only violate the law if he or she willfully endangered or injured the conceptus in the preimplantation stage by abuse, mutilation, extermination or destructive laboratory experimentation. The physician's decision not to reimplant, if done with the mother's permission, would be permissible as a lawful pregnancy termination (akin to the type protected in *Roe v. Wade*[4]).

The argument that a statute prohibiting in vitro fertilization is unconstitutional has also been made by various legal commentators. "Such a law would certainly infringe a fundamental interest of infertile women - their right to bear children," notes Reilly. "It might also infringe the first amendment rights of the clinical researchers by improperly restricting their freedom of inquiry."[30] The same argument could be made against any type of law that inhibits in vitro fertilization even if the law was designed for some other purpose, such as the restriction of fetal research. For if a fundamental privacy right to choose how to bear a child is recognized by the courts, then even laws adopted for other valid purposes will need to be amended so that they are narrow enough just to cover that purpose and not infringe upon in vitro fertilization. As the U.S. Supreme Court has said, the right to procreate is "one of the basic civil rights of man. Marriage and procreation are fundamental to the very existence and survival of the race."[2]

FEDERAL CONSIDERATIONS REGARDING IN VITRO FERTILIZATION

Although the federal regulations covering fetal research do not apply to the conduct of in vitro fertilization, there is a federal regulation that specifically covers proposals for federal funding of in vitro fertilization research. It provides that "No application or proposal involving human in vitro fertilization may be funded by the Department or any components thereof until the application or proposal has been reviewed by the Ethical Advisory Board and the board has rendered advice as to its acceptability from an ethical standpoint."[31] Pursuant to that regulation, an Ethics Advisory Board was appointed in 1977 and considered a proposal by Dr. Pierre Soupart. The Ethics Advisory Board held a series of public hearings during 1978 and 1979 and promulgated a report concluding that research in human in vitro fertilization and federal support of such research is ethically acceptable with certain stipulations. Nevertheless, to this date, no federal money has been awarded for human in vitro fertilization research.

In 1980, the Ethics Advisory Board ceased to exist. In view of the continuation of the requirement that any proposal for research in this area must be reviewed, a de facto moratorium on federally funded research is in place. This moratorium only prevents federal government support of research; it does not limit or regulate research otherwise supported and it does not limit clinical application of in vitro fertilization technology in the treatment of human infertility.

LEGAL CONSIDERATIONS REGARDING HOW IVF SHOULD TAKE PLACE

Even in states where in vitro fertilization is clearly permissible, there are various additional legal and regulatory considerations regarding how the procedure should take place. In addition, the issue of the control over the establishment and continued supervision of in vitro fertilization and embryo transfer clinical and research programs is likely to surface as more physicians and scientists become involved in the procedure. As somewhat of an analogy, human organ transplant programs are more or less self limited by the financial and personnel requirements as well as the fact that a bad outcome presents a substantial risk to the patient (e.g., an unsuccessful heart transplant results in death). Fortunately or unfortunately, in vitro fertilization may be done, or at least attempted, by personnel with little more expertise than the average obstetrical and gynecological training without prohibitive financial and personnel commitments. In this instance an unsuccessful outcome results in little or no physical risk to the patient. Yet concerns about the emotional and financial protection of the patient from improperly undertaken in vitro fertilization will likely lead to proposals to limit who may offer in vitro fertilization. Already, in England, the Royal College of Obstetricians and Gynaecologists (RCOG) Ethics Committee on In Vitro Fertilisation and Embryo Replacement has advocated a requirement that in vitro fertilization clinics be specially licensed and the directors of the facilities be registered.[32] Similarly, at least one American legal commentator has advocated the passage of statutes specifying "the degree of expertise and skill required of any physician undertaking the procedure."[33]

Currently, however, the most significant check on how in vitro fertilization may be undertaken is the Institutional Review Board (IRB) system. The Public Health Service Act requires that any institution that applies for a federal grant or contract involving any research with human subjects have established an Institutional Review Board to review the research in order to protect the rights of the human subjects.[34] Although federal regulations adopted pursuant to the Act[35] do not mandate the review of non-federally funded human research, most institutions require that all research involving human subjects be approved by its Institutional Review Board. In addition, some states have laws requiring the establishment of IRBs.[36] Thus, the fact that an in vitro fertilization project is not receiving federal funds will generally have no bearing on whether it needs to undergo institutional review.

Whether or not a physician's intended plans will need to be submitted to an Institutional Review Board will depend upon the substance of the project. The generally accepted definition of research is "a systematic investigation designed to develop or contribute to general knowledge."[37] If a physician merely wishes to apply the procedures developed elsewhere to the treatment of his infertile patients, probably no Institutional Review Board review would be required. On the other hand, if the physician wished to develop new treatment modalities, or to alter the currently accepted treatment protocols, in all likelihood, Institutional Review Board approval would be required. If the physician merely wished to be able to report the details of his treatment protocol with his outcome, Board approval may or may not be required.

The federal regulations specify what the IRB must consider and must not consider in reviewing a research proposal. Although these guidelines were designed to cover federally-funded research, the IRB probably will apply similar guidelines to a physician's proposal to undertake in vitro fertilization. The guidelines specify that research must be designed so that risks are minimized and are reasonable in relation to anticipated benefits, selection of subjects is equitable, informed consent is gained according to specific guidelines and is documented, the data is monitored to insure the safety of the subjects, and the privacy of the subjects and the confidentiality of the data is maintained.[38] The regulations also provide that in an in vitro fertilization proposal, there be additional protections such as adequate consideration to the selection of potential subjects and monitoring of the actual consent process.[39]

One provision of the federal regulations would discourage the IRB from debating the societal side effects of in vitro fertilization research. According to the regulations, "The IRB should not consider possible long-range effects of applying knowledge gained in the research (for example, the possible effects of the research on public policy) as among those research risks that fall within the purview of its responsibility."[40]

PHYSICIANS' LEGAL RESPONSIBILITIES

Once a program has been established within the bounds of the state statutes and, if applicable, according to the specification of an Institutional Review Board, the physician's main legal responsibilities concern his relationship with the patients, donors, and the embryo.

With respect to patient selection, a physician who is not affiliated with a governmental institution may generally legally turn down patients for any reason. However, an in vitro fertilization program affiliated with a city, county, or state facility must insure that the patient's constitutional rights are respected. Although the federal Ethics Advisory Board recommended that embryos be transferred only into married couples, such a limitation might be an unconstitutional deprivation of equal protection to unmarried infertile individuals. Since unmarried, infertile couples do not differ from married infertile couples on a medical basis, unmarried infertile couples could argue that such a limitation abridges their right of procreation. Already there has been an analogous case in which a 36-year-old woman sued Wayne State University's donor artificial insemination (AID) clinic because it restricted AID to married couples.[41] The suit was settled prior to trial with the University's agreement to drop this requirement.

In contrast to patient limitations based on social criteria, a limitation of program participants based on medical decisions is premissible. Specifically, this permits a program to deny treatment to patients with one diagnosis, for example, unexplained infertility, while treating couples with another factor, such as tubal damage, as the explanation for the infertility.

As women without oocytes, or without accessible oocytes and as men with azosperimia are medically separable from other individuals, it is permissible for an in vitro fertilization program to exclude couples in which the gametes cannot be obtained from the partners. However, there is nothing to prevent the program from utilizing donated oocytes and/or sperm if they so desire. There has already been one reported case in which pregnancy resulted from fertilization of a donated oocyte with frozen banked human sperm and reimplantation into an unrelated woman's uterus.[42]

After admitting patients into the program, the physician is obligated to obtain informed consent before initiating any procedures. The physician should explain to the couple what the process entails, what the risks are and if there are any alternatives to in vitro fertilization that would allow the couple to conceive. It is also important to give the couple a realistic estimate of the success rate of in vitro fertilization.

Physicians offering in vitro fertilization are not legally required to meet the federal regulations governing informed consent in governmentally funded research on pregnant women or fetuses,[43] but these regulations can provide a guideline for physicians who are trying to design adequate informed consent forms in this sensitive area. These requirements include a statement that the study involves research, an explanation of the purposes of the research and the expected duration of the subject's participation, a description of the procedures to be followed, and identification of any procedures which are experimental; a description of any reasonably foreseeable risks or discomforts to the subject; a description of any benefits to the subject or to others which may reasonably be expected from the research; a disclosure of appropriate alternative procedures or courses of treatment, if any, that might be advantageous to the subject; a statement describing the extent, if any, to which confidentiality of records identifying the subject will be maintained; and a statement that the particular treatment or procedure may involve risks to the subject (or to the embryo or fetus) which are currently unforeseeable. (An example of an IRB-approved informed consent form is given in Appendix B.)

In addition, special attention should be paid to the quality of the consent obtained from the donors. The RCOG Committee was particularly concerned that oocyte donors give informed consent about the particular use to which the oocyte will be put. Even if oocytes are removed in the course of another procedure such as a hysterectomy, the RCOG Committee advocated that the donor give informed consent because "as distinct from other tissues sometimes removed for research purposes, the egg cell carries the donor's genetic coding."[32]

It has also been suggested that counseling services be established to screen couples, donors, or surrogate carriers[44] who will participate in _in vitro_ fertilization (just as agencies screen those who participate in adoption).

Concern should also be paid to genetic counseling and screening of those people who will provide the gametes for the _in vitro_ fertilization and to awareness of any genetic risk to the embryo that may be due to the procedure. In 1978, Cohen suggested that children produced through _in vitro_ fertilization are subject to abnormally dangerous risks and the physicians involved should be held strictly financially liable if any risk materialized. Cohen wrote "if an experimenter is willing to subject an unborn child to an abnormally dangerous procedure, the experimenter should be willing to share the burden of support if the child is born with severe defects that are attributable to the technique."[33]

But until there is scientific evidence that _in vitro_ fertilization is significantly more likely to result in genetic defects like triploidy or trisomy-and there might _never_ be such evidence-penalizing physicians so harshly is not an appropriate legal remedy. After all, 4% of all normally conceived pregnancies result in a genetic defect, so even if a child conceived through _in vitro_ fertilization was born with an anomaly it would be impossible to say that the process itself was the cause. In addition, the births to date of children conceived in vitro do not indicate a higher rate of abnormality than normal procreation.[32] So at the current stage of in vitro fertilization practice, a physician's legal responsiblities with respect to genetic counselling should be much the same as in any pregnancy. He is legally required to tell a couple whether people of their age, ethnic group or occupation are particularly likely to be carriers of certain genetic defects and whether those defects can be screened for in the couple or through prenatal diagnosis.

A number of cases have been adjudicated that were brought by parents of children with genetic defects claiming that their physicians did not advise them that genetic screening could be done on them or on the developing fetus so that the parents would have had the option of not giving birth to an affected child. In other cases, the genetic testing of the couple or of the fetus was performed negligently and as a result the physician erroneously told the couple that they would not have an affected child.

Lawsuits on either cause of action, when brought by the parents of the child, are known as "wrongful birth" cases (the claim being that, had they known the child would be affected, they would never have given birth to him). Initially, these lawsuits were dismissed. Judges felt that physicians should not be held liable because, unlike someone who causes injury to a fetus in the womb, the physician does not "cause" the child's genetic defect.[45] On the other hand, the parents argued that, were it not for the physician's negligence, they would not have incurred the financial and emotional costs of bearing and raising an affected child.

In recent years, however, the parents have begun to prevail in such lawsuits. Examples have included a couple whose first child died of a fatal hereditary disease, yet who were erroneously told by their physician that there was no chance their next child would be similarly afflicted;[46] a 37-year-old woman who gave birth to a child with Down's Syndrome after her physician failed to advise her to undergo amniocentesis;[47] and parents of children with Tay-Sachs disease whose laboratory reports erroneously indicated that they were not carriers of the disease.[48] The success of parents in such cases has by no means been universal, however, and even in cases where parents have won, the courts have been split regarding what damages are recoverable. Some allow damages for emotional distress, others for the cost of special care for the child (which, in some cases is quite substantial - $250,000 for a child with Down's Syndrome, for example),[49] still others for the total cost of raising the child.

In addition to the "wrongful birth" cases initiated by parents, suits known as "wrongful life" cases have been brought in the name of the affected child. In those cases, the argument is essentially that the child would rather not have been born at all than been born with substantial defects. Until recently, such suits failed. In 1979, for example, the Pennsylvania Superior Court dismissed such a claim, saying, "Whether it is better to have never been born at all rather than to have been born with serious mental defects is a mystery more properly left to the philosophers and theologians, a mystery which would lead us into the field of metaphysics, beyond the realm of our understanding or ability to solve."[50]

In 1980, a California case changed the tide. The court ruled in favor of a Tay-Sachs child whose parents had been tested and erroneously told they were not carriers. The Court said it would be unfair to her if the justice system "retreat(ed) into meditation on the mysteries of life" rather than taking an objective view of the child's pain and suffering.[51]

These legal precedents will also cover in vitro fertilization pregnancies. Currently, there is an upper age limit of 35 for women who participate in some programs; as a result, it is probably not necessary to offer routine amniocentesis in those programs to detect Down's Syndrome. However, a genetic history of the couple should be obtained and they should be counseled about the availability of karyotyping, biochemical assays and amniocentesis for particular maladies for which they may be at risk.

Additional considerations come into play when a donor is used. Physicians are certainly not seen as providing a warranty with the donor sperm or donor oocyte they use in in vitro fertilization. Yet reasonable screening of donors must be done or the physician could be held negligent in choosing a donor. There probably would be a verdict against a doctor if he used the semen of a black donor to fertilize an oocyte of a black woman without testing either for a sickle cell trait.

Many artificial insemination clinics, especially those who use medical student donors, rely on the donor to disclose whether he has a genetic disorder or a family history of a particular abnormality. With fairly common disorders like sickle cell and Tay-Sachs, this self-report may not be enough to shield the physician from liability. Actual biochemical testing may be advisable. A court may feel it is negligent for a physician to merely rely on the word of a paid donor—especially in light of the research which shows that paid blood donors conceal health factors that would otherwise make them ineligible[52] as well as research that found that even medical student semen donors did not adquately recognize genetic disorders in their own families.

A physician using donor sperm should consult the guidelines of the American Assocation of Tissue Banks (AATB) or the American Fertility Society (AFS) to determine the standard medical practice for genetic screening of sperm donors.[53] The AATB standards, for example, list nineteen types of disorders that should prohibit men from being sperm donors. According to the standards, "A report of any condition in a prospective donor's family history which might put him at risk of more than one percent for producing a child with a birth defect and/or a genetic disease would disqualify him as a donor." The AATB also suggests rejecting donors who have been alcohol or drug abusers or who have worked at a job with any significant risk of radiation or chemical exposure. Similar considerations should come into play when oocyte donors are used. Selection of a surrogate carrier to gestate an IVF embryo for a couple should include an assessment of whether she is likely to undertake an activity during pregnancy (such as excessive drinking) that might harm the embryo or fetus.[54]

While courts are beginning to show more sympathy for the couples who give birth to a seriously ill child due to a physician's negligence, some legislatures are lending protection to the physicians. New laws in Minnesota, South Dakota, and Utah, for example, prohibit lawsuits charging wrongful birth or wrongful life.[55]

Once a physician has fertilized an oocyte in vitro, other legal principles cover the decision regarding implantation or termination of the fetus. There already has been one lawsuit based on the termination of an in vitro embryo. In 1973, an attempt was made by two doctors in New York to treat a woman's infertility by in vitro fertilization. But the department chairman at the hospital stopped the procedure by destroying the contents of the petri dish. The woman successfully sued the department chairman and the hospital, winning an award of $50,000 for having been the victim of an intentional infliction of emotional distress.[56]

Although the court in that particular case refused to hold that the embryo was the property of the woman and her husband, other precedents clearly emphasize the couple's rights to the embryo even while it is in the laboratory. The Australian Medical Research Council guidelines on in vitro fertilization emphasize this point, stating that the sperm and ova produced for in vitro fertilization are considered to belong to the donors and that their wishes in regard to the use, storage, and ultimate disposal of the sperm, ova, and embryo should be ascertained and as far as possible respected by the institution.[57] In the Illinois _in vitro_ fertilization case, the State's Attorney set forth the interpretation, accepted by the federal district judge, that an IVF patient is pregnant from the time her egg is fertilized, even though it is outside her body and she would not be deemed pregnant by any standard medical measures. That case held that a decision not to reimplant the embryo was subject to the same constraints as any other lawful pregnancy termination--primarily that the mother's permission be granted.

Accordingly, consent from both the sperm and egg donor should be sought when reimplantation of an embryo seems inadvisable (for example, if fertilization did not occur or has not proceeded normally) and specific consent should be obtained for study or disposal of the resulting product. It is particularly important that the physician allow the couple to make the decision regarding reimplantation since the physician is viewed as having a potential conflict of interest. Because physicians do not want their programs to look bad, they may "be overcautious in their judgments and refuse to implant or order the abortion of all but the most perfect blastocysts."[58] Yet if the physician wrongfully destroyed an embryo the parents wanted reimplanted, the parents might be able to sue to recover damages equal to "the value of the joys of parenthood minus the cost of raising the child."[33]

RIGHTS AND RESPONSIBILITIES OF OTHER PARTICIPANTS IN THE PROCESS

When a donor or surrogate carrier is used, questions arise regarding legal parenthood and the legal status of the resulting child. The Department of HEW Ethics Advisory Board studied the crazy quilt of laws that apply to the participants and recommended that a model law be drafted to clarify the right of IVF offspring, parents and others who participate in the process.[59]

Under existing law, the use of donor sperm to fertilize a woman's oocyte with resultant transfer of the embryo into her own uterus is analogous to the accepted process of donor artificial insemination and should present no additional legal questions. It would seem to fall within the artificial insemination by donor statutes enacted by 24 states that clearly provide that the legal father is the consenting husband of the woman who conceives with donor sperm.[60] The converse situation in which a donor oocyte is fertilized by a woman's husband's sperm with the embryo reimplanted in the woman's uterus should also present little legal difficulty. There is no legal basis for considering a woman who gives birth to a child to be anything other than the child's legal mother. Assuming appropriate informed consents were obtained from all parties, particularly acknowledgement of the termination of all potential rights by the donor of the oocyte, there should be no substantial legal questions.

The situation in which a woman is implanted with an embryo produced from another couple's oocyte and sperm in order to carry the child for the couple and turn it back over to them presents many legal questions. First, the woman who gives birth to the child (the surrogate carrier) will in all probability be considered the legal mother of the child and her husband, if any, the legal father. In many states, the man who provided the sperm could bring a paternity action to prove by blood testing that he rather than the women's husband is the child's legal father. However, in no state is there a specific provision for a woman to bring a maternity action to prove that she is the biological mother of a child born of another woman.[61] Thus, in this situation, a woman might have to legally adopt a child even though it is genetically hers. The scenario would then be legally analogous to the current situation in which a surrogate mother agrees (for a fee) to be artificially inseminated with the sperm from an infertile woman's husband, carry the pregnancy, give birth to the child and then turn it over to the infertile couple for their adoption.

The fee currently paid to a surrogate mother is anywhere from $5,000 to $20,000, and a surrogate carrier would probably charge a similar fee. But this exchange of money may be viewed by some courts as baby-selling, thus running afoul of a number of state statutes.[62] For example, some states have anti-slavery laws which prohibit buying or selling of "people". The California penal code provides that giving or receiving money or anything of value for the placement of one person in the custody of another is punishable by two to four years imprisonment.[63] Under such a law, the action of the physician, lawyer, surrogate and couple could be considered criminal.

The most extensive laws applicable to a surrogate mother arrangement, however, are the adoption laws. In 22 states, payment in connection with an adoption (other than for limited, enumerated medical and legal fees) is forbidden.[64]

A physician who acts as a matchmaker for a surrogate and couple and charges a fee for that service may find himself subject to potential legal penalties. In some states only the parent or guardian may assist in placing a child for adoption. Anyone else who gets involved must be licensed as a child placement agency. The Nevada version of this law specifically prohibits physicians from being involved with adoptions without that specialized license.[65] Such laws could apply to the surrogate/in vitro situation as well.

The surrogate parenting arrangement has been subject to legal criticism in several states. In Kentucky, the Attorney General issued an opinion likening the use of a surrogate to "baby-buying" and declaring that the procedure violated Kentucky law.[66]

In addition, legal action was commenced in Michigan.[67] In that state, a couple wants to pay the husband's secretary to be inseminated with the husband's sperm and bear a child for them. The payment will be $5,000 plus medical expenses, sick leave, pregnancy disability insurance, and medical insurance. Since Michigan law prohibits the payment of money in connection with an adoption, the couple's attorney brought suit to declare the law unconstitutional. However, both a trial court and an appellate court have ruled against him, stating that mercenary considerations like the payment of a surrogate mother should not figure into the creation of a parent-child relationship. The attorney for the state had also made the argument that courts should not sanction surrogate motherhood. He argued that "The integrity of the court system and the statutory adoption process demands that the court be absolutely prohibited from deciding what individual has a Saks-Fifth Avenue pricetag and what individual has a K-Mart pricetag."

In England, a couple hired a prostitute to be a surrogate mother. She was inseminated with the husband's sperm, got pregnant but refused to turn over the child. The couple sued, but the judge granted custody to the prostitute.[54] The judge said that the actions of the father and his wife in trying to create a child in this manner were "most selfish and irresponsible."[68] He refused to enforce what he felt was a pernicious agreement for the sale of a child.

Because of the legal uncertainties with respect to surrogate motherhood, legislatures in Alaska, California, Kansas, Michigan, North Carolina, Oklahoma, South Carolina, and Tennessee are considering surrogate legislation. However, all of these proposed laws deal with surrogate mothers who have been artifically inseminated (and thus provide a gamete as well as a uterus for gestation). None of the legislatures have had the foresight to consider the surrogate carrier arrangement.

The surrogate carrier has a stronger argument than does the surrogate mother that she is not selling a child. After all, she provides none of the genetic material, she just rents her womb. It is likely that additional laws governing surrogate carriers will be needed such as laws that exempt people who use surrogate carriers from the adoption process on the grounds that a surrogate carrier is not giving up her child but giving back the genetic child of the couple.

THE FUTURE OF IVF LAW

In the future, the legal landscape regarding *in vitro* fertilization may be clear. Agencies, similar to adoption agencies, may exist to screen and counsel couples and donors and fulfill much of the informed consent responsibility currently discharged by physicians. A system of licensing or accreditation may establish qualifications for the professionals offering *in vitro* fertilization to protect patients financially, physically and psychologically. The parental rights and responsibilities of the people choosing *in vitro* fertilization to create a family may be spelled out.

But for now, the physician offering *in vitro* fertilization must journey on a less clear path, carefully avoiding the barriers erected by the old cases and statutes that were generally developed long before *in vitro* fertilization was even conceivable.

REFERENCES

1. *Eisenstadt v. Baird*, 405 U.S. 438, 453 (1972).
2. *Skinner v. Oklahoma*, 316 U.S. 535 (1942).
3. *Griswold v. Connecticut*, 381 U.S. 479 (1965); *Carey v. Population Serv. Int'l.*, 431 U.S. 678 (1977).
4. *Roe v. Wade*, 410 U.S. 113 (1973).
5. *Maher v. Roe*, 432 U.S. 464 (1977).
6. The National Commission for the Protection of Human Subjects of Biomedical and Behavioral Research, Report and Recommendations: Research on the Fetus. 1975 DHEW Publication No. (OS) 76-127.
7. 45 C.F.R. 46 201 *et. seq.* (1982).
8. 45 C.F.R. 46 203 (c) (1982).
9. Ariz. Rev. Stat. Ann.§36-2302 (Supp. 1982-83);
   Cal. Health & Safety Code § 25956 (West Supp. 1983);
   Ill. Ann. Stat. ch. 38 § 81-26,-32,-32.1 (Smith-Hurd Supp. 1983-84);
   Ind. Code § 35-1-58.5-6 (1979);
   Ky. Rev. Stat. Ann. § 436.026 (1975);
   La. Rev. Stat. Ann. § 14:87.2 (West 1974);
   Me. Rev. Stat. Ann. tit. 22 § 1593 (West 1980);
   Mass. Ann. Laws ch. 112 § 12J (Supp. 1983);
   Mich. Comp. Laws Ann. §§ 333.2685 - .2692 (West 1980);
   Minn. Stat. Ann. § 145.421-.422 (West Supp. 1982);
   Mo. Ann. Stat. § 188.037 (Vernon Supp. 1983);
   Mont. Code Ann. § 50-20-108(3) (1981);
   Neb. Rev. Stat. § 28-342, 28-346 (1979);
   N.M. Stat. Ann. § 24-9 A-et seq. (1981);
   N.D. Cent. Code § 14-02.2-01 to -02 (Allen Smith 1981);

Ohio Rev. Code Ann. § 2919.14 (Baldwin 1982);
Okla. Stat. Ann. tit. 63 § 1-735 (West Supp. 1982-83);
Pa. Stat. Ann. tit. 18 § 3216 (Purdon Supp. 1983-83);
R.I. Gen. Laws § 11-54-2 (Supp. 1982);
S.D. Comp. Laws Ann. § 34-23A-17 (1977);
Tenn. Code Ann. § 39-308 (Supp. 1982);
Utah Code Ann. § 76-7-310 (Allen Smith 1978);
Wyo. Stat. 35-6-115 (1977);

10. Ariz. Rev. Stat. Ann. § 36-2302 (Supp. 1982-83);
Cal. Health & Safety Code § 25956 (West Supp. 1982);
Ill. Ann. Stat. ch. 38 § 81-22 (8), (9) (Smith-Hurd Supp. 1983-84);
La. Rev. Stat. Ann. § 14:87.2 (West 1974);
Mass. Ann. Laws chap. 112 § 12j (a) IV, § 12K (Supp. 1982);
Mich. Comp. Laws Ann. § 333.2685 (West 1980);
Minn. Stat. Ann. § 145.421 (subd. 2) (West Supp. 1982);
Mo. Ann. Stat. § 188.015 (5) (Vernon Supp. 1983);
N.M. Stat. Ann. § 24-9A-1 G. (1981);
N.D. Cent. Code § 14-02.2-02(3) (Allen Smith 1981);
Ohio Rev. Code Ann. 2919.14 (Baldwin 1982);
Okla. Stat. Ann. tit. 63 § 1-730(2) (West Supp. 1982-83);
Pa. Stat. Ann. § 3203 (Supp. 1982);
R.I. Gen. Laws § 11-54-2(f) (Supp. 1982);
Ky. Rev. Stat. Ann. § 311.720 (5) (1983);

11. Ind. Code § 35-1-58.5-6 (1979);
Me. Rev. Stat. Ann. tit. 22 § 1593 (West 1980);
Mont. Code Ann. § 50-20-108 (1981);
Neb. Rev. Stat. § 28-342, 28-346 (1979);
S.D. Comp. Laws Ann. § 34-23A-17 (1977;
Tenn. Code Ann. § 39-4-208 (1982);
Utah Code Ann. § 76-7-310 (Allen Smith 1978);
Wyo. Stat. 35-6-115 (1977).

12. Ariz. Rev. Stat. Ann § 36-2302 (Supp. 1982-83);
Cal. Health & Safety Code § 25956 (West Supp. 1983);
Ill. Ann. Stat. ch. 38 § 81-26, -32, -32.1 (Smith-Hurd Supp. 1983-84);
Ind. Code § 35-1-58.5-6 (1979);
Ky. Rev. Stat. Ann. § 436.026 (1975);
Neb. Rev. Stat. § 28-342, 28-346 (1979);
Ohio Rev. Code Ann. § 2919.14 (Baldwin 1982);
Okla. Stat. Ann. tit. 63 § 1-735 (West Supp. 1982-83);
Pa. Stat. Ann. tit. 18 § 3216 (Supp. 1983-84);
Tenn. Code Ann. § 39-308 (Supp. 1982);
Wyo. Stat. § 35-6-115 (1977);

13. See, e.g., N.M. Stat. Ann 24-9A-1H (1981).
14. Mich. Comp. Laws Ann. §§ 333.2685 (1) (West 1980).
15. Minn. Stat. Ann. § 145.421-422 (West 1983).
16. R. I. Gen. Laws § 11-54-1(a) (Supp. 1982).

17. J.E. Buster, M. Bustillo, I.H. Thornycroft, J.A. Simon, S.P. Boyers, J.R. Marshall, J.A. Louw, R.W. Seed, R.G. Seed, 1983, Non-surgical transfer of in vivo fertilized donated ova to five infertile women: Report of two pregnancies, Lancet, 2:223.
18. La. Rev. Stat. Ann. § 14-87.2 (West 1974).
19. Ariz. Rev. Stat. Ann. § 36-2302 (Supp. 1982-83);
Ind. Code § 35-1-58.5-6 (1979);
Ky. Rev. Stat. Ann. § 436-026 (1975);
Me. Rev. Stat. Ann. tit. 22 § 1593 (West 1980);
Mass. Ann. Laws ch. 112 § 12j (Supp. 1982);
Mich. Comp. Laws Ann. §§ 333.2685-.2692 (West 1980);
Minn. Stat. Ann. § 145-421-.422 (West Supp. 1982);
Mo. Ann. Stat. § 188.037 (Vernon Supp. 1983);
Mont. Code Ann. § 50-20-108(3) (1981);
Neb. Rev. Stat.§ 28-342, 28-246 (1979);
N.D. Cnet. Code § 14-02.2-01 to 02 (Allen Smith 1981);
Ohio Rev. Code Ann. § 2919.14 (Baldwin 1982);
Okla. Stat. Ann. tit. 63 § 1-735 (West Supp. 1983-84);
Pa. Stat. Ann. tit. 18 § 3216 (Purdon Supp. 1983-84);
R. I. Gen. Laws § 11-54-2 (Supp. 1982);
Utah Code Ann. § 76-7-310 (Allen Smith 1978);
Wyo. Stat. 35-6-115 (1977).
20. In Massachusetts, for example, pregnancy is "the condition of a mother carrying an unborn child" and an unborn child is "the individual human life in existence and developing from fertilization until birth." Abortion is "the knowing destruction of the life of an unborn child or the intentional expulsion or removal of an unborn child from the womb other than for the principal purpose of producing a live birth or removing a dead fetus." Mass. Ann. Laws ch. 12 § 12K (Supp. 1982).
21. Okla. Stat. Ann. tit. 63 § 1-730 (1), (2), (7) (West Supp. 1982-83).
22. Wyo. Stat. 35 6-101 (a)(i)(vi) (1977).
23. Minn. Stat. Ann. § 145.422 (subd. 3) (West Supp. 1982);
Ohio Rev. Code Ann. § 2919.14 (A) (Baldwin 1982).
24. Ky. Rev. Stat. Ann. § 436.026 (1975); Me. Rev. Stat. Ann. tit. 22 § 1593 (West 1980);
Mass. Ann. Laws chap. 112 § 12j (a) iv. (Supp. 1982);
Mich. Comp. Laws. Ann. § 333.2690 (West 1980);
Neb. Rev. Stat. § 28-342 (1979);
N.D. Cent. Code § 14-02.2-02(3) (Allen Smith 1981);
R.I. Gen. Laws § 11-54-2 (F) Supp. 1982);
Wyo. Stat. § 35-6-115 (1975).
25. The Minnesota statute makes it a gross misdemeanor for anyone to permit the use of a living human conceptus for any type of research. Minn. Stat. Ann. § 145.422 (Subd. 1) (West Supp. 1982).

26. Pa. Stat. Ann. tit. 18 § 3213(e) (Supp. 1983-4).
27. Ill. Ann. Stat. ch. 38 § 81-26(6)(7) (Smith-Hurd Supp. 1983-84).
28. McLaughlin, 1983, "Hub Hospitals Plan Test-Tube Fertilizations," Boston Globe, p 1, March 2,
29. Smith v. Fahner, No. 82 c4324 (D.Ct., Ill.).
30. Reilly, P., 1976, In Vitro Fertilization--A Legal Perspective, in "Genetics and Law", A. Milunsky and G. J. Annas, eds., Plenum Press, New York and London.
31. 45 C.F.R. § 46.204(d) (1982).
32. Report of the Royal College of Obstetricians and Gynaecologists Ethics Committee on In Vitro Fertilisation and Embryo Replacement or Transfer, 1983, Chameleon Press, London.
33. Lorio, K.V., 1982, In vitro fertilization and embryo transfer: Fertile areas for litigation, Southwestern Law Journal, 35:973. Similarly, Mark E. Cohen urged HEW to establish standards for federally funded in vitro fertilization research which could "define minimum qualifications for IVF experimenters, standardize the laboratory conditions that must be employed, develop safety standards necessary for conducting human IVF experimentation, and establish the circumstances in which an IVF conceptus may be destroyed." Cohen, M.E., 1978, The 'Brave new baby' and the law: Fashioning remedies for the victims of in vitro fertilization, American Journal of Law and Medicine, 4:319.
34. 42. U.S.C. § 2891-3 (1982).
35. 45 C.F.R. § 46.101 et. seq. (1982).
36. See, e.g. N.Y. Pub. H. Law §§ 2440-2446 (McKinney 1977).
37 This is the definition used in the federal regulations. 45 C.F.R. 46.102(e) (1982).
38. 45 C.F.R. § 46.111 (a) (1982).
39. 45 C.F.R. § 46.205(a)(2) (1982).
40. 45 C.F.R. § 46.111(a)(2) (1982).
41. Smedes v. Wayne State University (D.Ct., Mich.).
42. Trounson, A., Leeton, J. Besanko, M., Wood, C., Conti, A., 1983, Pregnancy established in an infertile patient after transfer of a donated embryo fertilised in vitro, Brit Med J. 286:835.
43. 45 C.F.R. § 46.116 (1982).
44. Comment, "Lawmaking and Science: A Practical Look at In Vitro Fertilization and Embryo Transfer," Detroit College of Law Review, III:429-456, (1979).
45. As recently as 1977, a court rejected an action based on a lack of informed consent to pregnancy in a situation where physicians failed to warn of the risk of having a child with Down's Syndrome. The court distinguished the

traditional informed consent cases since they dealt with situations where the injury "arose from some affirmative violation of the patient's physical integrity." Karlson v. Guerinot, 57 App. Div. 2d 73, 82, 394 N.Y.S. 2d 933,939 (1977). See also the similar logic in Smith v. United States, 392 F. Supp. 654 (N.D. Ohio 1975), a case involving maternal rubella, in which the court found that the physician's failure to warn of the risks had not proximately caused the child's injury, since there was nothing the physician could have done to have caused the child to have been born healthy.

46. Becker v. Schwartz, 46 N.Y. 2d 401, 413 N.Y.S. 2d 8951, 386 N.E. 2d 807 (1978).
47. Berman v. Allan, 80 N.J. 421, 404 A. 2d 8 (1979).
48. Gildner v. Thomas Jefferson University Hospital, 451 F. Supp. 692 (E.D. Pa. 1978).
49. Reilly, supra. n. 30, citing U.S. Department of Health Education and Welfare, "What are the Facts About Genetic Disease," DHEW Publication (NIH) 74-370 (1974) pp. 27-28; Sister M. Newmann, ed., The Tricentennial People; Human Applications of the New Genetics 7-8 (1978).
50. Speck v. Finegold, 408 A. 2d 496, 508 (Pa. Super. 1979). The denial of the wrongful life cause of action was upheld in Speck v. Finegold, 439 A. 2d 110 (1981).
51. Curlender v. Bio-Science Laboratories, 165 Cal. Rptr. 477, 106 Cal. App. 3d 811 (1980).
52. Titmuss, R., 1971, "The Gift Relationship: From Human Blood to Social Policy," Panteon, New York, New York
53. "Reproductive Council Guidelines," American Association of Tissue Banks Newsletter, 4:37 (November 1980); American Fertility Society, Report of the Ad Hoc Committee on Artificial Insemination.
54. For information on how to assess surrogates, see Andrews, L.B., 1984, New Conceptions, St. Martin's Press, New York, New York.
55. Minn. Stat. Ann. § 145.424; (West suppl, 1983); S.D. Cod. Laws § 21-55-1 (1981 Supp.);Utah Code Ann. §§ 78-11-23 to 25 (1983).
56. Del Zio v. Presbyterian Hospital, 74 Civ 3588 (S.D.N.Y. 1976). See also Sweeney, W. J., III, and Goldsmith, L.S., 1980, Test Tube Babies: Medical and Legal Considerations, J. of Leg. Med. 2:1.
57. "In Britain and Australia, New In Vitro Guidelines" 13(2) Hastings Center Report (February 1983).
58. Flannery, D.M., Weisman, C. D., Lipsett, C.R., Braverman, A.N., 1979, Test tube babies: Legal issues raised by in vitro fertilization, Georgetown Law Journal, 67:1295.
59. Ethics Advisory Board of the U.S. Dept. of Health, Education, and Welfare, 1979, "Report and Conclusions: DHEW Support

of Research Involving In Vitro Fertilization and Embryo Transfer," Federal Register 44:35034.

60. Alaska Stat. § 25.20.045 (Supp. 1982);
Ark. Stat. Ann. § 61-141 (1971);
Cal. Civ. Code § 7005 (West Supp. 1983);
Colo. Rev. Stat. § 19-6-106 (1978);
Conn. Gen. Stat. §§ 45-69f to -69n (1981);
Fla. Stat. Ann. § 742.11 (West Supp. 1983);
Ga. Code Ann. §§ 74-101.1, -9904 (1982);
Kan. Stat. Ann. §§ 23-128 to -130 (1981);
La. Civ. Code Ann. art. 188 (West Supp. 1983);
Md. Est. & Trusts Code Ann. § 1-206(b) (1974); and Md. Ann. Code art. 20 § 212 and art. 43, § 556E (1980);
Mich. Comp. Laws Ann. § 333.2824 (1980) and § 700.111 (1980);
Minn. Stat. Ann. § 257-56;
Mont. Rev. Code Ann. § 40-6-106 (1981);
Nev. Rev. Stat § 126-061 (1979);
N. Y. Dom. Rel. Law § 73 (McKinney 1977);
N. C. Gen. Stat. § 49A-1 (1976);
Okla. Stat. Ann. tit. 10 §§ 551-553 (West Supp. 1982-1983);
Or. Rev. Stat. §§ 109.239, .243, .247, 677.355, .360, .365, .370 (1981);
Tenn. Code Ann. § 53-446 (Supp. 1981);
Tex. Fam. Code Ann. § 12.03 (Vernon 1975);
Va. Code 64/1-7.1 (1980);
Wash. Rev. Code Ann. § 26.26.050 (West Supp. 1983-1984);
Wis. Stat. Ann. § 767.47(9) (West 1981), § 891.40 (West Supp. 1982-1983);
Wyo. Stat. § 14-2-103 (1978).

61. Despite the absence of a "maternity" law, the genetic mother in some states may be able to assert a claim to the child. In California, for example, "Any interested party may bring an action to determine the existence or nonexistence of mother-child relationship." Cal. Civil Code § 7015 (1983).

62. Andrews, L. B., 1981, Removing the stigma of surrogate motherhood, Family Advocate, 4:21.

63. Cal. Penal Code § 181 (West Supp. 1983).

64. Ala. Code § 26-10-89 (1975);
Ariz. Rev. Stat. Ann. § 8-126 (c) (1974);
Cal. Penal Code § 273 (a) (West Supp. 1983);
Colo. Rev. Stat. § 19-4-115 (1978);
Del. Code Ann. tit. 13 § 928 (1981);
Fla. Stat. Ann. § 63-212 (1) (b) (West Supp. 1983);
Ga. Code Ann. § 74-418 (b) (Supp. 1982);
Idaho Code § 18-1511 (1979);
Ill. Ann. Stat. ch. 40 §§ 1526, 1701, 1702 (Smith-Hurd 1980);
Iowa Code Ann. § 600.9 (West 1981);
Ky. Rev. Stat. § 199.590 (2) (1982);

Md. Ann. Code art. 16 § 83 (Supp. 1982);
Mass. Ann. Laws ch. 210 § 11A (1981);
Mich Comp. Laws Ann. § 710.54 (Supp. 1982-83);
Nev. Rev. Stat. § 127-290 (1981);
N.J. Stat. Ann. § 9.3-54 (West Supp. 1982-83);
N.Y. Soc. Serv. Law § 374(b) (McKinney Supp. 1982-83);
N.C. Gen. Stat. § 48-37 (Supp. 1981);
Okla. Stat. Ann. tit. 10 § 60.12 (g) (West Supp. 1982-83);
S.D. Codified Laws Ann. § 25-6-4.2 (Supp. 1982);
Tenn. Code Ann. § 36-136 (Supp. 1982);
Utah Code Ann. § 76-7-203 (1978);
Wis. Stat. Ann. § 946.716 (1982).

65. Nev. Rev. Stat. § 127.240(1) (1979).
66. "Surrogate Motherhood Contracts Declared Illegal by Kentucky A.G.," Fam. L. Rep. (BNA) 7:2246 (1981).
67. Doe v. Kelley, No. 7-8-815-531 (Cir. Ct., Wayne County, Mich., January 28, 1980), reported at 6 Fam. L. Rep. (BNA) 3011, aff'd. 106 Mich. App. 169 (1981), cert. denied, U.S. Supreme Court.
68. Scott, R. 1978, "The Body as Property," Viking Press, New York, New York.

3

PATIENT SCREENING AND SELECTION

Martin M. Quigley

In vitro fertilization and embryo transfer (IVF-ET) is an actual or potential treatment for many different types of infertility. Ultimately, the choice for treatment by IVF-ET will result from considerations of the couple's desires, the capacity of the treatment center and the particular orientation of the treatment team. However, at no time, either now or in the future, should a patient be treated with IVF-ET unless there is no other reasonable treatment available. A reasonable alternative is a treatment which offers either a greater chance of success than that available with IVF-ET or a comparable chance of success with substantially less risk or expense to the patient. Therefore, pretreatment screening of the couple should insure that 1) there is no alternative therapy available, and 2) that they are treatable by IVF-ET.

TYPES OF PATIENTS

Absolute Tubal Disease

IVF-ET represents the only realistic hope for a couple to have their own genetic child when the wife has absolute tubal disease (bilateral absence or irreparable obstruction of Fallopian tubes). It is these patients who should have first priority in any *in vitro* fertilization program as there is no other therapy available and no chance of spontaneous conception occurring.

Most groups should confine their efforts to patients with absolute tubal disease when initially establishing their IVF-ET program, as any pregnancy achieved in these patients is unequivocally due to the *in vitro* fertilization process. The repeated initiation of pregnancies in this group of patients will establish the credentials of a treatment program.

Other Tubal Factors

Patients who have undergone a surgical tuboplasty and have not conceived within one year after surgery, regardless of whether or not the tubes remain open, are considered appropriate candidates for IVF-ET in view of the low rate of spontaneous pregnancy after this time. In addition, patients with repeat tubal obstruction following a tuboplasty are considered for treatment by IVF-ET and, in fact, should be counselled against repeat surgical tuboplasty in view of the greatly reduced chance of success of a second tubal operation (Lauritsen et al., 1982).

Other Patient Groups

Infertile couples with male factors, endometriosis, unexplained infertility, cervical and/or immunologic factors do not generally have an absolute barrier to the establishment of a spontaneous pregnancy. Sporadic spontaneous pregnancies do occur in all of these patient groups, at times with a frequency estimated to approximate that currently associated with IVF-ET. For example, Leeton and Trounson (1982) cite a study performed by Drs. Gordon Baker and Brian Hudson in which they calculate that a couple with ideopathic infertility, defined as two years infertility in the presence of normal fertility parameters, have a 15% chance of conceiving in any given cycle. Accordingly, the chances of spontaneous conception need to be discussed with and understood by the prospective patients before they enter into an IVF-ET treatment cycle.

Among the tubal factor infertility couples on our waiting list we have had at least nine pregnancies before initiation of a treatment cycle. We had two patients with spontaneous tubal ectopic pregnancies following a single unsuccessful treatment cycle, one patient with a spontaneous tubal ectopic pregnancy between two unsuccessful treatment cycles, and three patients with ongoing intrauterine pregnancies following the completion of one, two, and three, respectively, unsuccessful treatment cycles. Although it is impossible to determine the exact denominator, our experience with spontaneous conceptions approaches the pregnancy rates reported by some established IVF-ET teams.

Male factors. As relatively few sperm are required to effect fertilization *in vitro* compared to *in vivo*, the application of IVF-ET to the treatment of couples in which the only etiology for infertility is marked oligospermia in the husband seems logical.

As the chances of spontaneous conceptions decrease with decreasing sperm count and percentage motility (Van Zyl et al., 1976), the worse that the husband's semen parameters are, the more appropriate IVF-ET seems to be. Obviously, these same couples are also suitable for treatment by means of donor artificial insemination (AID), with an expected overall pregnancy rate of 80% to 85% (Aiman, 1982; Albrecht et al., 1982). This fact needs to be discussed with the couple prior to selection of IVF-ET as a treatment. IVF-ET should only be recommended for couples with a major male factor who are unable or unwilling to accept AID as a treatment. Although 50,000 motile sperm per oocyte is our current insemination number for "normal" semen, 500,000 motile sperm per oocyte are required in the oligospermic group to achieve comparable levels of fertilization (See chapters 12 and 13). In addition, we have been unsuccessful in consistently obtaining fertilizations unless we have a minimum motility of grade 2 + or better. Accordingly, at the present time, our minimum semen quality for accepting an oligospermic male is 2,500,000 motile sperm in the entire ejaculate, with an average motility of grade 2+ or better.

Endometriosis. Patients who have failed to conceive following conservative surgery and a full course of hormonal suppresive therapy for endometriosis may be considered for IVF-ET, whether or not there is visible persistent endometriosis or resultant tubal obstruction. IVF-ET would not be an appropriate choice at this time for couples who have not received both conservative surgical treatment and hormonal suppression, and who have not been given a reasonable opportunity to conceive following each treatment.

Unexplained Infertility. The longer the duration of the couple's infertility, the lower are the chances of a spontaneous conception (Jones, 1965). Infertile couples in this category should have their infertility evaluation thoroughly scrutinized and/or repeated to ensure that there are no correctable explanations for the infertility. The results of IVF-ET for each particular couple in this group should be evaluated carefully before multiple repetitive IVF-ET treatment cycles are instituted. As some unexplained infertility is probably due to defects in the sperm's fertilizing ability, the oocyte's ability to be fertilized, or the ability of the embryo to implant in the uterus, repetitive failures in this group should lead to a cessation of attempts. The use of the cross-species oocyte penetration test (see chapter 14) may assist in evaluating these patients.

Cervical, Immunological, and Other. Patients in these groups, who have not conceived following treatment with the current modalities (e.g., supplemental estrogen, intrauterine AIH, immunosuppresive therapy) or for whom no therapy is available are appropriately treated by IVF-ET. However, as in the previous group of patients, repeated failures should lead to a discontinuation of treatment by this technique.

PATIENTS NOT TREATABLE BY IVF-ET

Anovulation

A woman who fails to ovulate (as opposed to failure to become pregnant) after treatment with menopausal gonadotropins, clomiphene and/or bromocryptine is not a candidate for *in vitro* fertilization, as there must be spontaneous or induced preovulatory follicular development for this technique to be applied. A patient who is anovulatory but responds to ovulation inducing drugs with normal follicular development, but who has not conceived, may be considered for treatment by IVF-ET, particularly if there are other infertility factors.

Lack of Available Gametes

Couples in which the husband is azoospermic or the wife has ovaries which are not accessible for laparoscopic follicular aspiration, or couples in which the wife has no functioning ovarian tissue are obviously not candidates for IVF-ET in the conventional fashion. Follicular aspiration under ultrasonographic guidance without laparoscopy may become available for women with obscuring pelvic adhesions which make laparoscopic aspiration impossible (Lenz and Lauritsen, 1982). Pregnancies have been reported in infertile couples following artificial insemination of an "embryo donor" with the husband's sperm, recovery of the embryo with subsequent transfer to the wife's uterus (Buster et al., 1983). The decision to use donated sperm, oocytes or embryos raises additional ethical and legal questions and is discussed elsewhere in this book (Chapters 2 and 20). The situation in which the wife has no functioning ovarian tissue not only includes the same ethical and legal questions cited above, but also requires that external hormonal therapies be given, first to prepare the endometrium for implantation and second, to sustain an established pregnancy until there is sufficient placental function for pregnancy maintenance. The types, dosages and durations of hormonal therapy necessary for these functions are not established at present, but in all probability will become known in the future.

PRETREATMENT SCREENING

Excluding the situation in which sperm or oocyte donation is required for *in vitro* fertilization and embryo transfer, the woman must first either spontaneously ovulate with normal ovarian hormone production, or respond to clomiphene or menopausal gonadotropins. The ovaries must be physically accessible for laparoscopic follicular aspiration (unless aspiration is to be done under ultrasonographic guidance), and there must be a normal uterus with functioning endometrium. The decision whether or not to treat patients with developmental uterine anomalies is a personal one between the physician and the couple. Anomalies (such as uterus didelphus), which are not associated with extremely high rates of pregnancy wastage, or situations such as a unicollis uterus, with no hope of surgical repair, may reasonably be considered for treatment. However, patients with anomalies associated with high pregnancy losses (such as a major uterine septation) should, perhaps, be treated by metroplasty prior to an attempt at *in vitro* fertilization. In addition, as mentioned above, the husband's semen analysis must indicate the possibility of recovering sufficient motile sperm for insemination.

Practical Considerations

Pretreatment screening involves a review of relevant medical records, a semen analysis, and screening for normal ovulation and normal corpus luteum function. Unless there is a suspicion from the previous evaluations or menstrual history that the woman may be anovulatory or have inadequate luteal function, screening involves a serum progesterone between cycle days 20 and 22 of a spontaneous cycle. If the serum progesterone six to eight days prior to the onset of the next menses is over 12 ng/ml, the woman is presumed to ovulate normally.

Microbiologic screening of semen or cervical mucus is not performed routinely unless there is an excess number of white cells in the ejaculate or preovulatory mucus. A hysterosalpingogram is not routinely required prior to treatment.

Place of Screening Laparoscopy

We still require most of our patients in the tubal factor group to undergo a preliminary screening laparoscopy prior to the initiation of a treatment cycle. Due to the expenses involved in a treatment cycle, the professional time and effort required during follicular monitoring, and the emotional strain on the couple during the monitoring program, we wish to maximize the chances that there will be accessible follicles for aspiration at the time of laparoscopy. This requires that we know before the treatment cycle whether or not there is access to either ovary, and gives us the opportunity to abort the follicular monitoring program and cancel the laparoscopy if it appears by ultrasonography that there are few or no follicles developing in the only accessible ovary, (if there is access on only one side). For treatment by IVF-ET, we require that a minimum of 50% of the total ovarian surface of at least one ovary is accessible to the aspirating needle. Figure 1 demonstrates a totally accessible ovary, ovaries with limited access to ovarian surfaces, and an example of an inaccessible ovary. Our experience with screening laparoscopies during the period July 1981 through June 1982 is summarized in Table 1. Of the patients in the tubal factor group, we have consistently had 15% to 20% who did not meet our criteria for minimum ovarian accessibility.

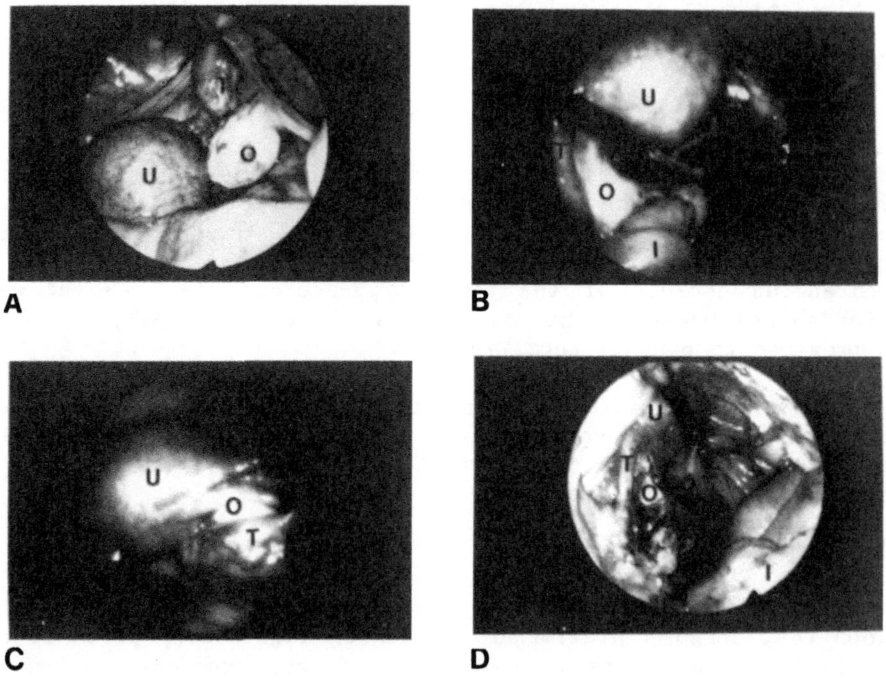

Figure 1

Laparoscopic visualization of ovarian access at the time of screening laparoscopy. A. Completely accessibble right ovary. B. Left ovary with approximately 50% of the ovarian surface accessible. C. Right ovary with adherent Fallopian tube limiting access. Only about 40% of the ovarian surface could be visualized. D. Severe left adnexal adhesions with less than 10% of the ovarian surface seen. O = ovary, T = tube, U = uterus, I = intestine.

Table 1. Results of screening laparoscopies, July 1981 through June 1982.

Number of ovaries present	Number of accessible ovaries*	Patients #	Patients %
2	2	38	80.9
	1	3	6.4
	0	6	12.8
		47	100.0
1	1	14	70.0
	0	6	30.0
		20	100.0
TOTALS	2	38	56.7
	1	17	25.4
	0	12	17.9
		67	100.0

* An accessible ovary has a minimum of 50% of the total ovarian surface visible at laparoscopy

As a rule, we do not require screening laparoscopies for patients in the oligospermic, unexplained, cervical factor, or other infertility groups, unless there is something in the history or physical exam which leads us to suspect there may be limited access to one or both ovaries. Similarly, we do not require a screening laparoscopy in patients who have undergone elective tubal ligation unless there has been an unsuccessful attempt at surgical reanastomosis. We consider waiving the screening laparoscopy in patients who have had bilateral salpingectomies for tubal ectopic pregnancies if the second salpingectomy was uncomplicated, and the operative report from that salpingectomy specifically notes the absence of obscuring pelvic adhesions on the contralateral ovary. Lastly, we do not require a repeat laparoscopy in patients who have undergone laparoscopy without an intervening laparotomy, as long as the full operative report is available, and there is a clear description of the lack of obscuring ovarian adhesions.

At the time of the screening laparoscopy (for statistical purposes only) we introduce a dilute solution of indigo carmine by means of a transcervical Foley catheter in patients with Fallopian tubes to document the presence or absence of tubal patency.

Age and Reproductive Performance

There is an age-associated decrease in reproductive capability due to unknown factor(s). A recently published report on a series of patients undergoing artificial insemination, due to azoospermia in their husbands, has shown that women over the age of 35 had an overall pregnancy rate of approximately 55% per year as opposed to 70% in women under the age of 35, and those that did become pregnant required approximately twice as many inseminations to do so (Federation CECOS, 1982). The decrease in reproductive capability with age (in the absence of discernible hormonal or anatomical factors) has been attributed by at least one author to age-associated changes in the endometrium (Berniske, 1978).

Although there is no absolute reason to exclude any premenopausal woman from an *in vitro* fertilization program, the decreased reproductive performance with age needs to be discussed with the couple. In view of the study by Tietze (1957) of the fertility of a group of women not using contraception, showing an 11% infertility rate over age 34, 33% by age 40, and 87% by age 44, most groups have made a pragmatic decision not to treat women over a certain age, which is usually 40 (Webster, 1983; Szalay, 1983).

Marital Status

Although the report and conclusions of the Ethics Advisory Board of the Department of Health, Education, and Welfare (1979) recommended that *in vitro* fertilization be restricted to married couples, with the sperm obtained from the husband, the oocytes from the wife, and the embryos transferred into the wife's uterus, there is apparently some legal question (see Chapter 2) about denying services to single women based merely on their marital status, particularly in institutions receiving governmental support. The decision whether or not to treat unmarried couples needs to be made by each institution on an individual basis.

SUMMARY AND CONCLUSIONS:

IVF-ET may soon become an acceptable and available treatment for all couples with infertility not otherwise treatable. Until these techniques are widely available, however, couples in which the wife has absolute tubal infertility, and thus, who have no other hope for having a child of their own, should be given first priority. Newly established programs should consider restricting the patients treated to these couples in order to prove to themselves and the medical community that the pregnancies established are, indeed, due to *in vitro* fertilization and embryo transfer and not spontaneously occurring ones. Patients should not be considered for IVF-ET unless there is no other reasonable therapy, or until all other therapies have been unsuccessfully attempted. The use of donated gametes and embryos for transfer into another woman's uterus is an ethical and legal, rather than a medical, decision.

REFERENCES

Aiman, J., 1982, Factors affecting the success of donor insemination, *Fertil. Steril.*, 37:94.

Albrecht, B.H., Cramer, D., and Schiff, I., 1982, Factor influencing the success of artificial insemination, *Fertil. Steril.*, 37:792.

Benirschke, K., 1978, The Endometrium, *in* "Reproductive Endocrinology: Physiology, Pathophysiology and Clinical Management", S.S.C. Yen and R.B. Jaffee, eds., W.B. Saunders, Philadelphia.

Buster, J.E., Bustillo, M., Thorneycroft, I.H., Simon, J.A., Boyers, S.P., Marshall, J.R., Louw, J.A., Seed, R.W., and Seed, R.G., 1983, Non-surgical transfer of in vivo fertilized donated ova to five infertile women: Report of two pregnancies, *Lancet*, 2:223.

Department of Health Education and Welfare, Office of the Secretary: Protection of Human Subjects; HEW Support of Human In Vitro Fertilization and Embryo Transfer: Report of the Ethics Advisory Board, 1979, *Federal Register*, 44:35033.

Federation CECOS, Schwartz, D., Mayaux, M.J., 1982, Female fecundity as a function of age: Results of artificial insemination in 2193 nulliparous women with azoospermic husbands, *New Eng. J. Med.*, 306:404.

Jones, G.S., 1965, Prognosis for the infertile couple, *Obstet-Gynec. Surv.*, 20:646.

Lauritsen, J.G., Pagel, J.D., Vangsted, P., and Starup, J., 1982, Results of repeated tuboplasties, *Fertil. Steril.*, 37:68.

Leeton, J.F., and Trounson, A.O., 1982, Application of *in vitro* fertilization to ideopathic infertility, *in* "Human Conception In Vitro", R.G. Edwards and J.M. Purdy, eds., Academic Press, London.

Lenz, S. and Lauritsen, J.G., 1982, Ultrasonically guided percutaneous aspiration of human follicles under local anesthesia: A new method of collecting oocytes for *in vitro* fertilization, *Fertil. Steril.*, 38:673.

Szalay, S., 1982, Discussion on patient selection and monitoring, in "Human Conception In Vitro", R. G. Edwards, J. M. Purdy, eds., Academic Press, London.
Tietze, C., 1957, Reproductive span and rate of reproduction among Hutterite women, Fertil. Steril., 8:89.
van Zyl, J.A., Menkreld, R., Retief, A.E., van Niekerk, W.A., 1976, Oligospermia, in "Human Semen and Fertility Regulation in Men", E.S.E. Hafez, ed., C.V. Mosby, St. Louis.
Webster, J., 1982, Discussion on patient selection and monitoring, in "Human Conception In Vitro", R.G. Edwards, J.M. Purdy, eds., Academic Press, London.

4

HYPOTHALAMIC CONTROL OF THE MENSTRUAL CYCLE

Julane Hotchkiss

INTRODUCTION

The relation between ovarian function and menstruation did not become clear nor widely accepted until the early twentieth century, and the details of this relation as currently understood are amply covered in other chapters in this volume. The next conceptual step forward in reproductive physiology came when it became evident that the ovary did not function autonomously, but depended upon the presence of the anterior pituitary gland. The concept of anterior pituitary ommipotence could not survive, however, in the face of the clever experimental designs of Harris (1955) who showed that ovulation in the rabbit could be induced by sensory signals arising in the periphery which were translated by the hypothalamus into hormonal signals from the pituitary gland. The isolation, characterization, and synthesis of the hypothalamic gonadotropin-releasing hormone (GnRH) and a myriad of other hypothalamic hormones that regulate the secretion of other anterior pituitary hormones have added substance to the original theories of the hypothalamic control of pituitary function.

The Primate Reproductive Cycle

The reproductive cycles of all primates share three features: 1) a phase of follicular development occurring in response to relatively low and unchanging tonic secretion of FSH and LH and culminating in increasing blood levels of estrogens as the dominant follicle matures; 2) a midcycle surge of gonadotropins, elicited by the rising tide of estrogen, which heralds incipient ovulation; and 3) a post ovulatory phase of high circulating progesterone levels and low circulating gonadotropin levels which terminates in menses (in some primates) as progesterone levels fall to near zero.

This chapter will deal only with the special relations between the hypothalamus, anterior pituitary gland, and ovary which are responsible for these three events, and will attempt to construct the simplest plausible model for the control of cyclic ovarian function in the higher primate.

HYPOTHALAMIC CONTROL OF PITUITARY GONADOTROPIN SECRETION

Pulsatile Secretion of Gonadotropins

Pulsatile secretion of luteinizing hormone (LH) was first observed in 1970 in the ovariectomized rhesus monkey (Dierschke et al., 1970). Assay of blood samples taken every 10-20 minutes over 8-10 hours revealed a striking pattern of massive, short-lived elevations in circulating LH. In man, as in the rhesus monkey, the basic unmodulated pulse frequency, as observed in the absence of the gonads (in both sexes) or in the follicular phase of the menstrual cycle, is about one pulse per hour, a circhoral frequency (Fig. 1). The acquisition of testicular function (specifically testosterone secretion) or luteal function (progesterone secretion) is accompanied by a marked slowing of this pulse frequency as shown in Fig. 2 (Yen et al., 1972; Plant, 1982; Winters and Troen, 1983; Filicori and Crowley, 1983).

Pulsatile gonadotropin secretion has also been described in early infancy in man and the rhesus monkey. This pattern of secretion essentially disappears during the prepubertal period, reappearing during early puberty as intermittent nocturnal secretory bursts of gonadotropin secretion. These matters, though fascinating and potentially instructive, do not fall within the purview of this discussion of the control of the menstrual cycle and the interested reader is referred to a recent symposium on puberty (Grumbach and Sizonenko, in press).

Pulsatile Secretion of Hypothalamic GnRH

Compelling evidence indicates that pulsatile gonadotropin secretion by the pituitary gland must be the consequence of antecedant pulsatile secretion of GnRH by the hypothalamus. Three lines of evidence support this claim. First, administration of an antiserum to GnRH to ovariectomized rhesus monkeys immediately abolishes the circhoral LH pulses, circulating LH levels falling exponentially to undetectable levels (Knobil, 1980). Secondly, intermittent increases in the GnRH content have been found in serial samples of pituitary portal blood of both ovariectomized and fol-

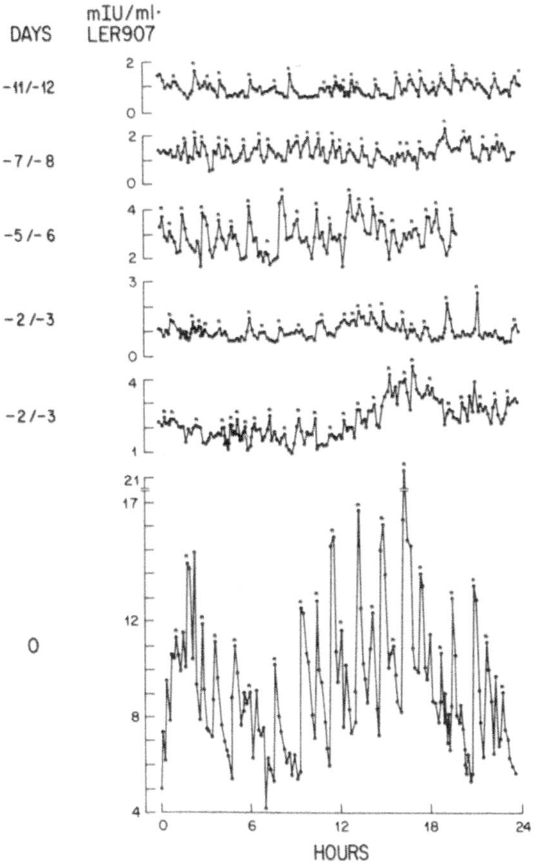

Figure 1

Patterns of circulating LH in women during the follicular phase of the menstrual cycle. Blood samples were taken every 7-10 min for 24 hr. Days indicates days from the midcycle LH surge. Asterisks indicate visually identified hormone pulses which are greater than 20% above the previous nadir and which last for at least two consecutive samples. The average pulse interval is 64 min. Reprinted with permission from Filicori and Crowley (1983).

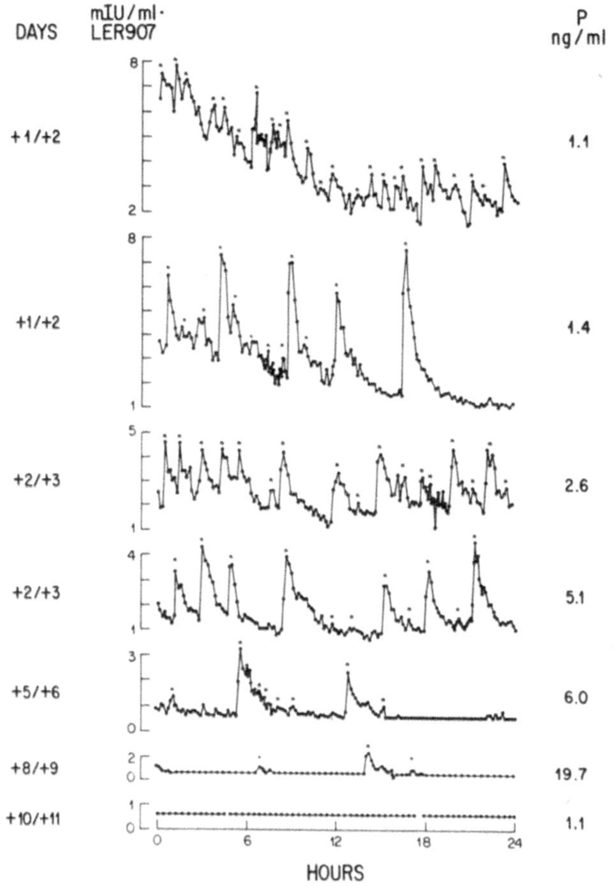

Figure 2

Patterns of circulating LH in women during the luteal phase of the menstrual cycle. Days indicates the time after the midcycle LH surge. P indicates the plasma progesterone concentration on the day of the study. Note that the pulse interval increases as the luteal phase progresses. See legend to Figure 1 for details. Reprinted with permission from Filicori and Crowley (1983).

licular phase rhesus monkeys (Carmel et al., 1976). The technique of blood sampling prevented any GnRH-enriched blood from reaching the pituitary gland however, so that no concommitant pituitary response to this hypothalamic activity could be recorded as incontrovertable proof of the causal relation between these phenomena. This problem has been overcome by elegant and novel surgical approaches to the pituitary portal vasculature in the ovariectomized ewe (Clarke and Cummins, 1982) where simultaneous sampling of a portion of the hypothalamic effluent (for GnRH measurments) and of the peripheral circulation (for LH measurements) proved the synchronous relation between these two events. Thirdly, chronic infusion of GnRH, while stimulating an acute elevation in circulating gonadotropin levels, cannot sustain this secretion, and circulating gonadotropins fall toward undetectable levels (Belchetz et al., 1978). The circhoral pattern, and high mean levels, of gonadoropins characteristic of the ovariectomized monkey can only be recreated in the hypothalamic-deficient ovariectomized monkey when GnRH is given hourly. The pituitary gland, then, can only remain responsive to GnRH if its presence is discontinuous.

The central nervous system mechanisms responsible for the intermittent release of GnRH are not completely clear. Isolation of the medial basal hypothalamus from the rest of the brain (but not from its intimate connections with the anterior pituitary gland) does not prevent circhoral gonadotropin secretion in the ovariectomized rhesus monkey, nor does it prevent ovulatory menstrual cycles from occurring in the otherwise intact monkey (Krey et al., 1975). In contrast, ablation of the area of the arcuate nucleus of the hypothalamus results in a cessation of pulsatile gonadotropin secretion in the ovariectomized rhesus monkey which can be restored if the animal is supplied with an intermittent GnRH source (a "hypothalamic prosthesis", Knobil, 1980). In short, while isolation of the hypothalamo-pituitary unit is compatible with normal gonadotropic function while severely compromising most other anterior and posterior pituitary functions, destruction of the small arcuate area of the medial basal hypothalamus causes only disruption of the gonadotropin-secretory functions of the pituitary gland, sparing the other endocrine functions of the hypophysis.

Recordings from electrodes placed deep within the hypothalamus show that huge bursts of electrical activity precede the appearance of the brisk elevations in circulating LH in the ovariectomized rhesus monkey (Knobil, 1981). Treatment of these animals with alpha adrenergic blocking agents causes an immediate cessation of this bursting electrical activity and of the circhoral pulses in circulating LH (Knobil, 1974). These data provide support for the idea that pituitary gonadotropin secretion is driven by a cascade of events which includes a sudden increase in specific hypothalamic electrical activity (a pacemaker ?) which results in the secretion of GnRH (from nerve terminals adjacent to the primary plexus of the pituitary portal system) and its humoral transport to the anterior pituitary gland where release of gonadotropins is stimulated. While the temporal relations between these three events are now clear, the initiating mechanism (and its modulation) is obscure and the cellular mechanisms at each level have yet to be described.

The Effect of Changing the Frequency of GnRH Pulses on Pituitary Gonadotropin Release

The frequency at which the pituitary gland is "driven" to discharge gonadotropins controls the ratio of FSH to LH in the circulation. In the ovariectomized rhesus monkey, with an arcuate lesion obliterating endogenous GnRH secretion and a hypothalamic prosthesis (1 µg GnRH/min for six minutes each hour), mean levels and temporal pattern of FSH and LH in the circulation approximate those seen in the original ovariectomized state. When GnRH pulse frequency is slowed to 1 every three hours, mean FSH rises as LH falls, resulting in an increase in the FSH/LH ratio (Wildt et al., 1981). A simple explanation for this phenomenon is that a longer interpulse interval allows more gonadotropin to accumulate in the pituitary. The delayed GnRH signal then stimulates a larger than usual release of FSH and LH. The slower $t_{1/2}$ for FSH (about 220 min) in comparison to that of LH (about 66 min) means that FSH tends to accumulate in the circulation while LH is almost entirely cleared from the blood during the protracted pulse interval.

The Effect of Changing Pituitary Gonadotropin Output on Ovarian Function

While the effects of changing GnRH frequency on circulating gonadotropin levels are most easily observed in the ovariectomized subject, it becomes relevant to inquire what effect this changing gonadotropin output might have on ovarian function. It was found that, in the arcuate-lesioned (but otherwise intact) rhesus monkey with a hypothalamic prosthesis, continued invariant GnRH administration (1 µg/min for 6 minutes each hour) resulted in prompt follicular development, a midcycle LH surge, ovulation, and a normal luteal phase (Knobil et al., 1980). In short, unremitting hourly pulsatile GnRH administration supported normal 28-day menstrual cycles. Similar regimens have been used successfully in women with amenorrhea of hypothalamic origin and uneventful pregnancies resulted (Leyendecker et al., 1980). When GnRH pulse frequency is slowed to one every 2 hours in the rhesus monkey, only limited follicular development and estrogen secretion occur, and follicular maturation and ovulation fail (Pohl et al., 1983). The ovary then is extremely sensitive to changes in gonadotropin delivery, although it is not clear yet whether the quality of follicular development depends upon the frequency at which gonadotropins are delivered, or upon the resultant ratio of FSH and LH in the circulation which is a function of GnRH pulse frequency.

REGULATION OF GONADOTROPIN SECRETION BY OVARIAN STEROIDS

Effects of Estradiol

The day-to-day secretion of gonadotropins throughout the menstrual cycle in the rhesus monkey and in women shows two distinct patterns: 1) relatively low and relatively stable serum concentrations of LH and FSH are characteristic of most of the follicular and luteal phases, while 2) an abrupt preovulatory discharge of LH and FSH occurs in the late follicular phase. It appears that these two different patterns of gonadotropin secretion are both controlled by the actions of estradiol directly upon the pituitary gland. Again, using the ovariectomized rhesus monkey with a lesioned nonfunctional hypothalamus replaced with a hypothalamic prosthesis, the administration of estradiol caused an abrupt fall in circulating gonadotropin levels to those seen in the normal intact animal (the negative feedback effect of estradiol), followed about 36 hours later by a surge of gonadotropins in the circulation mimicking the normal preovulatory surge (the positive feedback effect of estradiol). Since both of these estradiol-dependent phenomena can be observed without any change in the output of the hypothalamic prosthesis, it follows then that 1) these actions of estradiol must be directly at the pituitary level and 2) the midcycle gonadotropin surge does not require a midcycle GnRH surge (Knobil, 1980). In fact, the gonadotropin surge elicited by estradiol benzoate treatment will occur even when total GnRH support has been stopped for 24 hours (Wildt et al, 1981a).

The mechanisms by which estradiol exerts its effects on gonadotropin secretion are a mystery. Estradiol receptors in the cytosol of rhesus anterior pituitary cells migrate promptly to the nucleus when exposed to estradiol (a phenomenon characteristic of all steroid-sensitive cells), and remain there (as long as circulating estradiol remains high) during the negative feedback suppression and subsequent positive feedback surge secretion of LH. It is difficult to relate this unidirectional movement of estradiol receptors to the nucleus to a biphasic action of estradiol on gonadotropin secretion (Attardi et al., 1980).

Effects of Progesterone

Progesterone exibits many effects on gonadotropin secretion depending on the prior steroid milieu of the subject, the amount of steroid that is given, and the time frame in which it is given (see Pohl and Hotchkiss,1983). Some of these effects are catalogued below:

1) Progesterone synergizes with estradiol to suppress circulating gonadotropins below detectable levels in the ovariectomized monkey. This synergism is not seen in the normal intact animal in the luteal phase where identical levels of progesterone and estradiol may be found in the circulation, but where gonadotropin levels are still measureable. A synergism which can appear only when the ovaries are removed raises the possibility of a role for other ovarian factors which may modulate gonadotropin secretion.

2) In women, and other species as well, high luteal phase levels of progesterone are associated with a slowing of the endogenous gonadotropin pulse frequency. Mean circulating LH and FSH levels do not fall very much however, as the slower pulse frequency is partially compensated for by the larger pulse amplitude.

3) While estradiol benzoate treatment will elicit gonadotropin surges when given in the follicular phase, this treatment is no longer effective in the luteal phase, or if large amounts of progesterone are given (mimicking the luteal phase) in the follicular phase. This inhibitory action of progesterone may take place in the hypothalamus as it can no longer be demonstrated in animals whose hypothalamus has been lesioned and whose gonadotropin secretion is being maintained by a hypothalamic prosthesis. In addition, these inhibitory effects of progesterone cannot be demonstrated in the ovariectomized monkey.

4) In certain conditions in estrogen-primed women and monkeys, the administration of progesterone will advance the onset of the LH surge, increase peak concentrations of LH, and cause a more abrupt termination of the LH surge. In fact, the presence of small amounts of progesterone are required for the full development of the LH and FSH surge in humans. The locus of action of this facilitatory action of progesterone may be at the pituitary, as the facilitation persists in animals without hypothalamic function but receiving GnRH from a hypothalamic prosthesis. But other evidence shows that this facilitatory action disappears in the presence of anesthesia, arguing for a possible locus of action within the central nervous system. Regardless of how the effects of progesterone are viewed, it must be remembered that it is the continually rising levels of estradiol which are required for the generation of the gonadotropin surge, the effects of progesterone

on this event being, in the main, modulatory.

5) The presence of progesterone in the luteal phase inhibits follicular development.

Out of this confusing and admittedly incomplete list of the effects of progesterone on reproductive function emerges the conclusion that the absence of progesterone allows gonadotropin oscillations to occur more frequently and permits follicular development, estradiol secretion, and the development of the preovulatory gonadotropin surge. The creation of a corpus luteum and attendant progesterone secretion after ovulation is responsible then for a quiescent period in which gonadotropin pulse frequency is low, follicular development is held in check, and no gonadotropin surges can be elicited.

A MODEL OF THE MENSTRUAL CYCLE

The foregoing information, when taken together with the information that ovulatory menstrual cycles of normal duration and hormonal profile can be produced in rhesus monkeys with arcuate lesions or in women with amenorrhea of hypothalamic origin when pulsatile GnRH infusion is maintained for at least 14 days, allows us to draw the following conclusions about the regulation of the menstrual cycle in primates.

1) GnRH secretion, and consequent gonadotropin secretion in the adult, is and must be pulsatile in character, with an unmodulated frequency of about one pulse per hour. This obligate GnRH secretion plays a permissive role in that it allows the complex interactions between ovarian estradiol and pituitary gonadotropin secretion to take place. The importance of this permissive role of pulsatile GnRH secretion is underscored by the finding that pulsatile GnRH administration will elicit normal 28-day menstrual cycles with ovulation in the prepubertal rhesus monkey, showing that the ovary and the pituitary gland of the immature animal are capable of adult reproductive function when the pulsatile hypothalamic function characteristic of the adult is reproduced (Wildt et al., 1980).

2) The maintenance of low circulating gonadotropin levels during the major part of the menstrual cycle is an expression of the negative feedback effects of estradiol at the pituitary level to control the magnitude of gonadotropin release with each pulse, and, during the luteal phase, of the additional effect of progesterone on decreasing the frequency of gonadotropin pulses.

3) The elicitation of the midcycle preovulatory surge of gonadotropins a) is a natural sequel to increases in circulating estradiol produced by the maturing follicle, b) occurs independently of any changes in hypothalamic GnRH output, and c) leads to follicular rupture, ovulation, and corpus luteum formation and progesterone secretion. In the nonfertile cycle, the presence of progesterone merely seems to delay the reinitiation of follicular development. Thus, in the simplest of terms, the control of the primate reproductive cycle is vested in the ovarian secretion of estradiol which determines the response characteristics of the pituitary gonadotrophs to the permissive pulsatile secretion of GnRH by the hypothalamus.

REFERENCES

Attardi, B., Hotchkiss, J., and Knobil, E., 1980, Monkey pituitary oestrogen receptors and the biphasic action of oestradiol on gonadotropin secretion, Nature, 285:252.

Belchetz, P.E., Plant, T.M., Nakai, Y., Keogh, E.J., and Knobil, E., 1978, Hypophysial responses to continuous and intermittent delivery of hypothalamic gonadotropin-releasing hormone, Science, 202:631.

Carmel, P.W., Araki, S., and Ferin, M., 1976, Pituitary stalk portal blood collection in rhesus monkeys: evidence for pulsatile release of gonadotropin releasing hormone (GnRH), Endocrinology, 99:243.

Clarke, I.J., and Cummins, J.T., 1982, The temporal relationship between gonadotropin releasing hormone (GnRH) and luteinizing hormone (LH) secretion in ovariectomized ewes, Endocrinology, 111:1737.

Dierschke, D.J., Bhattacharya, A.N., Atkinson, L.E., and Knobil, E., 1970, Circhoral oscillations of plasma LH in the ovariectomized rhesus monkey, Endocrinology, 87:850.

Filicori, M., and Crowley, W.F., Jr., 1983, Hypothalamic regulation of gonadotropin secretion in the human female, in "Neuroendocrine Aspects of Reproduction", R.L.Norman, ed., Academic Press, New York, in press.

Grumbach, M.M., and Sizonenko, P.C., eds., "Control of the Onset of Puberty,II", Academic Press, New York, in press.

Harris, G.W., 1955, "Neural Control of the Pituitary Gland", Edward Arnold, Ltd., London.

Knobil, E., 1974, On the control of gonadotropin secretion in the rhesus monkey, Rec. Prog. Horm. Res., 30:1.

Knobil, E., 1980, The neuroendocrine control of the menstrual cycle. Rec. Prog. Horm. Res., 36:53.

Knobil, E., 1981, Patterns of hypophysiotropic signals and gonadotropin secretion in the rhesus monkey, Biol. Reprod., 24:44.

Knobil, E., Plant, T.M., Wildt, L., Belchetz, P.E., and Marshall, G., 1980, Control of the rhesus monkey menstrual cycle: permissive role of hypothalamic gonadotropin-releasing hormone, Science, 207:1371.

Krey, L.C., Butler, W.R., and Knobil, E., 1975, Surgical disconnections of the medial basal hypothalamus and pituitary function in the rhesus monkey, Endocrinology, 95:1073.

Leyendecker, G., Wildt, L., and Hansmann, M., 1980, Pregnancies following chronic intermittent (pulsatile) administration of GnRH by means of a portable pump ("Zyklomat") - A new approach to the treatment of infertility in hypothalamic amenorrhea. J. Clin. Endocrinol. Metab., 51:1214.

Plant, T.M., 1982, Effects of orchidectomy and testosterone replacement on pulsatile luteinizing hormone secretion in the adult rhesus monkey (Macaca mulatta), Endocrinology, 110:1905.

Pohl, C.R., and Hotchkiss, J., 1983, Neural control of reproductive function in primates, in "Reproductive Physiology, IV", Int. Rev. Physiol., Vol. 27, R.O. Greep, ed., University Park Press, Baltimore.

Pohl, C.R., Richardson, D.W., Hutchison, J.S., Germak, J.A., and Knobil, E., 1983, Hypophysiotropic signal frequency and the functioning of the pituitary-ovarian system in the rhesus monkey, Endocrinology, 112:2076.

Wildt, L., Hausler, A., Hutchison, J.S., Marshall, G., and Knobil, E., 1981a, Estradiol as a gonadotropin releasing hormone in the rhesus monkey, Endocrinology, 108:2011.

Wildt, L., Hausler, A., Marshall, G., Hutchison, J.S., Plant, T.M., Belchetz, P.E., and Knobil, E., 1981b, Frequency and amplitude modulation of gonadotropin-releasing hormone stimulation and gonadotropin secretion in the rhesus monkey, Endocrinology, 109:376.

Wildt, L., Marshall, G., and Knobil, E.,1980, Experimental induction of puberty in the infantile rhesus monkey, Science, 207:1373.

Winters, S.J., and Troen, P., 1983, A reexamination of pulsatile luteinizing hormone secretion in primary testicular failure, J. Clin. Endocrinol. Metab. 57:432.

Yen, S.S.C., Tsai, C.C., Naftolin, F., Vandenberg, G., and Ajabor, L., 1972, Pulsatile patterns of gonadotropin release in subjects with and without ovarian function, J. Clin. Endocrinol. Metab., 34:671.

5

MATURATION OF THE FOLLICULAR MICROENVIRONMENT

Cecilia L. Schmidt

Over the past decade, the orchestration of the menstrual cycle, formerly attributed to the hypothalamic-pituitary axis, has been properly ascribed to the dominant follicle. It is the microenvironment of the follicle destined to ovulate that determines the circulating hormonal milieu and impinges upon the fate of the selected oocyte. The purpose of this chapter is to survey the factors basic to follicular development and achievement of dominance in the spontaneous menstrual cycle. Understanding these events is mandatory to those who attempt hormonal manipulation of the ovarian cycle to ensure oocyte retrieval for _in vitro_ fertilization.

OVARIAN MORPHOLOGY FROM CONCEPTION TO THE PRESENT CYCLE

Embryological Development of the Gonad

Between 3 and 5 weeks after fertilization, the primitive germ cells derived from the endoderm of the yolk sac migrate to the mesonephric or urogenital ridge (Edman, 1983). Coelemic surface epithelial cells surround the primordial germ cells and encompass an inner core of medullary mesenchymal tissue. By the sixth week of fetal life, the indifferent stage of the primitive gonad has been completed and mitosis has resulted in a total of 100,000 germ cells (Baker, 1972).

The genotype of the fetus dictates further development into either an ovary or a testis. The absence of a Y chromosome, rather than the presence of 2 X chromosomes, probably allows oocyte formation (Haseltine, 1983). Unlike the male, female internal and external genitalia differentiation is initiated before gonadal maturation. Therefore, a female fetus is identified by the absence of testicular development. The apparently inactive ovary, however, exhibits cortical dominance over the medulla and nascent estradiol synthesis. At 6 to 8 weeks, marked mitotic division of oogonia is initiated and culminates in a zenith of 6 to 7 million germ cells by 20 weeks (Baker, 1972). The process of atresia, first evident at approximately 15 weeks gestation, will eliminate about 80% of the germ cell stores by the time of birth. At menarche only 400,000 germ cells will remain (Baker, 1972). Atresia, rather than ovulation, will be the fate of 99.9% of all germ cells (Rebar, 1983) as seen in Figure 1.

Ovarian Differentiation

Differentiation of oogonia and the primitive gonad involve changes in both the germ cells and the highly vascularized cortex. Between the eighth and thirteenth week of fetal life, penetrating blood vessels arising from the deeper medullary area of

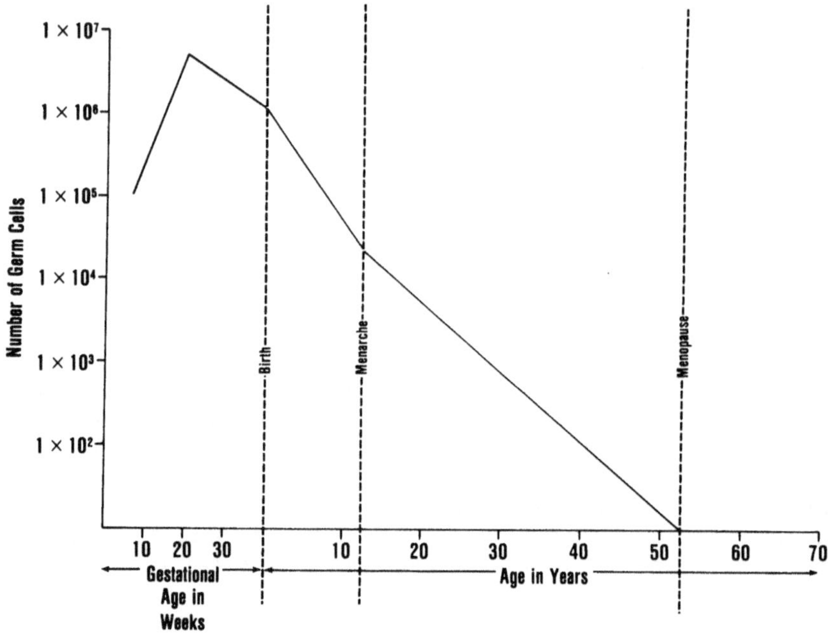

Figure 1

Changes in germ cell stores in the human ovary over time (Based on data summarized in Baker, 1972).

the ovary populate the cortex with perivascular mesenchymal and epithelial cells that surround the oogonia. These epithelial cells differentiating from mesonephric precursors constitute the innermost single layer of pre-granulosa cells. The mesenchymal cells form the less defined matrix of pre-thecal cells and the primitive ovarian stroma between the primitive follicles.

Concomitantly, the oogonia begin the first meiotic division and are arrested in the diplotene stage of prophase to become primary oocytes. Further progression beyond the prophase of meiosis I, with extrusion of the first polar body, occurs in the 36 hours prior to ovulation secondary to the LH surge or in spontaneous maturation preceding atresia. The inhibition of meiosis appears dependent upon the follicular environment. A polypeptide substance responsible for this inhibition has been identified in porcine follicular fluid and extracts of granulosa cells (Tsafriri and Channing, 1975). This oocyte maturation inhibitor (OMI) would explain the observation that oocytes aspirated from medium-size follicles will spontaneously resume meiosis in vitro when placed in a balanced salt solution. Furthermore, involvement of granulosa cells in the intrafollicular inhibition of meiosis is supported by the resumption of meiosis in the presence of degenerating granulosa cells, i.e., in the atretic follicle (Ingram, 1962). Oocyte maturation inhibitor thus appears to be present in all follicles except pre-ovulatory and atretic ones (Channing et al., 1982). For a further discussion of OMI, see Chapter 12.

In the fetal ovary, 5 types of follicles are found as a result of oocyte growth and granulosa - theca cell organization and proliferation: primordial, primary, pre-antral, antral and atretic follicles. The primordial follicle is a unit comprised of a primary oocyte arrested at prophase of meiosis I and surrounded by a single layer of pre-granulosa cells defined by a spindle-shaped epithelial morphology (Baker and Franchi, 1967; Mossman and Duke, 1973). The basal lamina separates the primordial follicle from the surrounding stroma.

Although mitotic divisions of oogonia have ceased by the seventh month of gestation, incorporation of all viable cells into primordial follicles is not completed until 6 months postpartum (Potter, 1961; Lintern-Moore et al., 1974; Peters et al., 1976). Primary follicles first appear between the fifth and sixth months of gestation (Van Wagenen and Simpson, 1965). The pre-granulosa cells differentiate into a single layer of cuboidal cells equivalent to granulosa cells. Cytoplasmic processes from the granulosa cells abut closely upon the oocyte. The pre-antral follicle houses an enlarging oocyte whose diameter has increased from 25 μm to a maximum of approximately 80 μm (Baca and Zamboni,

1967). Proliferation of granulosa cells results in a multi-layered population, originally thought to produce the mucopolysaccharides that form the zona pellucida around the oocyte (Chiquoine, 1960). However, characterization of zona pellucida components in the mouse, coupled with radiolabel incorporation studies, have revealed that denuded oocytes can synthesize these glycoproteins (Wassarman, 1983). Hence, biochemical evidence supports the idea that the growing oocyte, not the surrounding granulosa cells, produces the zona pellucida (Chapter 12).

Intimate contact between the granulosa cells and the plasma membrane of the oocyte is maintained across the zona pellucida through cytoplasmic processes of the granulosa cells (Zamboni, 1972). Outside the basal lamina, the pre-theca cells organize concentrically to form the theca cells, laced by lymphatics and blood vessels that do not traverse the basal lamina. Accumulation of cytoplasm and differentiation into steroid-secreting cells separates the inner theca interna cells from the outer spindle-shaped theca externa cells.

Further proliferation of granulosa cells is accompanied by localized accumulation of fluid among rosettes of granulosa cells, Call-Exner bodies. Coalescence of these Call-Exner bodies produces a central fluid-filled body called the antrum. Antrum formation forces the oocyte into a more eccentric position surrounded by several layers of granulosa cells that constitute the cumulus oophorus and transforms the pre-antral follicle into a Graafian follicle. The antrum is lined by mural granulosa cells which, in contrast to the granulosa cells of the cumulus oophorus, are not expelled with the oocyte at the time of ovulation. Rather, the mural granulosa cells, together with the theca interna, will luteinize to form the corpus luteum after oocyte extrusion. Antral fluid is rich in mucopolysaccharides produced by the granulosa cells, proteins and electrolytes diffusing from vascular spaces and sex steroids jointly produced by granulosa and theca cells. Virtually all ovaries examined between the fourth to sixth months after birth exhibit antral follicles. However, further growth of any Graafian follicle to the size characteristic of pre-ovulatory follicles in menstruating women has not been detected during fetal life (Polhemus, 1953; Potter, 1961; Peters et al., 1976).

The fifth type of follicle found in the fetal ovary is the atretic follicle. Degeneration and death of the oocyte is inevitable in the atretic follicle. However, as already mentioned, the first polar body may be extruded by the oocyte during the initial stages of atresia (Himelstein-Braw et al., 1976). Granulosa cells undergo reduction in mitotic index and cytolysis preceded by pyknosis, karyorrhexis and karyolysis.

Frequently, this sequence of cellular degeneration proceeds from layers of granulosa cells farthest from the ovary toward the zona pellucida. Ultimately, the granulosa cells are replaced by fibrocytes that form avascular scars. The thecal cells outside the basal lamina hypertrophy and then dedifferentiate, returning to the pool of interstitial stromal cells. It is the follicular development preceding atresia that accounts for mid-gestational estrogen production by the female fetus.

Pubertal and Adult Ovary

The 5 types of follicles described in the fetal ovary are also found in the pubertal and adult ovary. However, the emergence of the pre-ovulatory Graafian follicle occurs only in the pubertal or adult ovary (Figure 2). Once growth of the primary follicle is initiated, maturation can proceed to the antral stage if gonadotropins are present, without the need for hormonal cyclicity. However, formation of the large pre-ovulatory follicle requires orderly exposure to gonadotropins. Therefore, the growth spurt of most follicles will terminate in atresia. The maturation of the hypothalamic-pituitary axis is essential to the first and subsequent ovulations.

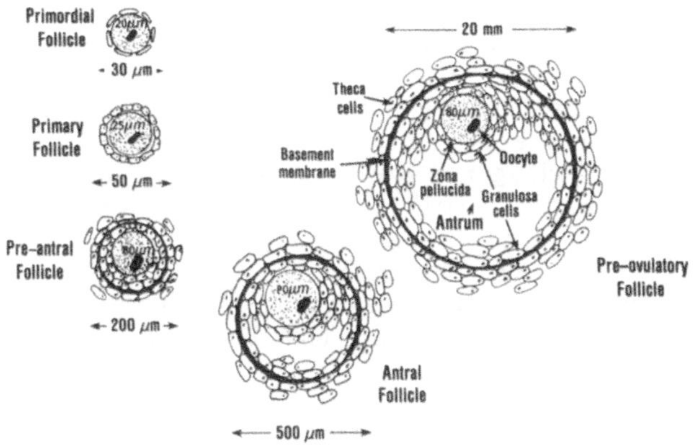

Figure 2

Morphological characteristics of ovarian follicles (Modified from Speroff et al., 1983).

FOLLICULAR MATURATION DURING THE MENSTRUAL CYCLE

Now familiar with the morphology of the adult ovary, it is advantageous to consider the sequence of events in a normal 28-day cycle from the viewpoint of the dominant follicle.

The Cohort Stage

Between menstrual cycle days 1 and 5, a group of follicles begins to respond to increasing gonadotropins in a manner quite distinct from follicular growth unrelated to hormonal cyclicity. This cohort of follicles responds to increasing levels of FSH with growth of the primary oocyte and mitotic proliferation of granulosa cells. The total number of FSH receptors in granulosa cells is enhanced by both this proliferation of cells and an increase in the number of FSH receptors in each granulosa cell (Richards, 1979). FSH, working via an adenylate cyclase system, induces the aromatase enzyme system. Aromatization of androgens to estrogens by granulosa cells regulates follicular estrogen production, best explained by the two-cell/two-gonadotropin theory of intrafollicular estrogen biosynthesis (Ryan et al., 1968). In the pre-antral and antral follicle, FSH receptors are found only on the granulosa cells and LH receptors are present only on the thecal cells. Although both granulosa cells and thecal cells have the ability to synthesize all 3 classes of steroids as demonstrated in vitro (McNatty et al., 1979), thecal cells respond to LH with androgen production while granulosa cells, via an FSH-stimulated aromatase system, convert these androgens to estrogens. This interaction between the granulosa and thecal cells is most prominent in the larger antral follicles.

Estrogens synergize with FSH in further enhancing the FSH receptor content of the follicle. Hence, the follicles comprising the cohort are propelled to the pre-antral and antral stages of development during the beginning of the cycle. In the absence of FSH, follicular androgens are predominant. This situation is evident in pre-antral follicles of patients with polycystic ovarian syndrome whose defect can be reversed by in vitro administration of FSH (Erickson et al., 1979). Hence, an estrogenic microenvironment acting in concert with FSH enhances the sensitivity of follicles to FSH by increasing the number of FSH receptors.

Selection of the Dominant Follicle

The earliest sign of selection of the dominant follicle is asymmetrical ovarian estrogen secretion noted between days 6 and 8 of the menstrual cycle (diZerega et al., 1980a and 1981). This asymmetry signals the establishment, by the dominant follicle, of a self-perpetuating estrogenic microenvironment to the detriment of other follicles. The conversion of androgens to estrogens through the FSH-dependent aromatase system of the granulosa cells is amplified in the dominant follicle. The elevated circulating estradiol levels resulting from the escalating estrogen production of the dominant follicle exerts a negative central feedback on FSH production by the pituitary. Declining FSH plasma concentrations limit the amount of FSH available to the less mature follicles. Consequently, in all but the dominant follicle, aromatase decreases and an androgenic microenvironment pervades, resulting in atresia. The antral morphology of the dominant follicle further fosters perpetuation of this estrogenic milieu. Follicular fluid bathes the granulosa cells, sequestering estradiol and FSH for the dominant follicle. To compound the discrepancy in FSH availability between the dominant follicle and those slated for atresia, a follicular fluid non-steroidal inhibitor of FSH has been cited. Folliculostatin, alternately donned "ovarian inhibin", has been postulated as the component of porcine follicular fluid responsible for a central decrease in FSH secretion when this fluid is administered to intact animals (Grady et al., 1981).

Evidence for folliculostatin in the human female is somewhat circumstantial. Increasing levels of FSH contrast with the steady LH levels during the late luteal phase, a stage of decreased follicular fluid secondary to a relative dearth of antral follicles. A decrease in estrogen alone does not adequately explain this disparate rise in FSH. Similarly, a decreased number of developing antral follicles may explain the increase in FSH which hallmarks the peri-menopause and precedes the rise in LH levels after the menopause (Sherman et al., 1976). Adequate estrogen replacement of post-menopausal women lowers circulating FSH values but fails to suppress FSH levels to pre-menopausal values. Since charcoal-treated (steroid-free) follicular fluid from several species, including the human, is capable of this inhibition in rats and lower primates (Channing et al., 1982), a comparable role of folliculostatin is postulated in the human.

It has been shown that FSH and estradiol induce LH/hCG receptors (Channing et al., 1978). Although the affinity of the granulosa cell receptors for LH is not altered with follicular maturation, the number of LH/hCG receptors in the granulosa cells is increased by estrogen and FSH (Richards and Midgley, Jr., 1976). In the midst of FSH deprivation and decreasing estradiol levels, only the dominant follicle continues to produce significant estradiol. Hence, the dominant follicle controls the timing of the LH surge according to its own specific estrogen microenvironment. The teleologic purpose of this control is to prevent the havoc which would be wrought by a premature LH surge.

An inadequate aromatase system would fail to convert androgens produced by the theca into estrogens. The resulting androgenic environment would lead to atresia. Furthermore, even an LH surge occurring merely 1 to 2 days before adequate FSH-estradiol priming would find granulosa cells with only few LH/hCG receptors.

The supremacy of this dominant follicle after selection has been completed is supported by experimental evidence in monkeys. After ablation of the dominant follicle between cycle days 7 and 9, no follicles remain that are able either to respond to administered gonadotropins or to develop to the point of ovulation within the time frame of that cycle. Rather, ovulation occurs 14 days after destruction of the dominant follicle, and hence, from a newly recruited cohort of follicles (Hodgen et al., 1983).

Development of the Dominant Follicle

The mid-follicular rise of circulating estradiol, reflecting the milieu of the dominant follicle, proceeds along a linear escalation by day 9 of the menstrual cycle (Figure 3). Estradiol maintenance above 200 pg/ml for at least 36 to 50 hours will exert a positive feedback upon LH secretion, culminating in the LH surge. The site of this regulatory action appears to be the pituitary, since replacement of hypothalamic function with pulsatile administration of GnRH permits this positive feedback in both monkeys (Knobil, 1980) and women (Crowley and McArthur, 1980; Leyendecker et al., 1980) (See Chapter 4).

Since the dominant follicle employs estradiol secretion to coordinate the timing of the LH surge with the development of LH receptors on the granulosa cells, luteinization of granulosa cells is initiated with the escalating LH levels. It should be noted that many authors have found a marked discrepancy between the prodigious elevation of bioassayable LH and lower RIA levels (Marut et al., 1981; Williams et al., 1982). The notorious heterogeneity of gonadotropins may explain the different affinity of pre-ovulatory LH for various antisera used in different RIA's.

Luteinization denotes the imbibition of lipids and lutein pigment by the granulosa cells and signals progesterone secretion into both follicular fluid and the circulation in response to LH. It is thought that the limited surge of progesterone may be responsible for the FSH peak. Premature luteinization is further thought to be prevented by a third ovarian non-steroidal follicular regulator, luteinization inhibitor (LI; Channing et al., 1978). These authors have noted that charcoal-treated follicular fluid from half of the small and medium porcine follicles, in contrast to large follicles, inhibited progesterone secretion by cultures of granulosa cells from large pre-ovulatory

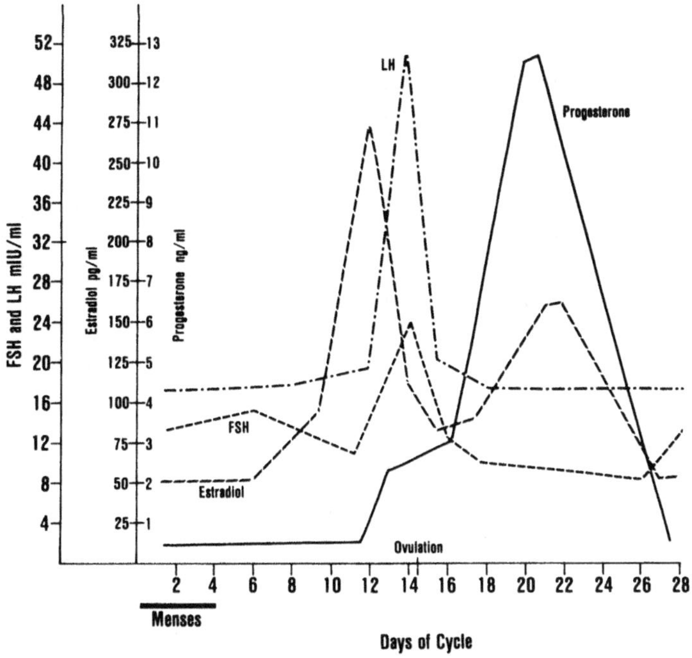

Figure 3

Circulating gonadotropin and steroid concentrations typified in a normal 28-day cycle.

follicles and prevented morphological luteinization. Similar extracts of human follicular fluids from all but larger follicles inhibited rat ovarian cyclic AMP accumulation (Lunenfeld et al., 1977). It is theorized that luteinization occurs only through antagonism of LI by a luteinization stimulator, yet to be characterized.

Concomitant with the developing sensitivity of granulosa cells to LH is the continued stimulation of theca cells by increasing LH. Androgen production by the theca of all growing follicles steadily increases. These androgens, particularly androstenedione and testosterone, serve as enhanced substrates for estrone and estradiol production in the dominant follicle, which is rich in aromatase. As summarized in Table 1, follicular fluid estradiol levels in healthy pre-ovulatory follicles have ranged between 1000 ng/ml (Edwards et al., 1980) and 1800 ng/ml (Brailly et al.,

Table 1 Summary of steroid concentrations (mean ± SEM) of human follicular fluids (ng/ml) as cited in the literature.

Reference Source	Time of Aspiration	Estradiol	Estrone	Androstenedione	Progesterone	Testosterone
Edwards et al.,1980	Onset of LH surge to ovulation	1081 ± 173 (45)	---	28 ± 8 (45)	15323 ± 1115 (45)	---
McNatty et al.,1976	"Late Follicular Phase"	1570 ± 289 (23)	136 ± 39 (4)	266 ± 86 (23)	---	37.6 ± 10.5 (12)
Brailly et al.,1981	Estradiol peak to ovulation	1779 ± 204 (22)	---	159 ± 31 (22)	5360 ± 679 (22)	17.7 ± 2.9 (22)
	LH peak to ovulation	1109 ± 142 (12)	---	69 ± 19 (12)	7773 ± 643 (12)	10.1 ± 2.2 (12)

Numbers in parentheses refer to the number of follicles analyzed.

1981), dependent upon the time of aspiration. The androstenedione/estradiol ratio was found to be less than 1 in large follicular phase follicles, ranging from 0.05 to 0.6. The lowest ratios were found in large follicles from the late follicular phase (McNatty et al., 1976). Testosterone concentrations within follicular fluid were found to be approximately 1/12 that of androstenedione while dihydrotestosterone was approximately 0.4 to 0.8% that of androstenedione (Brailly et al., 1981). A correlation has been noted between follicular fluid with high 17β estradiol and high progesterone levels and healthy, fertilizable oocytes (Wramsby et al., 1981).

The mid-cycle androgen peak arising from LH-stimulated thecal components of the recruited non-dominant follicles enhances atresia of these follicles. Evidence supporting the atretogenic potential of testosterone and other androgens includes the increased follicular atresia in the rat after injections of these hormones (Ross and Lipsett, 1978). Channing et al., (1978) noted that the addition of testosterone to cultures of granulosa cells from human pre-ovulatory follicles resulted in decreased progesterone secretion, compatible with atresia (Channing et al., 1978). Furthermore, the elevated serum androgen levels stimulate libido at a fortuitous point in preparation for ovulation.

Ovulation

The focal point of ovulation is the LH surge, artfully timed by the dominant follicle. By day 14 of the cycle, this pre-ovulatory follicle has enlarged to as much as 30mm in diameter, containing up to 8 ml of follicular fluid. Hence, ovulation, denoting physical extrusion of the oocyte, can be induced in response to the series of events initiated by the LH surge. By frequent serum sampling of peri-ovulatory spontaneously cycling women, ovulation has been most reliably noted to occur approximately 28 to 32 hours after the onset of the LH surge (Pauerstein et al., 1978; Garcia et al., 1981). Similarly, the peak of the LH surge predicts follicular rupture approximately 10 to 12 hours later. Using a rapid, double-antibody radioimmunoassay for LH in serum; Quigley et al. (1982) demonstrated a separation at 30 mIU/ml between basal and surge levels of LH in 12 periovulatory women (Figure 4). Basal levels were 14.5 ± 6.8 mIU/ml (mean $\pm$ SEM), while peak levels were 120.7 ± 16.5 mIU/ml. These time sequences are true of spontaneous cycles. In cycles stimulated with clomiphene citrate, ovulation usually occurs 38 to 40 hours after administration of exogenous hCG (Edwards and Steptoe, 1975).

The mechanisms by which the LH surge results in ovulation involve several modifications of the follicular unit. It is

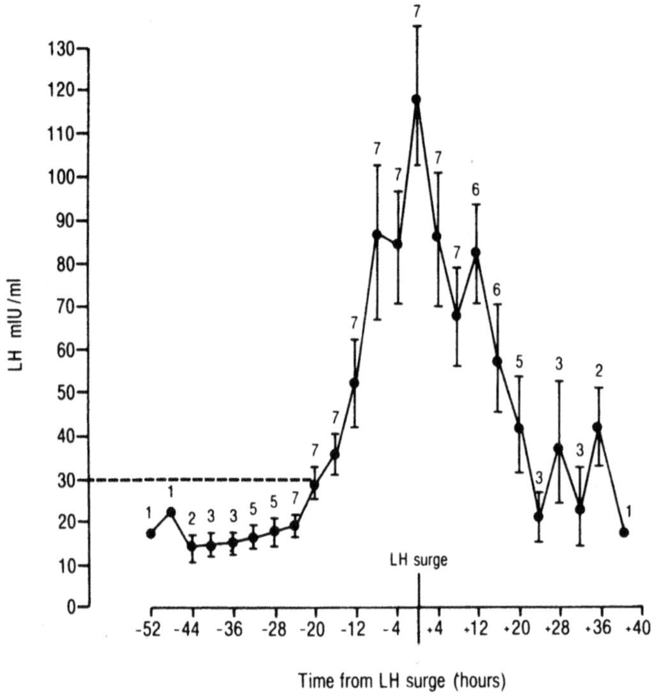

Figure 4

LH concentrations as determined by rapid double-antibody assay in 12 peri-ovulatory women. Samples were taken at 4-hourly intervals and normalized in relation to the LH surge. Numbers above data points indicate the number of women sampled at each time point. (Data from Quigley et al., 1982).

postulated that the magnitude of the LH surge overcomes the locally inhibiting non-steroidal follicular factors preventing premature oocyte maturation (OMI) and luteinization (LI). Hence, in vivo resumption of oocyte maturation from prophase of meiosis I at approximately 20 hours after the LH surge results in the extrusion of the first polar body between 25 and 35 hours after the LH surge (Steptoe and Edwards, 1970; Testart et al., 1982). Cytological analysis of the oocyte after pre-ovulatory aspiration has temporally related the resumption of meiosis with the expansion of the cumulus oophorus (Testart et al., 1982).

Granulosa cells produce increasing amounts of progesterone in response to the LH surge. The impact of this rising progesterone includes enhanced distensibility of the follicular wall through degenerative changes in the collagen framework by increased levels of collagenase and plasminogen activator. Granulosa cell proliferation is halted. The FSH surge is initiated and appears to facilitate detachment of the cumulus and oocyte from the follicle wall. FSH promotes production of plasminogen activator, converting plasminogen into the proteolytic enzyme plasmin (Stickland and Beers, 1976). Incorporation of hyaluronic acid into the cumulus oophorous, permiting cumulus expansion and mobility, has been stimulated in vitro by FSH (Eppig, 1979 and 1980). LH also induces marked increases in follicular fluid prostaglandin concentrations, highest at ovulation (LaMaire et al., 1975). Although follicular rupture is blocked by inhibition of prostaglandin synthesis in rodents, the exact role of prostaglandins in oocyte extrusion is unknown (O'Grady et al., 1972; Tsafriri et al., 1973). Possible explanations include digestion of the follicular wall by released lysosomal enzymes and prostaglandin-stimulated contractions of smooth muscle fibers present in the theca externa (Amsterdam et al., 1977).

Luteal Phase

The stage of corpus luteum dominance intimately reflects pre-ovulatory follicular development. Hormonal inadequacies during the 2 weeks following ovulation and failure to be rescued by hCG are directly related to follicular granulosa and thecal deficiencies.

After extrusion of the oocyte, capillaries originating in the thecal layers penetrate the granulosa cell layer and fill the former antral cavity with blood. Cholesterol transported by low density lipoproteins is thus allowed to reach the granulosa cells to augment progesterone production. Early luteal function is dependent upon basal levels of LH as observed in ovulation induction in hypogonadotropic hypogonadal patients. These women exhibit shortened luteal phases when a single dose of LH is employed to create the pre-ovulatory gonadotropin surge, since LH levels are not maintained. In contrast, hCG, with a functional half-life of approximatley 30 hours, or repeated doses of LH, allow basal gonadotropin support of the corpus luteum (Jewelwicz et al., 1973).

Progesterone secretion affects both ovarian and endometrial development. In concert with estrogen, progesterone exerts a negative feedback on gonadotropin secretion. New follicular growth is further suppressed by antagonism of estrogen dependent mitogenic effects of other follicles. McNatty et al., (1983) have shown that 94% of luteal phase follicles greater than 1 mm in diameter are atretic by oocyte viability and granulosa cell number assessment. Biochemical criteria of decreased aromatase activity do not distinquish between atretic and healthy luteal phase follicles. Although these authors claim corpus luteum suppression of bilateral luteal follicular growth in women, Goodman and Hodgen (1977 and 1979) have noted that ovulation occurs in monkeys in the contralateral ovary about 70% of the time in normal, unperturbed menstrual cycles. Furthermore, regardless of the site of the former corpus luteum, the subsequent dominant follicle will develop in the ovary releasing the lowest amount of progesterone into the venous system during the antecedent luteal phase (Goodman and Hodgen, 1977 and 1979; and diZerega and Hodgen, 1982). Hence, intraluteal progesterone affects future follicular development.

Progesterone is vital to secretory alterations made upon the estrogen-primed endometrium. Restraint of endometrial height is probably a function of progesterone. However, the continued estrogen-induced growth of glands and spiral vessels within this fixed framework results in tortuosity of the glands and coiling of the spiral vessels. In glandular cells, vacuoles migrate from the subnuclear to the intraluminal position. These changes are most prominent at the height of progesterone secretion from the corpus luteum and coincident with implantation in a conception cycle. Inadequate levels of progesterone will be reflected in an asynchronous endometrium lacking progesterone-induced stability.

It is at the high point of luteal activity, approximately 8 days after ovulation, that hCG from a developing trophoblast can rescue the corpus luteum. A two-week prolongation of the lifespan of the corpus luteum and, hence, the menstrual cycle can be elicited experimentally with exogenous hCG administration approximately 8 to 10 days after ovulation (Quagliarello et al., 1980). Since hCG alone cannot simulate pregnancy maintenance of the corpus luteum beyond this two-week interval, other factors must be intrinsic to luteal function. Furthermore, it is known that the sensitivity of the corpus luteum to LH/hCG stimulation progressively decreases as a non-steroidal LH receptor binding inhibitor (LHRBI) increases (Channing et al., 1982). Progesterone secretion *in vitro* can be inhibited by LHRBI. Maintenance of the corpus luteum in early pregnancy may result from a non-hCG mediated antagonism of the effect of LHRBI.

Progesterone and relaxin are actively secreted by the corpus luteum throughout pregnancy (Quagliarello et al., 1979). However, luteal function is necessary for pregnancy maintenance until approximately 7 weeks of gestation. Luteectomy prior to this time necessitates administration of large doses of progestagens for continuation of the pregnancy (Csapo et al., 1973). This pharmacological progesterone replacement may mimic the high levels of progesterone delivered to the endometrium via ovarian-uterine circulatory anastomoses. Alternatively, the uterine quiescence synergistically effected by relaxin and progesterone (Sarosi et al., 1983) may be duplicated by higher levels of exogenous progesterone alone after luteectomy.

Failure of the corpus luteum to be "rescued" by the developing trophoblast results in luteolysis. The mechanisms proposed for termination of luteal function have been elucidated in lower primates but have not been verified in the human cycle. Luteal production of estradiol has been touted as the pivotal luteolytic trigger since intraovarian injections of estradiol induce luteolysis only when the ovary containing the corpus luteum is treated (Karsch and Sutton, 1976). In vitro studies have extended estradiol inhibition of hCG-induced progesterone production by luteal cells from rhesus monkeys (Stouffer et al., 1977) to those obtained from the human menstrual cycle (Williams et al., 1979). The site of estradiol inhibition has been hypothesized to be at the LH receptor. The number of LH receptors has been decreased in cultured human luteal tissue by diethylstilbestrol (Nakano et al., 1981) and in intact corpora lutea by estradiol administered to rhesus monkeys (Sotrel et al., 1981).

Estrogen administered early in the luteal cycle increases the ratio of PGF to PGE (Balmaceda et al., 1980), an event occurring physiologically late in the luteal phase (Balmaceda et al., 1979). It has also been noted that PGF_2 inhibits progesterone production while PGE_2 stimulates progesterone synthesis (Sotrel et al., 1981; Peters and McNatty, 1980). Hence, it is speculated that luteal estradiol fosters the decline of the corpus luteum via alteration of this prostaglandin balance. Since hCG inhibits prostaglandin synthesis (Balmaceda et al., 1981), the elevation of PGF:PGE may be prevented in the corpus luteum by the intervening pregnancy.

The role of prolactin in maintenance of the human corpus luteum has not been completely elucidated, although it is well known that prolactin is luteotropic in the rat (Goldsmith et al., 1981). In vitro data from human granulosa cells suggests that physiologic concentrations of prolactin may be instrumental in luteal support, while higher levels of prolactin inhibit progesterone synthesis (McNatty et al., 1974).

The consequences of luteolysis and, hence, of waning progesterone include increasing circulatory levels of FSH, secondary to the release from feedback inhibition (Ross et al., 1970). The significance of the pre-menstrual serum FSH elevation was investigated by diZerega et al. (1980b) by serial ablation of the presumed dominant follicle at approximately day 10 in 2 subsequent cycles. Folliculogenesis during the third cycle resulted in a normal appearing spontaneous ovulation and luteal phase. These results in monkeys suggest that the intercycle FSH rise may not be obligatory for the subsequent folliculogenesis but do not minimize the significance of FSH levels during the cohort stage.

Having examined the normal spontaneous development of the dominant follicle, we recognize the sublime coordination that is effected by this structure and which is responsible for transition to an adequate luteal function. It is these principles of normalcy which must be held foremost as we attempt surpassing the usual quota of one dominant follicle per cycle in in vitro fertilization programs.

REFERENCES

Amsterdam, A., Lindner, H.R., and Groschel-Stewart, U., 1977, Localization of actin and myosin in the rat oocyte and follicular wall by immunofluorescence, Anat. Rec., 187:311.

Baca, M. and Zamboni, L., 1967, The fine structure of human follicular oocytes, J. Ultrastruct. Res., 19:354.

Baker, T.G., 1972, Oogenesis and ovulation, in: "Reproduction in Mammals. I. Germ Cells and Fertilization," C.R. Austin and R.V. Short, eds., Cambridge University Press, Oxford.

Baker, T.G., and Franchi, L.L., 1967, The fine structure of oogonia and oocytes in human ovaries, J. Cell. Sci., 2:213.

Balmaceda, J.P., Asch, R.H., Fernandez, E.O., Valenzuela, G., Eddy, C.A., and Pauerstein, C.J., 1979, Prostaglandin production by rhesus monkey corpora lutea in vitro, Fertil. Steril., 31:214.

Balmaceda, J., Valenzuela, G., Eddy, C.A., and Asch, R.H., 1980, Prostaglandin production by rhesus monkey corpora lutea in vitro: effects of estrogen administration, Int. J. Gynaecol. Obstet., 18:15.

Balmaceda, J.P., Valenzuela, G., Eddy, C.A., and Asch, R.H., 1981, Effects of hCG on prostaglandin synthesis and function of corpus luteum, Obstet. Gynecol., 57:505.

Brailly, S., Gougeon, A., Milgrom, E., Bomsel-Helmreich, O., and Papiernik, E., 1981, Androgens and progestins in the human ovarian follicle: differences in the evolution of preovulatory, healthy nonovulatory, and atretic follicles, J. Clin. Endocrinol. Metab., 53:128.

Channing, C.P., Anderson, L.D., and Batta, S.K., 1978, Follicular growth and development, Clin. Obstet. Gynaecol., 5:375.

Channing, C.P., Anderson, L.D., Hoover, D.J., Kolena, J., Osteen, K.G., Pomerantz, S.H., and Tanabe, 1982, The role of nonsteroidal regulators in control of oocyte and follicular maturation, Recent Prog. Horm. Res., 38:331.

Chiquoine, A.D., 1960, The development of the zona pellucida of the mammalian ovum, Am. J. Anat., 106:149.
Crowley, W.F., and McArthur, J.W., 1980, Stimulation of the normal menstrual cycle in Kallman's syndrome by pulsatile administration of luteinizing hormone-releasing hormone (LHRH), J. Clin. Endocrinol. Metab., 51:173.
Csapo, A.I., Pulkkinen, M.O., and Wiest, W.G., 1973, Effects of luteectomy and progesterone replacement therapy in early pregnant patients, Am. J. Obstet. Gynecol., 115:759.
diZerega, G.S., and Hodgen, G.D., 1982, The interovarian progesterone gradient: a spatial and temporal regulator of folliculogenesis in the primate ovarian cycle, J. Clin. Endocrinol. Metab., 54:495.
diZerega, G.S., Lynch, A., and Hodgen, G.D., 1981, Initiation of asymmetrical ovarian estradiol secretion in the primate ovarian cycle after luteectomy, Endocrinol., 108:1233.
diZerega, G.S., Marut, E.L., Turner, C.K., and Hodgen, G.D., 1980a, Asymmetrical ovarian function during recruitment and selection of the dominant follicle in the menstrual cycle of the rhesus monkey, J. Clin. Endocrinol. Metab., 51:698.
diZerega, G.S., Nixon, W.E., and Hodgen, G.D., 1980b, Intercycle serum FSH elevations: significance in recruitment and selection of the dominant follicle and assessment of corpus luteum normalcy, J. Clin. Endocrinol. Metab., 50:1046.
Edman, C.D., 1983, Testicular regression syndrome, Semin. Reprod. Endocrinol., 1:129.
Edwards, R.G., and Steptoe, P.C., 1975, Induction of follicular growth, ovulation and luteinization in the human ovary, J. Reprod. Fert., Suppl. 22:121.
Edwards, R.G., Steptoe, P.C., Fowler, R.E., and Baillie, J., 1980, Observations on preovulatory human ovarian follicles and their aspirates, Br. J. Obstet. Gynaecol., 87:769.
Eppig, J.J., 1979, FSH stimulates hyaluronic acid synthesis by oocyte-cumulus cell complexes from mouse preovulatory follicles, Nature, London, 281:483.
Eppig, J.J., 1980, Role of serum in FSH stimulated cumulus expansion by mouse oocyte-cumulus cell complexes in vitro, Biol. Reprod., 22:629.
Erickson, G.F., Hsueh, A.J.W., Quigley, M.E., Rebar, R.W., and Yen, S.S.C.,1979, Functional studies of aromatase activity in human granulosa cells from normal and polycystic ovaries, J. Clin. Endocrinol. Metab., 49:514.
Garcia, J.E., Jones, G.S., and Wright, G.L., 1981, Prediction of the time of ovulation, Fertil. Steril., 36:308.
Goldsmith, L.T., Grob, H.S., Scherer, K.J., Surve, A., Steinetz, B.G., and Weiss, G., 1981, Placental control of ovarian immunoreactive relaxin secretion in the pregnant rat, Endocrinol., 109:548.
Goodman, A.L., and Hodgen, G.D., 1977, Systemic versus

intraovarian progesterone replacement after luteectomy in rhesus monkeys: differential patterns of gonadotropins and follicle growth, J. Clin. Endocrinol. Metab., 45:837.

Goodman, A.L., and Hodgen, G.D., 1979, Between-ovary interaction in the regulation of follicle growth, corpus luteum function, and gonadotropin secretion in the primate ovarian cycle. II. Effects of luteectomy and hemiovariectomy during the luteal phase in cynomolgus monkeys, Endocrinol., 104:1310.

Grady, R.R., Savoy-Moore, R.T., and Schwartz, N.B., 1981, Selective suppression of follicle-stimulating hormone by folliculostatin: a proposed ovarian hormone, in: "Bioregulators of Reproduction," G. Jagiello and H.J. Vogel, eds., Academic Press, Inc., New York.

Haseltine, F.P., 1983, Defects in H-Y antigen expression and related gonadal failure, Semin. Reprod. Endocrinol., 1:113.

Himelstein-Braw, R., Byskov, A.G., Peters, H., and Faber, M., 1976, Follicular atresia in the infant human ovary, J. Reprod. Fertil., 46:55.

Hodgen, G.D., Goodman, A.L., Stouffer, R.L., Williams, R.F., diZerega, G.S., Kreitman, O.L., Marut, E.L., and Schenken, R.S., 1983, Selection and maturation of the dominant follicle and its ovum in the menstrual cycle, in: "Fertilization of the Human Egg In Vitro," H.M. Beier and H.R. Lindner, eds., Springer-Verlag, Berlin.

Ingram, D.L., 1962, Atresia, in: "The Ovary," S. Zuckerman, A.M. Mandl and P. Eckstein, eds., Academic Press, London.

Jewelwicz, R., Dyrenfurth, I., Warren, M., Joshi, U., and Vande Wiele, R.L., 1973, Factors involved in the maintenance and regression of the corpus luteum of women, in: "Le Corps jaune. Rapporteurs generaux," R. Denamur, ed., Masson, Paris.

Karsch, F.J., and Sutton, G.P., 1976, An intra-ovarian site for the luteolytic action of estrogen in the rhesus monkey, Endocrinol., 98:553.

Knobil, E., 1980, The neuroendocrine control of the menstrual cycle, Recent Prog. Horm. Res., 36:53.

LeMaire, W.J., Leidner, R., and Marsh, J.M., 1975, Pre and post ovulatory changes in the concentration of prostaglandins in rat Graafian follicles, Prostaglandins, 9:221.

Leyendecker, G., Wildt, L., and Hansmann, M., 1980, Pregnancies following chronic intermittent (pulsatile) administration of Gn-RH by means of a portable pump ("Zyklomat")-a new approach to the treatment of infertility in hypothalamic amenorrhea, J. Clin. Endocrinol. Metab., 51:1214.

Lintern-Moore, S., Peters, H., Moore, G.P.M., and Faber, M., 1974, Follicular development in the infant human ovary, J. Reprod. Fertil., 39:53.

Lunenfeld, B.I., Ben-Aderet, N., Michael, R.B., Griistein, S., Kraiem, Z., Potashek, G., Shalit, A., Tikotzky, D., and Rofehh, C., 1977, Correlation of hormonal profile and ovarian morphological features during the preovulatory peroid in the human, in: "Endocrinology of the Ovary," R. Scholler, ed., Editions Sepe, Paris.

McNatty, K.P., Baird, D.T., Bolton, A., Chambers, P., Corker, C.S., and McLean, H., 1976, Concentrations of oestrogens and androgens in human ovarian venous plasma and follicular fluid throughout the menstrual cycle, J. Endocrinol., 71:77.

McNatty, K.P., Hillier, S.G., van der Boogaard, A.M.J., Trimbos-Kemper, T.C.M., Reichert, L.E., and van Hall, E.V., 1983, Follicular development during luteal phase of the human menstrual cycle, J. Clin. Endocrinol. Metab., 56:1022.

McNatty, K.P., Makris, A., DeGrazia, C., Osathanondh, R., and Ryan, K.J.,1979, The production of progesterone, androgens, and estrogens by granulosa cells, thecal tissue, and stromal tissue from human ovaries in vitro, J. Clin. Endocrinol. Metab., 49:687.

McNatty, K.P., Sawers, R.S., and McNeilly, A.S., 1974, A possible role for prolactin in control of steroid secretion by the human Graafian follicle, Nature, London, 250:653.

Marut, E.L., Williams, R.F., Cowan, B.D., Lynch, A., Lerner, S.P., and Hodgen, G.D., 1981, Pulsatile pituitary gonadotropin secretion during maturation of the dominant follicle in monkeys: estrogen positive feedback enhances the biological activity of LH, Endocrinol., 109:2270.

Mossman, H.W., and Duke, K.L., 1973, "Comparative Morphology of the Mammalian Ovary," University of Wisconsin Press, Madison.

Nakano, R., Yamoto, M., and Iwasaki, M., 1981, Effects of oestrogen and prostaglandin F_2 on luteinizing hormone receptors in human corpora lutea, J. Endocrinol., 88:401.

O'Grady, J.P., Caldwell, B.V., Auletta, F.J., and Speroff, L., 1972, The effects of an inhibition of prostaglandin synthesis (indomethacin) on ovulation, pregnancy, and pseudopregnancy in the rabbit, Prostaglandins, 1:97.

Pauerstein, C.J., Eddy, C.A., Croxatto, H.D., Hess, R., Siler-Khodr, T.M., and Croxatto, H.B., 1978, Temporal relationships of estrogen, progesterone, and luteinizing hormone levels to ovulation in women and infrahuman primates, Am. J. Obstet. Gynecol., 130:876.

Peters, H., and McNatty, K.P., 1980, Corpus luteum function, in: "The Ovary," University of California Press, Los Angeles.

Peters, H., Himelstein-Braw, R., and Faber, M., 1976, The normal development of the ovary in childhood, Acta. Endo., 82:617.

Polhemus, D.W., 1953, Ovarian maturation and cyst formation in children, Pediatrics, 1:588.

Potter, E.L., 1961, "Pathology of the Fetus and the Newborn," Yearbook Publishers, Chicago.

Quagliarello, J., Goldsmith, L., Steinetz, B., Lustig, D.S., and Weiss, G., 1980, Induction of relaxin secretion in nonpregnant women by human chorionic gonadotropin, J. Clin. Endocrinol. Metab., 51:74.

Quagliarello, J., Szlachter, N., Steinetz, B.G., Goldsmith, L.T., and Weiss, G., 1979, Serial relaxin concentrations in human pregnancy, Am. J. Obstet. Gynecol., 135:43.

Quigley, M.M., Kendall, J.Z., and Wilbourn, S.D., 1982, Application of a rapid serum RIA for LH in a clinical human in vitro fertilization (IVF) Program, Endocrinol., 110:411.

Rebar, R.W., 1983, Premature menopause, Semin. Reprod. Endocrinol., 1:169.

Richards, J.S., 1979, Hormonal control of ovarian follicular development: a 1978 perspective, Recent Prog. Horm. Res., 35:343.

Richards, J.S., and Midgley, A.R., Jr., 1976, Protein hormone action: a key to understanding ovarian follicular and luteal cell development, Biol. Reprod., 14:82.

Ross, G.T., and Lipsett, M.B., 1978, Hormonal correlates of normal and abnormal follicle growth and atresia after puberty in humans and other primates. Clin. Endocrinol. Metab., 7:561.

Ross, G.T., Cargille, C.M., Lipsett, M.B., Rayford, P.L., Marshall, J.R., Strott, C.A., and Rodbard, D., 1970, Pituitary and gonadal hormones in women during spontaneous and induced ovulatory cycles, Recent Prog. Horm. Res., 26:1.

Ryan, K.J., Petro, Z., and Kaiser, J., 1968, Steroid formation by isolated and recombined ovarian granulosa and thecal cells, J. Clin. Endocrinol. Metab., 28:355.

Sarosi, P., Schmidt, C.L., Essig, M., Steinetz, B.G., and Weiss, G., 1983, The effect of relaxin and progesterone on rat uterine contractions, Am. J. Obstet. Gynecol., 145:402.

Sherman, B.M., West, J.H., and Korenman, S.G., 1976, The menopausal transition: analyses of LH, FSH, estradiol and progesterone concentrations during menstrual cycles of older women. J. Clin. Endocrinol. Metab., 42:629.

Sotrel, G. Helvacioglu, A., Dowers, S., Scommmegna, S., and Auletta, F.J., 1981, Mechanisms of luteolysis: effect of estradiol and prostaglandin F_2 on corpus luteum luteinizing hormone/human chorionic gonadotropin receptors and cyclic nucleotides in the rhesus monkey, Am. J. Obstet. Gynecol., 139:134.

Speroff, L., Glass, R.H., and Kase, N.G., 1983, Regulation of the menstrual cycle, in: "Clinical Gynecologic Endocrinology and Infertility," Williams and Wilkins, Baltimore.

Steptoe, P.C., and Edwards, R.G., 1970, Laparoscopic recovery of preovulatory human oocytes after priming of ovaries with gonadotropins, Lancet, 1:683.

Stoufer, R.L., Nixon, W.E., and Hodgen, G.D., 1977, Estrogen inhibition of basal and gonadotropin-stimulated progesterone production by rhesus monkey luteal cells in vitro, Endocrinol., 101:1157.

Strickland, S., and Beers, W.H., 1976, Studies on the role of plasminogen activator in ovulation, J. Biol. Chem., 251:5694.

Testart, J., Thebault, A., and Frydman, R., 1982, Timing of ovulation and oocyte maturity after LH surge in women, in : "In Vitro Fertilization and Embryo Transfer," E.S.E. Hafez and K. Semm, eds., M.T.P. Press Ltd., Lancaster.

Tsafriri, A., and Channing, C.P., 1975, An inhibitory influence of granulosa cells and follicular fluid upon porcine oocyte meiosis in vitro, Endocrinol., 96:922.

Tsafriri, A., Koch, Y., and Lindner, H.R., 1973, Ovulation rate and serum LH levels in rats treated with indomethacin or prostaglandin E_2, Prostaglandins, 3:461.

Van Wagener, G., and Simpson, M.E., 1965, "Embryology of the Ovary and Testis: Homo sapiens and macaca mulatta", Yale University Press, New Haven.

Wassarman, P.M., 1983, Oogenesis: synthetic events in the developing mammalian egg, in: "Mechanism and Control of Animal Fertilization," J.F. Hartmann, ed., Academic Press, New York.

Williams, M.T., Roth, M.S., Marsh, J.M., and LeMaire, W.J., 1979, Inhibition of human chorionic gonadotropin-induced progesterone synthesis by estradiol in isolated human luteal cells, J. Clin. Endocrinol. Metab., 48:437.

Williams, R.F., Turner, C.K., and Hodgen, G.D., 1982, The late pubertal cascade in perimenarchial monkeys: onset of asymmetrical ovarian estradiol secretion and bioassayable LH release, J. Clin. Endocrinol. Metab., 55:660.

Wramsby, H., Kullander, S., Liedholm, P., Rannevik, G., Sundstrom, P., and Thorell, J., 1981, The success rate of in vitro fertilization of human oocytes in relation to the concentrations of different hormones in follicular fluid and peripheral plasma, Fertil. Steril., 36:448.

Zamboni, L., 1972, Comparative studies on the ultrastructure of mammalian oocytes, in: "Oogenesis," J.D. Biggers and A.W. Schuetz, eds., University Park Press, Baltimore.

6

ENHANCED FOLLICULAR DEVELOPMENT WITH CLOMIPHENE CITRATE AND HUMAN CHORIONIC GONADOTROPIN

Cecilia L. Schmidt

The unifying goal of pregnancy underlies diverse strategies to monitor and/or control the ovulatory cycles of women undergoing *in vitro* fertilization and embryo transfer (IVF-ET). This goal requires either stringent surveillance of an unperturbed spontaneous follicular phase, as detailed in the previous chapter, or hormonal regulation of the cohort stage. Edwards et al. (1980b) credited their change from stimulated cycles to spontaneous cycles as the major breakthrough responsible for their first (Steptoe and Edwards, 1978) and subsequent pregnancies. They cautioned other investigators about the derangements of follicular steroidogenesis caused by ovarian hyperstimulation (Edwards and Steptoe, 1975). However, Trounson et al. (1981) and Johnston et al. (1981) proved that clomiphene citrate given daily from days 5 through 9 of the menstrual cycle within the context of an IVF-ET program could result in viable pregnancies. We have elected to follow the latter approach in an attempt to achieve maturation of multiple pre-ovulatory follicles and to intervene in the biologic clock of ovulation.

The rationale of inducing maturation of several follicles for an IVF-ET cycle is to maximize the number of recoverable oocytes. Our successful retrieval of oocytes from approximately 60% of follicles aspirated (Quigley et al., 1982) agrees with that of others (Johnston et al., 1981; Renou et al., 1981). Between 60 and 70% of these oocytes are fertilized and cleaved (Tables 1 and 2). However, less than 20% of these concepti result in recognizable pregnancies. Limited data is available from the various IVF-ET programs characterizing the relationship between the establishment of intrauterine gestations and the number of embryos transferred (Edwards et al., 1980b; Trounson, 1983;

Table 1. Oocyte recovery, fertilization and cleavage rates of all follicles ≥ 15mm in mean diameter. (Adapted from Quigley et al., 1982).

	#	%
Oocyte recovery rate/aspirated follicle	39/69	57
Fertilization rate/ recovered oocyte	23/35*	66
Normal cleavage rate/fertilized oocyte	21/23	91
Fertilization and normal cleavage rate/recovered oocyte	21/35	60

*Four oocytes were not inseminated (one was lost; no sperm were available for the other 3).

Jones, 1983). However, certain tenets have been accepted by the most experienced centers. It appears that replacement into the donor's uterus of 2 embryos results in a higher pregnancy rate than the transfer of a single conceptus. Trounson (1983) has noted a threefold increase in pregnancy rate when 2 embryos, rather than a single embryo, are transferred. Although the transfer of 3 or 4 concepti may further enhance the pregnancy rate and the risk of multiple pregnancies (Kerin et al., 1983), a linear relationship between the number of embryos transferred and the pregnancy rate has not been demonstrated (See Chapter 12). More basic than these observations, however, is the fact that failure to transfer an embryo consistently effects a zero pregnancy rate. Using the stepwise success rates cited in Table 1, it can be calculated that 2.5 accessible 15mm follicles are necessary to ensure, on the average, transfer of one embryo to each patient. In fact, we recommend that patients with only one developing accessible follicle not undergo laparoscopy during that cycle (Quigley et al., 1982). We have found that when clomiphene citrate is used for follicular stimulation (Table 3), only 4/96

Table 2. Summary of oocyte observations using 2 clomiphene citrate dosage regimens. (Adapted from Quigley et al., 1983b).

Clomiphene citrate dose in mg/day (n=patient treatment cycles)	Oocyte recovery rate/ aspirated follicle		Fertilization rate/ recovered oocyte		Cleavage Rate/ fertilized oocyte	
	#	%	#	%	#	%
50 (n=54)	88/142	62.0	61/84*	72.6	59/60**	98.3
150 (n=34)	62/102	60.9	39/58***	67.2	36/39	92.3

* Excludes 4 immature oocytes (matured *in vitro*) inseminated and transferred without evidence of fertilization.

** Excludes 1 immature oocyte (matured *in vitro*) transferred at pronuclear stage before cleavage.

*** Excludes 3 oocytes not inseminated (no sperm sample) and 1 oocyte not assessed (technical difficulties).

All comparisions are not significantly different.

patients (4.2%) have had laparoscopy postponed for this reason (Quigley et al., 1983b).

The clomiphene citrate-induced cycle further allows the logistical feasibility of scheduling hospital personnel. Both laparoscopy for oocyte retrieval and embryo transfer can be scheduled with the cooperation of a "daytime" nursing and anesthesia staff in lieu of an "emergency" crew. Attempts to exert comparable temporal control over spontaneous cycles with human chorionic gonadotropin (hCG) administered acccording to ultrasonographic and clinical criteria result in a high percentage of pre-laparoscopy ovulations or aspiration of immature ooctyes (Wentz et al., 1983).

MECHANISM OF ACTION OF CLOMIPHENE CITRATE

Clomiphene citrate was first described by Kistner and Smith (1960) and Greenblatt (1961) as a non-steroidal estrogen antagonist capable of ovulation induction. Over the past 16 years of its commercial availability, numerous studies have characterized the therapeutic and diagnostic uses of clomiphene citrate without completely defining the mode of gonadotropin stimulation and the extent of ovarian and uterine effects.

The structure of clomiphene citrate vaguely resembles that of the non-steroidal estrogen diethylstilbestrol as depicted in Figure 1. Hence, its weak estrogenic effect is comprehensible on the basis of this morphological relation to an orally active potent estrogen. The binding affinity of clomiphene citrate to uterine estrogen receptors has been determined to be lower than that of estradiol (Ruh and Ruh, 1974). Clomiphene citrate has not been found to exert any progestational, androgenic or anti-androgenic biologic activity (Owman and Hafez, 1980). However, clomiphene citrate has been found to persist in body tissues for up to 3 months (Trounson, 1981).

The pivotal augmentation of gonadotropins by clomiphene citrate has not been localized specifically to either a hypothalamic or pituitary event. It has been suggested that clomiphene citrate depletes estrogen receptors in the hypothalamus, stimulating GnRH release and a subsequent rise in LH and FSH. Alternatively, or concomitantly, clomiphene citrate may decrease the cytosol estrogen receptor content of pituitary cells, allowing an interruption of tonic gonadotropin suppression by estrogen. The specific cellular action of clomiphene citrate resulting in the diminished estrogen receptor content of target cells has been shown in endometrial tissue to be the result of the inhibition of replenishment of cytosol receptors (Clark et al., 1974).

Table 3. Treatment outcome by patient treatment cycles in 2 clomiphene citrate dose regimens. (Reproduced with permission from Quigley et al., 1983b).

	Clomiphene citrate dose			
	50 mg/day		150 mg/day	
	No.	%	No.	%
No laparoscopy	6[a]	9.8	2[b]	5.6
No oocyte recovered	9[c]	15.7	3[d]	8.3
No oocyte fertilized	9	15.7	8	22.2
No implantation	27	49.0	22	61.1
Biochemical pregnancy	2	3.3	1	2.8
Clinical pregnancy	7[e]	11.7	0[e]	0
TOTAL	60	100	36	100

[a] One follicle, 4 patients; premature LH surge, 1 patient; acute asthma, 1 patient.

[b] Premature LH surge, 2 patients.

[c] Follicles aspirated, no oocytes recovered, 6 patients; ovulated prior to laparoscopy, 1 patient; no follicles at laparoscopy, 1 patient; follicle ruptured during aspiration, no oocyte recovered, 1 patient.

[d] Follicles aspirated, no oocytes recovered, 2 patients; ovulated prior to laparoscopy, 1 patient.

[e] $p < 0.05$. All other comparisons are not significantly different.

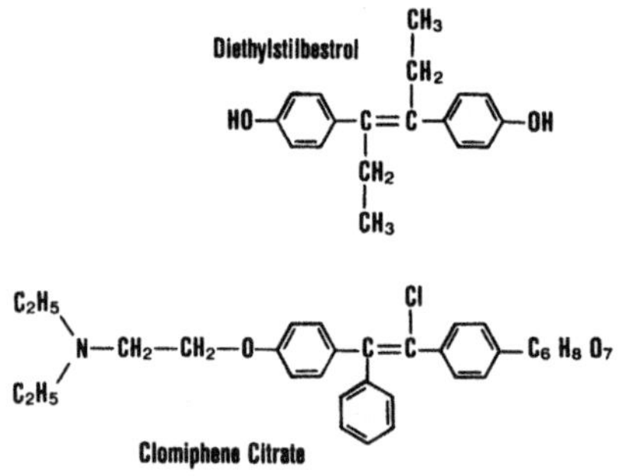

Figure 1

Chemical structures of diethylstilbestrol and clomiphene citrate

During the 5 day course of treatment, the FSH elevation in response to clomiphene citrate is thought to allow follicles other than the dominant follicle to become pre-ovulatory by increasing the amount of FSH available to them (Chapter 5). Those follicles recruited in the cohort prior to clomiphene citrate administration continue to be exposed to enhanced FSH levels through at least day 10 of the cycle. This situation contrasts with the spontaneous cycle in which the estradiol production of the dominant follicle unopposedly exerts a negative feedback upon gonadotropin secretion. Hence, the concurrent development of several follicles may result from this increased accessibility of FSH. The resultant enhancement of FSH-induced granulosa cell aromatase allows maintenance by the follicle of an estrogenic milieu and, thus, escape from atresia.

In anovulatory women treated with clomiphene citrate, multiple-follicle development occurs in over 50% of cycles (Smith et al., 1983), while multiple gestations are seen in only 8% of the pregnancies resulting from these cycles (Goldfarb et al., 1968). The discrepancy between the rate of supernumerary follicular development and the rate of multiple gestations demonstrates the possible antagonistic effects of clomiphene citrate on pregnancy establishment. These negative effects have also been evoked to explain the disparity between ovulation and conception rates in treated patients. Kase et al. (1967) contrasted an ovulation rate of 60.5% with a conception rate of 25.9% and Garcia et al. (1977) reported a failure to conceive in 52% of their patients who ovulated on clomiphene citrate.

The anti-estrogenic effects of clomiphene citrate upon the hypothalamic-pituitary axis have been hypothesized to result in the blunting of the endogenous LH peak in response to estradiol as observed in many clomiphene citrate-induced cycles (Garica et al., 1977). Experimentally, a dose-related anti-estrogenic effect of clomiphene citrate has been defined in endometrial tissue. Clomiphene citrate administered to estrogen-primed post-menopausal women decreased the endometrial cytosol progesterone receptor content by approximately 50% and was associated with increased endometrial atrophy (Kokko et al., 1981). Similarly, Garcia et al. (1977) found that 50% of 86 anovulatory patients treated with clomiphene citrate had endometrial biopsies consistent with a luteal phase defect. In 19 of 27 of these patients with defective endometrial patterns, adjuvant administration of hCG and/or intravaginal progesterone suppositories (50 mg daily) corrected the defect. The latter therapy directly supplements inadequate progesterone secretion by the corpus luteum, while the former therapy attempts to induce a normally functioning corpus luteum by mimicking the spontaneous LH surge. In either case, the final outcome is to prevent a progesterone deficiency from impeding implantation. These studies must be reviewed critically in relation to the possible anti-estrogenic effects of clomiphene citrate on the endometrium of spontaneously ovulatory women. The pathology underlying anovulation may be responsible for the luteal phase defects in the clomiphene citrate-treated anovulatory women. Only comparable studies of endometrial sampling in the normally ovulating women given clomiphene citrate will clarify the direct effects, if any, of this drug on the endometrium.

Examination of the cervical mucus in anovulatory women treated with clomiphene citrate often demonstrates clomiphene citrate's anti-estrogenic properties. While poor mucus production is not detrimental to IVF-ET techniques, similar anti-estrogenic effects of clomiphene citrate may affect the endometrium. Finally, similar dose-related antagonism directly upon the follicle is suggested by a comparison of a 150 mg-dosage schedule and 50 mg-dosage regimen in our program (Quigley et al., 1983b). When follicles were first ultrasonographically examined after completion of clomiphene citrate administration, the largest follicle in the 150 mg group was smaller than that in the 50 mg group (Table 4). Hence, follicular growth may have been inhibited by the presence of higher concentrations of clomiphene citrate in the 150 mg group, despite the high levels of estradiol. Similarly, Mandelbaum et al. (1983) found that in patients treated during the follicular phase with 100 to 150 mg/day of clomiphene citrate, 50 to 80% of the follicles were immature or atretic on the day of aspiration. Interestingly, this high incidence of follicles containing non-fertilizable oocytes was reduced to 23% by adding IM injections of 150 to 225 IU of FSH to the clomiphene citrate protocol on cycle days 6, 8 and 10.

CLOMIPHENE CITRATE IN IVF-ET PROGRAMS

The earliest attempts in an IVF-ET program to stimulate follicular development with clomiphene citrate and to effect pre-ovulatory maturation with hCG did not result in the establishment of normal pregnancies. Edwards and Steptoe (1975) found no evidence of implantation in patients undergoing IVF-ET after having received 100 mg of clomiphene citrate/day over a period of 5 days beginning on cycle day 2 or 3 and 5000 IU of hCG IM on cycle day 12 or 13. In 2 of 27 patients treated with 50 to 100 mg clomiphene citrate on 5 consecutive days ranging from cycle days 3 to 11, a transient post-embryo transfer increase in hCG excretion was detected (Lopata et al., 1978). In 1981, Trounson et al. disproved the dictum that natural ovulatory cycles were mandatory for successful IVF-ET cycles by reporting 4 clomiphene citrate-induced intrauterine pregnancies. The dosage schedule had been altered to 150 mg daily on cycle days 5 through 9. In 3 of the 4 women achieving pregnancy, 4000 IU of hCG had been administered 36 hours before laparoscopy predetermined by the "follicle growth rate and availability of the operating room" (Trounson et al., 1981). Ultrasonographic and hormonal evidence was offered to attest to the "normalcy" of the first 9 pregnancies established with this 150 mg clomiphene citrate protocol. Seven of these pregnancies, including 2 twin gestations, were reported to have progressed between 16 and 31 weeks of gestation while 2 had aborted at 8 weeks (Wood et al., 1981). Other early reports of pregnancies established with clomiphene citrate in IVF-ET programs (Johnston et al., 1981) have supported the feasibility of utilizing clomiphene citrate.

The maturational status of the retrieved oocytes in clomiphene citrate/hCG-stimulated cycles has been compared to that obtained during the monitored spontaneous cycle. The scheduling of laparoscopy approximately 36 hours after hCG injection reduces the occurrence of pre-operative ovulation (Edwards and Steptoe, 1975) but may do so at the expense of vital in vivo maturation. However, the retrieval of mature, pre-ovulatory oocytes with cumulus masses indistinguishable from mature oocytes recovered in spontaneous cycles (Wood et al., 1981) argues against lengthening the hCG-laparoscopy interval. The same dilemma exists in choosing the time of laparoscopy based upon the initiation of the spontaneous LH surge in an unstimulated cycle. Furthermore, pre-insemination oocyte maturation in vitro, tailored to the maturity of the oocyte, undoubtedly minimizes these concerns (See Chapter 12). At laparoscopy, pre-ovulatory follicles in clomiphene citrate-stimulated cycles appear identical to those in spontaneous cycles in the protrusion of the follicle beyond the smooth ovarian contour. The appearance of fine blood vessels through the transparent distended follicular wall suggests

Table 4. Summary of ultrasonographic observations (mean ± SEM) from 2 clomiphene citrate regimens. (Reproduced with permission from Quigley et al., 1983b).

Clomiphene citrate dose in mg/day	# foll. 15–19mm	# foll. ≥20mm	Total # foll.	Cycle Day for 20 mm follicle	Dia. largest foll. (mm) 1st U/S day	Dia. largest foll. (mm) on 20mm day	Follicular growth rate in mm/day
50 (n=60)	1.1±0.1	1.3±0.1	2.3±0.1	12.7±0.2	13.9±0.3*	21.2±0.2	3.2±0.2**
150 (n=36)	1.2±0.2	1.2±0.1	2.4±0.2	12.6±0.2	12.5±0.3*	21.3±0.2	4.2±0.4**

* $p < 0.02$.

** $p < 0.01$.

All other comparisons are not significantly different.

imminent ovulation (Wood et al., 1981). The ease of collecting the oocyte of a mature follicle with this appearance bespeaks cumulus mobility acquired through incorporation of hyaluronic acid as described physiologically in the spontaneous cycle (See Chapter 5). Testart et al. (1983b) found that the average number of retrieved oocytes with fully expanded, homogenous cumulus masses did not differ significantly between spontaneous and clomiphene citrate-stimulated cycles. However, there was an increase in the number of fertilizable, although less mature, oocytes exhibiting limited expansion of a heterogenous, granular cumulus in the stimulated cycles. Overall, there were increased total numbers of recovered oocytes in the clomiphene citrate group which were able to be fertilized without prolonged pre-incubation. We have confirmed the presence of follicles containing oocytes of varying pre-ovulatory maturity in our clomiphene citrate-treated patients.

Trounson and Leeton (1981) noted several disturbing anomalies in a small number of patients undergoing IVF-ET who had received clomiphene citrate. These patients developed large cystic follicles which averaged approximately 3 cm in diameter and lacked a normal oocyte and normal granulosa cells. Such follicles had became atretic before aspiration. Other patients experienced premature ovulation or lengthened follicular phases. However, those patients who underwent laparoscopic aspiration of follicles did not exhibit short luteal phases even though they were not supplemented post-transfer with progesterone. Normal luteal function in clomiphene citrate-treated women undergoing follicular aspiration has also been documented by Trotnow et al. (1982) by monitoring BBT charts and plasma progesterone levels.

Data generated from studies of steroid concentrations of follicular fluids in clomiphene citrate-stimulated cycles has been confusing. Carson et al. (1982) found that follicles from which oocytes were retrieved contained significantly higher concentrations of both estradiol and progesterone compared with those from which no oocytes were obtained. Normal embryo growth following <u>in vitro</u> fertilization was associated with significantly elevated levels of androstenedione, progesterone and estradiol; while establishment of pregnancy correlated with significantly higher concentrations of estradiol. According to these investigators, only clomiphene citrate-stimulated follicles containing high follicular fluid progesterone levels ($p < 0.05$) produced healthy, fertilizable oocytes. In contrast, Wramsby et al. (1981) had earlier made a correlation in spontaneous cycles between the fertilizability of retrieved oocytes and high follicular fluid concentrations of both estradiol and progesterone. In analyzing follicular fluid during both spontaneous and stimulated cycles, Testart et al. (1983a) defined the "normal" hormonal steroid concentrations of androstenedione as < 250 ng/ml, testosterone as < 13 ng/ml, estradiol as $\geq$ 100 ng/ml, progesterone as $\geq$ 6000 ng/ml and 17-hydroxyprogesterone as $\geq$ 100 ng/ml. Treatment with 100 to 150 mg clomiphene citrate on cycle days 5 through 9 reduced the proportion of follicles with "normal" steroid concentrations. Follicular fluid from 32 of 36 follicles (88.9%) from 36 untreated women fulfilled the criteria of "normalcy" compared to that from only 6 of 76 follicles (7.9%) from 41 women undergoing the clomiphene citrate regimen. Most often, the "abnormal" follicles exhibited androgen-rich or progestin-poor follicular fluid. It should be noted that these authors' estimation of "normal" pre-ovulatory follicular fluid estradiol is well below the range described by other investigators as summarized in Chapter 5. Hence, the "abnormal follicles" cited in this study may also be estrogen-poor and, therefore, either atretic or immature. Contrary to the study in spontaneous cycles (Wramsby et al., 1981), Testart et al. (1983a) found that the success rates of in vitro fertilization or embryo transfer were not significantly influenced by follicular fluid steroid concentrations of the pre-ovulatory follicles yielding the oocyte, provided that minimum levels had been reached. Based upon these conflicting findings, follicular fluid steroidal analysis may not be predictive of the outcome of either spontaneous or clomiphene citrate-stimulated cycles in IVF-ET.

Furthermore, follicular fluid concentrations of gonadotropins offer no greater tool for oocyte selection than do steroid levels. Testart et al. (1983a) noted FSH levels $\geq$ 0.3 mIU/ml in 100% of pre-ovulatory follicles aspirated during spontaneous cycles compared with only 75.9% of hormonally stimulated cycles. The problem with these findings is that results from both clomiphene citrate and human menopausal gonadotropin treatments with hCG were pooled. Also, the FSH concentrations did not influence cumulus dissociation (Testart et al., 1983b). The degree of cumulus expansion, closely related to hyaluronic acid synthesis, has been previously shown in vitro to be dependent upon FSH (Eppig, 1979 and 1980 and Testart et al., 1982). Hence, further characterization of follicular fluid gonadotropin and steroidal concentrations in relation to oocyte performance is mandatory before intelligent hypotheses can be drawn from these parameters.

Separate from the method of follicular stimulation, the underlying hypothetical concern about disruption of the steroidogenic potential of the resultant corpus luteum by the aspiration of granulosa cells has not been substantiated. Edwards et al. (1980a) could not detect differences in the excretion of pregnanediol during the luteal phase in relation to the number of granulosa cells removed. In fact, they cited a pregnancy established in a patient from whom a large number of cells had been aspirated. Similarly, Feichtinger et al. (1982) reported that only 2 of 32 patients who underwent laparoscopic oocyte aspiration after non-stimulated follicular phases had low progesterone values and shortened luteal phase lengths indicative of luteal phase deficiences. The remaining 30 women showed mean intervals between laparoscopy and the onset of menses of 13.5 $\pm$ 1.3 days. In comparison to the total complement of approximately 50 X 10^6 granulosa cells contained in a mature Graafian follicle (McNatty et al., 1979), the aspiration of an average of 3 X 10^6 granulosa cells (Jones et al., 1981) does not seem devastating. However, in 9 spontaneous cycles monitored with identification of the LH surge, multiple vigorous aspirations were performed in a futile effort to obtain oocytes. The amount of luteal progesterone secreted in these cycles was significantly less than in control cycles during which laparoscopy had not been performed (Jones et al., 1981). The difference was attributed to a decrease in granulosa cell number without a more disciplined consideration of intrinsic follicular development so vital to luteal function (See Chapter 5).

THE EXPERIENCE WITH CLOMIPHENE CITRATE IN IVF-ET AT HOUSTON

In our program, daily oral dosages of clomiphene citrate are administered on cycle days 5 through 9. Follicular diameters are monitored by daily ultrasonographic examination as described in Chapter 8, usually beginning on cycle day 10. On the day that the largest follicle reaches 20mm in diameter, 2500 IU of hCG are administered IM 36 hours before scheduled laparoscopy for follicular aspiration. Usually, all pre-ovulatory follicles at least 15mm in mean diameter are aspirated. A follicle is reaspirated or flushed with culture media only if an oocyte has not been retrieved from it. Transcervical embryo transfer is performed between 40 and 48 hours after insemination of the oocytes. In view of luteal phase inadequacy previously reported with clomiphene citrate-stimulated cycles (Garcia et al., 1977), all patients receive 5 daily IM injections of 12.5 mg of progesterone in oil commencing on the day of embryo transfer. Subsequent luteal phases, estimated by the interval between follicular aspiration and ensuing menses, have not been shortened relative to untreated controls and previous patient cycles.

In patients receiving 150 mg/day of clomiphene citrate, the estradiol values expressed as either serum estradiol levels or serum estradiol levels per large follicle agreed with those of other investigators employing clomiphene citrate in their IVF-ET programs (Vargyas et al., 1982). Figure 2 (Quigley et al., 1983a) depicts our laboratory's calculated mean $\pm$ 2 standard deviations of the mean for serum estradiol levels in these patients. Cycle day 0 is defined as the day the largest follicle equals or exceeds 20mm in mean diameter. The peak of the estradiol surge occurred on cycle day 0. Therefore, similar to the spontaneous cycle (See Chapter 5), the estradiol peak was reached shortly before the initiation of the exogenously created "LH surge." However, the absolute values of estradiol were higher in our clomiphene citrate-stimulated cycles than in spontaneous cycles. In a subgroup of 10 patients who were serially monitored with daily estradiol measurements, the mean ± SEM of serum estradiol concentration on the day of hCG administration was 1064 ± 169 pg/ml (538 ± 67 pg/ml/large follicle). Furthermore, individual profiles of estradiol levels of several patients exhibited patterns divergent from the spontaneous cycle in that estradiol levels continued to rise after hCG administration. The wide range of estradiol concentrations coupled with the idiosyncrasies of individual patterns under clomiphene citrate stimulation complicate estrogen monitoring as a method of correlating follicular maturation with appropriate administration of hCG. This topic is further discussed in Chapter 9.

Between August, 1981 and December, 1982, two daily dosages of clomiphene citrate, 150 mg or 50 mg, were administered on cycle days 5 through 9. Only the lower dose regimen resulted in clinical pregnancies in our program. In an attempt to evaluate the dose-related effects of this non-steroidal anti-estrogen on the stimulated cycle, we compared the 2 groups of treatment cycles (Quigley et al., 1983b). Relevant to interpretation of this comparison, it should be noted that the 150 mg regimen was studied in 36 patients between August, 1981 and June, 1982 while the 50 mg protocol was evaluated in 60 patients between May and December, 1982. Hence, the difference in pregnancy rate may not be related only to the clomiphene citrate schedules but also to other factors.

Although previous reports have found that 50 mg clomiphene citrate administered daily on cycle days 5 through 9 did not produce more than one large follicle (Trounson and Leeton, 1981), in our experience (depicted in Table 4), there were no statistical differences in the number or size of follicles as determined by ultrasound on the day of hCG administration in patients receiving either 50 or 150 mg/day of clomiphene citrate. The mean ± SEM number of follicles was 2.3 ± 0.1 in the 50 mg group and 2.4 ± 0.2 in the 150 mg group. Furthermore, the day (mean ± SEM) on which the largest follicle equalled or exceeded 20mm in mean diameter was 12.7 ± 0.2 in the 50 mg group and 12.6 ± 0.2 in the 150 mg group, again not statistically different. Although the mean diameters of the largest follicles on the day of hCG injection in the 50 mg group (21.2 ± 0.2mm) and the 150 mg group (21.3 ± 0.2mm) were comparable, the growth rate of the latter was significantly

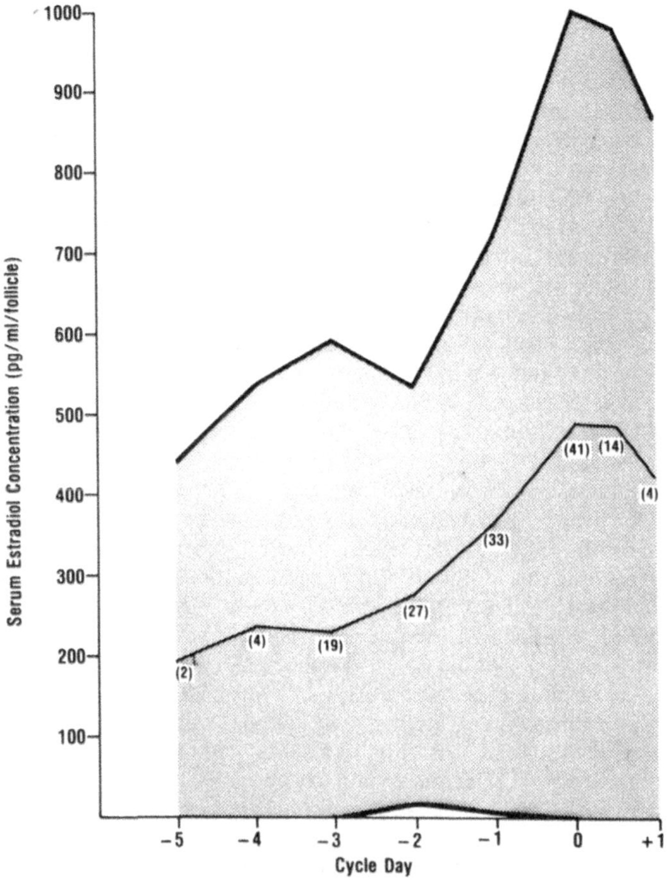

Figure 2

Serum estradiol concentrations in pg/ml/large follicle for patients receiving 150 mg/day of clomiphene citrate. The solid line represents the mean and the shaded area depicts $\pm$ 2 standard deviations of the mean. Cycle day 0 is defined as the cycle day on which the largest follicle equalled or exceeded 20mm mean diameter by ultrasonographic scanning. The number of measurements at each cycle day is indicated in parentheses. (Reprinted with permission from Quigley et al., 1983b.)

faster (4.2 ± 0.4mm/day in the 150 mg group versus 3.2 ± 0.2mm/day in the 50 mg group). As already discussed, this increased growth in the 150 mg group was secondary to the smaller size of the largest follicle in the 150 mg group on the first day of ultrasound (12.5 ± 0.3mm versus 13.9 ± 0.3mm) and may denote anti-estrogenic effects during clomiphene citrate administration.

The fates of the oocytes recovered from stimulated follicles in both the 50 mg group and 150 mg group after hCG injection did not differ significantly (Tables 2 and 3). In greater than 90% of all treatment cycles, patients underwent laparoscopy. The oocyte recovery rate/laparoscopy hovered around 60%, the fertilization rate/recovered oocyte approximated 70% and the cleavage rate approached 95% in both groups. Again, the only statistically significant difference between the 50 mg group and 150 mg group was the higher clinical pregnancy rate in the former (11.7% overall, 13.0%/laparoscopy, 19.4%/embryo transfer) than in the latter (none).

The results of this comparison suggest that there is no reason to utilize more than 50 mg clomiphene citrate daily to achieve pregnancies in an IVF-ET program. Furthermore, our experience attests the efficacy of this lower dose for stimulating multifollicular development and suggests the need to explore even lower dosages.

In summary, 10 pregnancies have resulted in our IVF-ET program through monitoring of clomiphene citrate/hCG-stimulated ovarian cycles ultrasonographically. In our hands, the 50 mg dosage regimen produces a higher pregnancy rate than the 150 mg schedule. However, the marked contrast between the retrieval of fertilizable oocytes which cleave normally and the low pregnancy rate warrants further modification of our hormonal stimulation. Our aim remains to emulate the endometrial milieu of a spontaneous luteal phase after promoting the maturation of more than one pre-ovulatory follicle.

REFERENCES

Carson, R.S., Trounson, A.O., and Findlay, J.K, 1982, Successful fertilisation of human oocytes in vitro: Concentration of estradiol- 17β , progesterone and androstenedione in the antral fluid of donor follicles, J. Clin. Endocrinol. Metab., 55: 798.

Clark, J.H., Peck, E.J., Jr., and Anderson, J.N., 1974, Oestrogen receptors and antagonism of steroid hormone action, Nature, London, 251: 446.

Edwards, R.G., and Steptoe, P.C., 1975, Induction of follicular growth, ovulation and luteinization in the human ovary, J. Reprod. Fert., Suppl., 22:121.

Edwards, R.G., Steptoe, P.C., Fowler, R.E., and Baillie, J., 1980a, Observations on preovulatory human ovarian follicles and their aspirates, Br. J. Obstet. Gynaecol., 87:769.

Edwards, R.G., Steptoe, P.C., and Purdy, J.M., 1980b, Establishing full-term human pregnancies using cleaving embryos grown in vitro, Br. J. Obstet. Gynaecol., 87:737.

Eppig, J.J., 1979, FSH stimulates hyaluronic acid synthesis by oocyte-cumulus cell complexes from mouse preovulatory follicles, Nature, London, 281:483.

Eppig, J.J., 1980, Role of serum in FSH stimulated cumulus expansion by mouse oocyte-cumulus cell complexes in vitro, Biol. Reprod., 22:629.

Feichtinger, W., Kemeter, P., Szalay, S., Beck, A., and Janisch, H., 1982, Could aspiration of the Graafian follicle cause luteal phase deficiency?, Fertil. Steril., 37:205.

Garcia, J., Jones, G.S., and Wentz, A.C., 1977, The use of clomiphene citrate, Fertil. Steril., 28:707.

Goldfarb, A.F., Morales, A., Rakoff, A.E., and Protos, P., 1968, Critical review of 160 clomiphene-related pregnancies, Obstet. Gynecol., 31:342.

Greenblatt, R.B., 1961, Chemical induction of ovulation, Fertil. Steril., 12:402.

Johnston, I., Lopata, A., Speirs, A., Hoult, I., Kellow, G., and du Plessis, Y., 1981, In vitro fertilization: The challenege of the eighties, Fertil. Steril., 36:699.

Jones, H.W., 1983, personal communication.

Jones, G.S., Garcia, J., and Acosta, A., 1981, Luteal phase evaluation in in-vitro fertilization, in: "Human Conception In Vitro," R.G. Edwards and J.M. Purdy, eds., Academic Press, London.

Kase, N., Mroueh, A., and Olson, L.E., 1967, Clomid therapy for anovulatory infertility, Am. J. Obstet. Gynecol., 98:1037.

Kerin, J.F., Warnes, G.M., Quinn, P.J., Jeffrey, R., Kirby, C. Matthews, C.D., Seamark, R.P., and Cox, L.W., 1983, Incidence of multiple pregnancy following human in vitro fertilization and embryo transfer, Lancet, 2:537

Kistner, R.W., and Smith, O.W., 1960, Observations on use of a non-steroidal estrogen antagonist: MER-25, Surg. Forum, 10:725.

Kokko, E., Janne, O., Kauppila, A., and Vihko, R., 1981, Cyclic clomiphene citrate treatment lowers cytosol estrogen and progestin receptor concentrations in the endometrium of postmenopausal women on estrogen replacement therapy, J. Clin. Endocrinol. Metab., 52:345.

Lopata, A., Brown, J.B., Leeton, J.F., Talbot, J.M., and Wood, C., 1978, In vitro fertilization of preovulatory oocytes and embryo transfer in infertile patients treated with clomiphene and human chorionic gonadotropin, Fertil. Steril., 30:27.

McNatty, K.P., Smith, D.M., Makris, A., Osathanondh, R., and Ryan, K.J., 1979, The microenvironment of the human antral follicle: interrelationships among the steroid levels in antral fluid, the population of granulosa cells, and the status of the oocyte in vivo and in vitro, J. Clin. Endocrinol. Metab., 49:851.

Mandelbaum, J., Plachot, M., Cohen, J., Junca, A.M., and Debache, C., 1983, The use of Clomid and hMG in human in vitro fertilization: Consequences for egg quality and luteal phase adequacy, in: "Fertilization of the Human Egg In Vitro," H.M. Beier and H.R. Lindner, eds., Springer-Verlag, Berlin.

Owman, C., and Hafez, E.S.E., 1980, Ovulation mechanisms, prediction, detection, and induction, in: "Human Reproduction, Conception and Contraception, E.S.E Hafez, ed., Harper and Harper, Cambridge.

Quigley, M.M., Kendall, J.Z., Maklad, N.F., and Wolf, D.P., 1983a, Monitoring follicular development in an IVF-ET program: serum estrogen versus ultrasonography, Fertil. Steril., 39:416.

Quigley, M.M., Maklad, N.F., and Wolf, D.P., 1983b, Comparison of two clomiphene citrate dosage regimens for follicular recruitment in an in vitro fertilization program, Fertil. Steril., 40:178.

Quigley, M.M., Wolf, D.P., Maklad, N.F., Dandekar, P.V., and Sokoloski, J.E, 1982, Follicular size and number in human in vitro fertilization, Fertil. Steril., 38:678.

Renou, P., Trounson, A.O., Wood, C., and Leeton, J.F., 1981, The collection of human oocytes for in vitro fertilization. I. An instrument for maximizing oocyte recovery rate, Fertil. Steril., 35:409.

Ruh, T.S, and Ruh, M.F., 1974, The effect of antiestrogens on the nuclear binding of the estrogen receptor, Steroids, 24:209.

Smith, D.H., Picker, R.H., Sinosich, M.J., Saunders, D.M., and Grudzinskas, J.G., 1983, Effects of clomiphene administration on ovarian function as measured by estradiol and ultrasound, Obstet. Gynecol., 61, 695.

Steptoe, P.C., and Edwards, R.G., 1978, Birth after the reimplantation of a human embryo, Lancet, 2:366.

Testart, J., Castanier, M., Feinstein, M.C., and Frydman, R., 1982, Pituitary and steroid hormones in the preovulatory human follicle during spontaneous or stimulated cycles, in: "Proceedings of the IVth Reiner de Graaf Symposium (Nijmegen)," Excertpa Medica, Amsterdam.

Testart, J., Frydmann, R., Castanier, M., Lassalle, B., and Belaisch, J., 1983a, Influence of ovarian stimulation on follicular fluid steroid levels and fertilization of the oocyte, in: "Fertilization of the Human Egg In Vitro," H.M. Beier and H.R. Lindner, eds., Springer-Verlag, Berlin.

Testart, J., Frydmann, R., DeMouzon, J., Lassalle, B., and Belaisch, J.C., 1983b, A study of factors affecting the success of human fertilization in vitro. I. Influence of ovarian stimulation upon the number and condition of oocytes collected, Biol. Reprod., 28:415.

Trounson, A.O., 1983, Factors controlling normal embryo development and implantation of human oocytes fertilized in vitro, in: "Fertilization of the Human Egg In Vitro," H.M. Beier and H.R. Lindner, eds., Springer-Verlag, Berlin.

Trounson, A.O., and Leeton, J.F., 1981, The endocrinology of clomiphene stimulation, in: "Human Conception In Vitro," R.G. Edwards and J.M. Purdy, eds., Academic Press, London.

Trounson, A.O., 1981, Discussion on clomiphene stimulation, in: "Human Conception In Vitro," R.G. Edwards and J.M. Purdy, eds., Academic Press, London.

Trounson, A.O., Leeton, J.F., Wood, C., Webb, J., and Wood, J., 1981, Pregnancies in humans by fertilization in vitro and embryo transfer in the controlled ovulatory cycle, Science, 212:681.

Trotnow, S., Becker, H., Kniewald, T., Al-Hasani, S., and Mulz, D., 1982, Luteal phase following oocyte aspiration, in vitro fertilization, and embryo transfer in clomid/HCG-stimulated cycles, Arch. Gynecol. 231:171.

Vargyas, J.M., Marrs, R.P., Kletzky, O.A., and Mishell, D.R.,1982, Correlation of ultrasonic measurement of ovarian follicle size and serum estradiol levels in ovulatory patients following clomiphene citrate for in vitro fertilization, Am. J. Obstet. Gynecol. 144:569.

Wentz, A.C., Torbit, C.A., Daniell, J.F., Fleischer, A.C., Garner, C.H., Pittaway, D.E., Christianson, C.D., Repp, J.E., and Maxson, W.S., 1983, Combined screening laparoscopy and timed follicle aspiration for human in vitro fertilization, Fertil. Steril., 39:270.

Wood, C., Trounson, A., Leeton, J., Talbot, J.M., Buttery, B., Webb, J., Wood, J., and Jessup, D., 1981, A clinical assessment of nine pregnancies obtained by in vitro fertilization and embryo transfer, Fertil. Steril., 35:502.

Wramsby, H., Kullander, S., Liedholm, P., Rannevik, G., Sundstrom, P., and Thorell, J., 1981, The success rate of in vitro fertilization of human oocytes in relation to the concentrations of different hormones in follicular fluid and peripheral plasma, Fertil. Steril., 36:448.

7

HUMAN MENOPAUSAL GONADOTROPINS FOR FOLLICULAR RECRUITMENT IN *IN VITRO* FERTILIZATION AND EMBRYO TRANSFER

Pedro J. Beauchamp

The initiation of follicular development is a continuous process which occurs throughout the menstrual cycle. At the beginning of a new cycle (or in the last few days of the previous cycle) a cohort of those follicles beginning development are recruited to further development by rising levels of follicle stimulating hormone (FSH). These follicles grow to the antral stage and require the continued availability of FSH and Luteinizing Hormone (LH) for further growth and maturation, culminating in ovulation (Fritz and Speroff, 1982). Usually one follicle (seldom more) escapes atresia and is selected to become the dominant, preovulatory follicle (Hodgen, 1982; Chapter 5.) This natural sequence of events is sub-optimal for IVF-ET. The development of multiple preovulatory follicles increases the probability of recovering at least one fertilizable oocyte by laparoscopy (Edwards et al., 1980; Jones et al., 1982). As higher pregnancy rates are obtained when more than one embryo is transferred to the patient (Spiers et al., 1983; Jones et al., 1983), increasing the number of follicles by providing an excess of gonadotropins directly by human menopausal gonadotropins (hMG) administration or indirectly with clomiphene citrate or Gonadotropin Releasing Hormone (GnRH) will increase the patient's chances of achieving pregnancy. This chapter will discuss the use of hMG for follicular recruitment.

HISTORICAL BACKGROUND

HMG has been available for ovulation induction since 1960. During the preceding years, gonadotropins isolated from pregnant mare's serum (PMSG) were successfully used for ovulation induction in humans, but their clinical use was later abandoned because of their antigenicity in humans (Buxton, 1953). Human pituitary gonadotropins (hPG) followed by human chorionic gonadotropin (hCG) was also effective in inducing ovulation but the use of hPG has been restricted by limited supply (Gemzell et al., 1958). Lunenfeld et al. (1960) reported successful induction of ovulation and pregnancy with gonadotropins extracted from the urine of postmenopausal women (hMG) and hCG. Since then, the experience from several thousand treatment cycles has been collected and reviewed (Schwartz and Jewelewicz, 1981; Schenker et al., 1981).

Recruitment and maturation of multiple follicles is desirable for <u>in vitro</u> fertilization for the reasons discussed above. During the early work of Edwards and Steptoe (Edwards and Steptoe 1975; Edwards et al., 1980), hMG and hCG were utilized to enhance oocyte recovery and to avoid difficulties associated with identifying the time of ovulation during a natural cycle. In these studies, five ampules per day of hMG were given on days 6, 8 and 10 of the cycle. When urinary estrogens rose to 75 μg/day or more, 5,000 IU of hCG were administered (usually on days 11 or 12 of the cycle). Laparoscopy was performed 32 hours after the hCG injection. Using this protocol, no pregnancies were established and almost all of these patients had a short luteal phase. Edwards and coworkers (1980) noticed an inverse correlation between the preovulatory urinary estrogen levels and the duration of the luteal phase; i.e., patients with higher estrogen levels had shorter luteal phases. Endometrial biopsies performed during the luteal phase in patients who did not have an embryo transfer were abnormal and frequently out of phase. They also observed that follicular development was asynchronous; oocytes at various stages of maturation were recovered during laparoscopy. Based on the assumption that high preovulatory estrogen levels were disrupting the luteal phase, attempts were made to modify the follicular recruitment protocol and to support the luteal phase. Three pregnancies were established in cycles supplemented with progesterone and hCG during the luteal phase, but none of them continued beyond the first trimester. In an effort to eliminate the endocrinopathies observed during stimulated cycles, Edwards and co-workers attempted oocyte recovery during natural cycles and four pregnancies resulted (two of which delivered at term) from 78 patients (Steptoe et al., 1980).

Other groups have reported pregnancy establishment from oocytes recovered during natural cycles (Lopata et al., 1980) or during cycles stimulated with clomiphene citrate (Wood et al., 1981; Johnston et al., 1981). In the United States, Jones and co-workers, after a disappointing experience attempting oocyte retrieval during natural cycles, reported successful pregnancies with hMG-hCG stimulated cycles (Wortham et al., 1981; Jones et al., 1982; Garcia et al., 1983a and b). Pregnancies have recently been reported from combined clomiphene citrate-hMG-hCG protocols (Vargyas et al., 1983; Johnston et al., 1983; Kerin et al., 1983).

PHARMACOLOGY

Human menopausal gonadotropin (Pergonal-Serono Laboratories, Randolph, Mass.) is a purified preparation of FSH and LH extracted from the urine of postmenopausal women. Urinary FSH has a molecular weight of 28,000 daltons, 208 amino acids, and a biologic activity of 780 IU/gm. In spite of the dissimilarity between urinary FSH and pituitary FSH (molecular weight 41,000 daltons, 254 amino acids and biologic activity of 14,000 IU/gm), there is no clinically significant difference in ovarian stimulation when these preparations are given in biologically equivalent dosages (Schwartz and Jewelewicz, 1981). The half life of FSH is 3 hours and LH is 30-45 minutes.

Each Pergonal package costs $20 to $30 and contains two glass ampules: one ampule with lyophilized powder containing 75 IU of FSH and 75 IU of LH (based on the Second International Reference Preparation for Human Menopausal Gonadotropins) and the second contains 2 ml of diluent. HMG is inactive orally and therefore, must be given by intramuscular injection. The medication needs to be reconstituted immediately prior to injection. If more than one ampule of hMG is to be administered, up to 4 ampules of hMG may be reconstituted with one ampule (2 ml) of diluent.

EFFECT OF HMG ON THE OVARIAN FOLLICLE

The mechanism by which follicles initiate growth is poorly understood but appears to be independent of gonadotropin stimulation. However, in order to prevent early atresia, a timely increase in FSH is necessary. During the menstrual cycle, FSH begins to rise 2-3 days before the onset of menses and remains elevated for 4 to 5 days into the new cycle. As previously described in Chapters 4 and 5, FSH is essential to: (1) increase the number of granulosa cells; (2) increase the number of FSH and later LH receptors on granulosa cells; and (3) increase the aromatase activity of these granulosa cells. The main purpose of FSH is to stimulate follicular growth to the pre-ovulatory stage and to facilitate conversion from an androgenic to an estrogenic follicular microenvironment.

Selection and dominance of the pre-ovulatory follicle is believed to occur as a result of progressive withdrawal of the gonadotropin support (FSH in particular) to other less developed follicles (Fritz and Speroff, 1982; Hodgen, 1982). FSH levels decline progressively from day 5 or 6 of the cycle to nadir levels just prior to the pre-ovulatory LH and FSH surge. Decreasing the support of FSH-dependent follicular events in the non-dominant follicles results in their atresia.

The mechanism determining follicular selection and atresia may be influenced by altering the gonadotropin patterns of the menstrual cycle. By preventing the decline in FSH (or actually increasing its level) while follicular selection and dominance is occuring, several extra follicles may be rescued from atresia and go on to develop to the pre-ovulatory stage. These increased gonadotropin levels may be accomplished directly with hMG administration or indirectly by clomiphene citrate or GnRH administration.

MONITORING FOLLICULAR RESPONSE TO HMG

Ovarian response to hMG administration is monitored by clinical, ultrasonographic and laboratory methods. The use of clinical parameters (cervical mucus response, vaginal cytology, palpation of ovarian size) is unreliable at higher levels of follicular estradiol (E_2) production, is somewhat subjective in nature and is not readily reproducible by other observers. Nonetheless, the group at the Eastern Virginia Medical School has defined and utilized the "clinical estrogen shift" to monitor hMG response (Garcia et al., 1983a and b).

Monitoring follicular response with ultrasound and estradiol is discussed further in Chapters 8 and 9. The size of pre-ovulatory follicles, as determined by ultrasound, is smaller with hMG stimulation when compared to clomiphene citrate stimulated or natural cycles (Renaud et al., 1980; Mantzavinos et al., 1983; Buttery et al., 1983). A mature, fertilizable oocyte can usually be obtained from 15-17 mm diameter follicles during hMG stimulation (Garcia et al., 1983a). In clomiphene stimulated or natural cycles, mature oocytes are usually obtained only from follicles $\geq$ 20mm in diameter. Possible explanations for this discrepancy are either: (a) inhibition of endogenous LH by hMG; (b) inhibition of follicular growth by a fixed FSH/LH ratio during hMG therapy; (c) accelerated oocyte maturation with hMG; and (d) decreased number of granulosa cells or follicular fluid volume with hMG. Further research is needed to evaluate the pathogenesis and significance, if any, of smaller follicular size with hMG.

The circulating levels of E_2 are derived primarily from developing follicles (Fritz and Speroff, 1982; Spiers et al.,

1983). Measurements of serum or urinary estradiol concentrations have been utilized to monitor follicular development in patients undergoing ovulation induction. Studies have shown that, during hMG stimulation, plasma E_2 levels correlated well with total follicular volume (Haning et al., 1982). Three patterns of estrogen response to hMG stimulation have been identified by Jones and co-workers: Low, normal, and high E_2 responses corresponding to E_2 levels of < 300, 300-600 and > 600 pg/ml, respectively (Garcia et al., 1983a). The estrogen response is classified on the day of the "clinical estrogen shift" (defined as $\geq 30\%$ superficial cells on vaginal cytology, cervical mucus volume ≥ 0.2 ml, spinnbarkeit ≥ 10 cm and 4+ ferning). This classification further demonstrates the biologic variation of target tissue response to circulating levels of E_2. In other words, some women require higher E_2 levels than others to induce a response in cervical mucus and vaginal cytology. Such a classification may, in experienced hands, be a clinically useful parameter for monitoring a hMG protocol (Garcia et al., 1983b) and it may correlate with pregnancy rates (see below; Acosta et al., 1983; Jones et al., 1983b).

Studies on anovulatory women undergoing ovulation induction with hMG show that the duration of the active phase of follicular maturation and the rate of exponential E_2 rise may be as important as absolute E_2 levels in determining normalcy of the luteal phase, conception and multiple pregnancy rates (Bergquist et al., 1983a; Bergquist et al., 1983b). Even though the ovulatory dose of hCG was given at a standard E_2 level (2000 pmol/l), a short active phase (≤ 6 days from baseline to threshold levels) was associated with a defective luteal phase or anovulation. Furthermore, conceptual cycles were associated with lower E_2 levels during the follicular phase and higher progesterone levels during the luteal phase. It appears that rapid follicular development by hMG (as evidenced by rapid rise of E_2 levels), results in lower pregnancy rates and abnormal luteal phases probably due to ovulation of immature oocytes or abnormal corpus luteum formation (Yuen et al., 1981). We have observed similar results when high doses of hMG are used for follicular recruitment (see below).

Duration of the hMG administration to anovulatory women (number of days necessary to increase E_2 from baseline to threshold levels) may also influence follicular recruitment. Singleton pregnancies were associated with treatments of ≤ 7 days duration while multiple pregnancies had longer (8-10 days) active phases. It appears that the longer ovarian exposure to hMG predisposes to multiple follicular development (Bergquist et al., 1983a).

The ovarian response to hMG depends on at the least two factors; the amount of gonadotropins administered and the state of the follicles at the beginning of therapy (Insler and Potashnik, 1983). Each patient appears to have her own sensitivity to hMG, accounting for the variation observed in E_2 response and in follicular development.

HMG ALONE IN FOLLICULAR RECRUITMENT: PROTOCOLS AND RESULTS

The pioneering work of Edwards and Steptoe (Edwards and Steptoe, 1975; Edwards et al., 1980) has been described earlier in this chapter.

Initially, the group at Eastern Virgina Medical School used a protocol similar to that used for ovulation induction in anovulatory, infertile women (Garcia et al., 1983a). Two ampules of hMG (150 IU FSH and 150 IU LH) was administered starting on the 1st, 3rd or 5th day of the cycle depending on cycle length, < 25 days, 25-35 days or >35 days, respectively. After 3 days of treatment, the dose was lowered to one ampule of hMG daily. With the appearance of the "estrogen clinical shift", hMG was discontinued and 10,000 IU hCG was administered 2-3 days later, depending on when the largest follicle reached 18mm in diameter as determined by ultrasound. Garcia et al. (1983a) noticed that none of the patients in this series had an endogenous LH surge. They recovered oocytes in all but one patient (31 cycles in 25 patients) with 60 oocytes recovered in all (1.94 oocytes/cycle; Table 1). Eighty precent of those oocytes were pre-ovulatory, 15% were immature and 5% were atretic. Only 16 of the 48 (33%) pre-ovulatory oocytes fertilized and cleaved, and two pregnancies resulted from embryos transferred to 12 patients (Wortham et al., 1983).

During phase II of their program, the hMG protocol was individualized according to the estrogen level at the time of the clinical estrogen shift (Garcia et al., 1983b). Two ampules of hMG were administered starting on the 3rd or 5th day in patients who had 28 ± 3 and 35 ± 3 day cycles, respectively. Further management was based on serum E_2 levels and the occurrence of the "clinical shift". For low responders (E_2 < 300 pg/ml on the day of the clinical shift) hMG was continued for 3 additional days after the shift. In the normal E_2 responders (E_2 300-600 pg/ml) hMG was discontinued if the shift had occurred, or the dose was lowered to one ampule daily until the shift occurred. In the high estrogen responders, hMG was discontinued once the E_2 exceeded 600 pg/ml, even if the clinical estrogen shift had not occurred. The ovulatory dose of hCG (10,000 IU) was administered

Table 1. In vitro fertilization program at Eastern Virginia Medical School: Comparison of phases I and II, 1981. (Modified from Jones et al., 1982; Garcia et al., 1983a, 1983b).

	Phase I	Phase II
Number of pregnancies	2	5
Pregnancy rate/laparoscopy	6%	21%
Pregnancy rate/transfer	17%	26%

50 hours after the last hMG injection (Jones et al., 1982). A normal E_2 response was observed in 17 patients, 3 patients had a low and 4 had a high E_2 response.

These twenty four patients underwent laparoscopy; no oocytes were obtained in one patient and only immature oocytes were obtained in another. Ninety eight follicles were aspirated (4.1 follicles per patient) and 57 oocytes were recovered (2.4 oocytes per patient). Forty oocytes (70%) were considered mature. One patient had one follicle ruptured prior to laparoscopy but mature oocytes were aspirated from other follicles. Of the mature oocytes, 30 out of 33 fertilized and cleaved; seven of 10 immature oocytes matured in vitro fertilized and cleaved. Five pregnancies resulted after transfer of 37 embryos to 19 patients.

Besides an overall improvement in outcome, there were two differences between phases I and II. First, oocyte post-maturity (aging) was observed in seven patients during phase I. Fragmentation of the oocytes and darkening of granulosa cells (lipid inclusions from excessive luteinization) were observed, most frequently in the high E_2 responders. This phenomenon is probably the result of prolonged hMG stimulation and failure of the E_2 from the developing follicles to elicit an endogenous LH surge. Post-maturity was decreased by shortening the duration of hMG therapy and by shortening the interval from the last hMG dose to the time of hCG administration to 26 hours in the high E_2 responders.

Second, serum progesterone levels were three times higher at the time of hCG injection and laparoscopy in the high E_2 responders compared to normal or low E_2 responders. Higher serum progesterone (P) values were seen at the time of laparoscopy in follicles with dark granulosa cells and fragmented oocytes. It appears that excessive, premature elevation of P values (seen mainly in high E_2 responders) is detrimental to the follicle and oocyte.

Further analysis of their data on E_2 response was recently reported by Acosta et al. (1983). In 17 low E_2 responders, 1.58 oocytes were recovered per patient, 77.7% cleaved and one pregnancy was established. Forty-five patients had a normal E_2 response; 1.75 oocytes were recovered per patient, 68.3% cleaved and 15 pregnancies resulted. A high E_2 response occurred in 25 patients, 2.04 oocytes were obtained per patient, 66.6% cleaved and 5 pregnancies were established. These data showed that the quality of the oocytes, as judged by cleavage rates, was similar in all three groups. Nonetheless, pregnancy rates were significantly lower in the low E_2 responders, which probably indicates deficient implantation rather than oocyte defects. The highest pregnancy rates were observed in normal E_2 responders (33%), followed by high E_2 responders (20%). Based on these data the authors felt that it might be possible to preselect patients with a lower probability of pregnancy in whom laparoscopy might be discouraged. Their data has been expanded and reported by Jones et al. (1983b). In 175 consecutive patients who underwent laparoscopy, 26 were classified as high responders, 109 as normal responders, and 40 as low responders. The number of follicles per cycle were 5.5, 4.26, and 4.1 for high, normal and low responders, respectively. An average of 1.69, 1.47 and 1.05 preovulatory oocytes were obtained per cycle producing a pregnancy rate of 23%, 19% and 15% for the high, normal and low E_2 responders.

Higher doses of hMG has been used by DeCherney and coworkers at Yale University (personal communication). Patients usually receive three or four ampules of hMG starting on the 3rd day of the cycle. Treatment is continued until two or more follicles reach 16mm diameter as determined by ultrasound. Successful pregnancies have been established with this regimen.

At the University of Texas, we recently finished a prospective, randomized study comparing clomiphene citrate and high dose hMG for follicular recruitment (Quigley et al., 1984). Half of the patients received 50 mg clomiphene citrate daily from days 5 to 9 of the cycle and hCG (2500 IU) on the evening of the day when the largest follicle reached or exceeded 20mm in mean diameter as determined by ultrasound (usually day 12 or 13 of the cycle). The other patients received hMG four ampules (300 IU FSH and 300 IU LH) beginning on the 3rd day of the cycle. Follicular response was monitored by ultrasound beginning on day 8 of the cycle. HMG was discontinued and 5,000 IU hCG were administered the evening of the day when two or more follicles reached or exceeded 16mm in diameter. In both groups, laparoscopy was performed 36 hours after hCG injection. Progesterone in oil (12.5 mg IM) was administered to all patients immediately after embryo transfer and for the following 4 days. Analysis of our data (Table 2) indicates that in the clomiphene citrate treated patients, the cycle length was 26.8 2.3 days (mean ± Standard Deviation) compared to 21.1 ± 1.5 days for the hMG cycle ($p < .001$). The duration of the luteal phase was significantly shorter in hMG cycles (11.6 ± 1.5 days) than in clomiphene citrate cycles (14.4 ± 2.3 days; $p < .001$) in spite of progesterone supplementation. Even though an increased number of embryos were transferred in the hMG group (3.5 vs. 1.8 embryos per patient undergoing embryo transfer for the hMG and clomiphene citrate group respectively; $p < 0.001$), no pregnancies were established in 18 patients in the hMG group. This observation is consistent with the earlier work of Edwards et al. (1980) and Bergquist et al. (1983a, 1983b) regarding poor pregnancy rates and short luteal phases in patients receiving high doses of hMG and ovarian hyperstimulation. A high incidence of fractured zonae pellucidae after follicular aspiration was observed by G.S. Jones et al. (personal communication) with high dose hMG; such phenomena was not observed by DeCherney et al. (personal communication) but we have noticed that such oocytes are fragile and the zona pellucida can rupture occasionally during the mechanical manipulation necessary to remove the corona radiata. It appears that modifications of the high dose hMG protocol, lowering the hMG dose or better supplementation of the luteal phase, will be necessary to improve pregnancy rates.

HMG PLUS CLOMIPHENE CITRATE COMBINATION THERAPY IN FOLLICULAR RECRUITMENT

Several studies have been performed comparing clomiphene citrate, clomiphene citrate augmented with hMG, clomiphene citrate followed by hMG, and hMG alone (Vargyas et al., 1983; Johnston, 1983; Lopata, 1983). Vargyas et al. (1983) compared four protocols: Group I consisted of clomiphene citrate 150 mg per day from days 3-7; group II received clomiphene citrate 150 mg days 5-9 followed by two ampules of hMG for 3-5 days until adequate follicular development; Group III patients received clomiphene citrate 150 mg days 3-7 as well as 2 ampules hMG on days 3, 5, 7, 8, 9, 10 and 11 of cycle; and group IV received two ampules of hMG starting on the 3rd day of the cycle and extending 6 to 8 days until adequate follicular maturation had occurred.

Table 2. Comparison of hMG and clomiphene citrate protocols for enhanced follicular recruitment at The University of Texas at Houston, 1983 (Quigley et al., 1984).

	Clomiphene Citrate N=18	hMG N=18	Significance
Cycle length (days)	26.8 ± 2.3	21.1 ± 1.5	$p<.001$
Duration of luteal phase (days)	14.3 ± 2.3	11.6 ± 1.5	$p<.001$
No. follicles $\leq$ 10mm diameter on day of hCG	4.9 ± 1.3	5.2 ± 1.4	NS
No. oocytes recovered/laparoscopy	1.7 ± 0.9	4.6 ± 2.7	$p<.001$
No. embryos transferred per patient	1.8 ± 0.9	3.5 ± 1.5	$p<.01$

NS = Not significant

The ovulatory dose of hCG (4,000 IU) was administered on the day that ultrasound revealed at least one follicle $\geq$ 18mm diameter. The mean number of follicles per patient was 3.3, 6.0, 4.5 and 4.3 for groups I, II, III and IV, respectively (Table 3). These numbers were significantly higher for group II. The development of only one follicle per patient was lowest in group II (10% patients) followed by group IV (20% patients). The mean number of embryos transfered per patient was 2.2, 3.0, 2.4, 1.5 for groups I, II, III and IV, respectively. Only values for group IV were significantly lower (due to two patients having no oocytes retrieved at laparoscopy). One patient from group II and another from group III achieved pregnancy. Preovulatory E_2 levels were lower in groups I and IV. Fertilization rates were highest in groups II and III, and slightly lower in groups I and IV. Only 3% of group II patients had a spontaneous LH surge prior to hCG administration as opposed to 33% of group IV patients. Even though their numbers were small (29 patients), the best overall results were observed in group II (clomiphene followed by hMG), followed by group IV (hMG alone).

Data presented by Johnston (1983) showed similar results regarding improved outcome with combination clomiphene citrate-hMG (Table 4). In his report, a group of patients received clomiphene citrate 100-150 mg/day, days 5-9 (group A). Patients in group B received the same dose of clomiphene citrate as group A followed by 4 ampules of hMG daily until adequate follicular development had occurred. In group C, clomiphene citrate 50-100 mg/day, days 5-9 was followed by an individualized dose of hMG depending on the follicular size and response to clomiphene. If the second-order follicles were 8-12mm as measured by ultrasound, 225 IU of hMG were given daily until follicular maturation ($\geq$ 18mm diameter); 150 IU hMG were given if follicular diameter was 12-16mm. The average number of follicles per patient were 3, 6.4 and 5.6 and the average numbers of oocytes recovered per laparoscopy were 1.7, 5.0 and 4.0 for groups A, B and C, respectively. Fertilization rates of 75%, 60% and 58% resulted in 9.3, 14.9 and 23.2% pregnancy rate per laparoscopy and 14.8, 18.5 and 38.1% pregnancy rate per transfer for groups A, B and C, respectively. Due to a high spontaneous abortion rate, the corresponding ongoing pregnancy rates per transfer were 7.4, 10.9 and 23.8%. Even though hMG alone was not used for comparison, these data suggest that clomiphene citrate followed by hMG may be superior to clomiphene citrate alone. Furthermore, an individualized hMG dose following clomiphene citrate results in higher ongoing pregnancy rates in spite of a lowered oocyte recovery rate per laparoscopy. The details of their data are discussed further in a recent review article by Lopata (1983).

Table 3. Comparison of clomiphene citrate, combined clomiphene citrate-hMG, and hMG for enhanced follicular recruitment. University of Southern California, 1982-83. (Vargyas et al., 1983).

	Group I (clomiphene) (N=7)	Group II (clomiphene followed by hMG) (N=3)	Group III (clomiphene with and followed by hMG) (N=13)	Group IV (hMG alone) (N=6)
Number follicles per patient	3.3	6.0*	4.5	4.3
Number embryos transferred per patient	2.2	3.0	2.4	1.5**

* Group II significantly higher than others ($p<.01$)
**Group IV significantly lower than others ($p<.02$)

At our institution, we performed a double blind, prospective, randomized study to compare clomiphene citrate, 50 mg/day, days 5-9 of the cycle, with the combination of the same clomiphene citrate regimen, plus 2 ampules of hMG on days 6, 8 and 10 (unpublished observations). The mean number of follicles per patient were significantly higher in the combination compared to the clomiphene citrate groups (5.1 vs 3.7 respectively; $p<.01$; Table 5). An increase in the number of follicles 10-14mm in size was responsible for the higher number of follicles observed in the combination group (2.1 vs 0.9; $p<.01$). No differences were observed in the number of follicles 15-19mm or $\geq$ 20mm in diameter. A significantly higher number of oocytes were recovered per patient in the combination (2.8) compared to the clomiphene citrate group (1.9; $p<.05$). Oocyte (mature and immature) fertilization and cleavage rates were similar in both groups. Even though more embryos were transferred per patient in the combination than in clomiphene citrate group (2.5 vs 2.0 respectively), this difference was not statistically significant. Two clinical pregnancies resulted from embryos transferred to 12 clomiphene citrate group patients and two other pregnancies (one twin) from transfers to 13 combination clomiphene citrate-hMG group patients. This study shows that a fixed combination of clomiphene citrate and hMG, as described above, results in greater follicular recruitment and increased number of fertilizable oocytes than clomiphene citrate alone. An increase in the overall

Table 4. Comparison of clomiphene citrate and combination clomiphene citrate-hMG for enhanced follicular recruitment (Johnston I, 1983; Lopata, 1983).

	Group A (Clomiphene citrate)	Group B (Clomiphene followed by fixed hMG)	Group C (Clomiphene followed by individual hMG)
Number of patients	43	148	69
Number follicles per patient	3	6.4	5.6
Number oocytes recovered per laparoscopy	1.7	5.0	4.0
Fertilization rate	75%	60%	58%
Laparoscopies in which at least one oocyte fertilized	72%	85%	72.5%
Pregnancy rate per laparoscopy	9.3%	14.9%	23.2%
Pregnancy rate per transfer	14.8%	18.5%	38.1%
Ongoing pregnancy rate per transfer	7.4%	10.9%	23.8%

pregnancy rate will probably be obtained in the combination vs clomiphene citrate group once larger numbers are obtained. In conclusion, clomiphene citrate plus hMG (in combination or in sequence) appears better than clomiphene citrate alone.

POTENTIAL COMPLICATIONS

The ovarian hyperstimulation syndrome (Schenker and Weinstein, 1978) (characterized by ovarian enlargement, ascitis, hydrothorax, weight gain, hemoconcentration, electrolyte imbalance, and possible renal failure) has not been observed during hMG stimulated IVF cycles. It appears that the aspiration of preovulatory follicles interfere with its development in spite of abnormally high preovulatory E_2 levels. One of our high dose hMG patients developed multiple follicles, had E_2 levels of 2800 pg/ml, received the ovulatory dose of hCG but withdrew from the program for personal reasons before laparoscopy was performed. A clinical ovarian hyperstimulation syndrome did not occur in this case.

Table 5. Comparison of clomiphene citrate and combination clomiphene citrate-hMG for enhanced follicular recruitment (unpublished observations).

	Clomiphene Citrate (N=16)	Combination Clomiphene Citrate + hMG (N=16)	Significance
Total No. follicles per patient	3.7 ± 1.2	5.1 ± 2.0	$p < .01$
Follicles 10 to 14 mm	0.9 ± 1.3	2.1 ± 1.1	$p < .01$
Follicles 15 to 19 mm	1.6 ± 0.9	1.8 ± 1.4	NS
Follicles ≥20 mm	1.2 ± 0.4	1.1 ± 0.3	NS
No. oocytes recovered per patient	1.9 ± 0.9	2.8 ± 1.9	$p < .05$
Fertilization rate	85%	83%	NS
Cleavage rate	96%	86%	NS
No. embryos transferred per patient	2.0 ± 0.4	2.5 ± 1.2	NS
No. of clinical pregnancies	2	2*	NS
Pregnancy rate per transfer	17%	15%	NS

* One twin pregnancy
NS = Not significant

The luteal phase of hMG stimulated cycles is frequently abnormal. Partly attributed to removal of granulosa cells during follicular aspiration (See Chapter 10) lowered post-ovulatory progesterone values and shortened luteal phases may be observed. The higher preovulatory E_2 levels seen with hMG may interfere with corpus luteum development and function (Edwards et al., 1980; Ben-Rafael et al., 1983; Olson et al., 1983). Studies in anovulatory women receiving hMG have shown that midluteal progesterone levels were significantly higher in conceptual cycles than in ovulatory non-conceptual cycles (36.8 ng/ml vs 23.0 ng/ml respectively; $p < .001$). Furthermore, mean midluteal progesterone levels in conceptual cycles which progressed to term were higher than in cycles which aborted or had a transient embryo implantation (36 ng/ml, 27.5 ng/ml, 19.6 ng/ml respectively (Insler and Potashnik, 1983). Garcia et al. (1983c) demonstrated the importance of an early rise in progesterone in the luteal phase to advance endometrial maturation with resultant increased implantation (pregnancy) rates during hMG stimulated IVF cycles. Endometrial dating on biopsies performed during the first four days after laparoscopy showed that advanced dating correlated positively with higher progesterone values. Progesterone values two days after laparoscopy (expected day of embryo transfer) were higher ($\sim$12 ng/ml) in patients with advanced endometrial development and in patients who had pregnancies established. Progesterone values of $\sim$ 4 ng/ml were observed during normal, non-stimulated cycles; intermediate progesterone values of 9-10 ng/ml were observed in a group of patients who had embryos transferred but did not become pregnant. After the second post ovulatory day, progesterone values were significantly higher in the pregnancy and advanced endometrial dating group compared to non-conceptual cycles after embryo transfer, which in turn were higher than normal, non-stimulated cycles.

The spontaneous abortion rate in anovulatory women undergoing ovulation induction with hMG has averaged 28-30% (Schwartz and Jewelewicz, 1981; Ben-Rafael et al., 1983). Possible etiologic factors are: increased E_2 levels during the follicular phase (biochemical hyperstimulation); higher multiple pregnancy rates (Schenker et al., 1981); shortened luteal phase (close to 20% of ovulatory cycles) (Olson et al., 1983); and oocyte dysmaturity-maldevelopment (Garcia et al., 1983a). With improvement in hMG treatment protocols and monitoring, the incidence of spontaneous pregnancy loss should decrease.

SUMMARY

Recruitment of multiple follicles is desirable in IVF to increase the probability of successfully recovering at least one fertilizable oocyte and to attain the higher pregnancy rates seen with transfer of multiple embryos. The administration of hMG provides an excess of gonadotropins (particularly FSH) which can stimulate several follicles to the preovulatory stage. Early experiences (Edwards and Steptoe, 1975; Edwards et al., 1980) using high doses of hMG were disappointing due to the high incidence of shortened luteal phases. A modified, low dose hMG protocol has been successfully implemented by Jones and co-workers. They monitor follicular response both clinically (cervical mucus, vaginal cytology) and with E_2. Patients who have a normal E_2 response (E_2 levels 300-600 pg/ml at the time of the clinical estrogen shift) have the highest pregnancy rate. In the high E_2 responders (E_2 levels $\geq$ 600 pg/ml at time of clinical estrogen shift), oocyte post-maturity and excessive luteinization of the granulosa cells were observed in some patients.

At our institution, high doses of hMG have resulted in more embryos transferred to the patients compared to clomiphene citrate alone or clomiphene-hMG combinations, but no pregnancies. Possibly related were the observations of a significantly shortened luteal phase and fragile zonae pellucidae.

Several combinations of clomiphene citrate and hMG have been reported. Two studies are available demonstrating that clomiphene citrate followed by hMG until follicular maturation is completed results in higher oocyte recovery rates, number of embryos transferred and pregnancy rate, when compared to clomiphene citrate alone, hMG alone, or clomiphene citrate-hMG in combination. The optimal follicular recruitment protocol, providing the highest number of mature oocytes with minimal disruption of the luteal phase, resulting in high pregnancy rates, is yet to be established.

REFERENCES

Acosta, A.A., Jones, G.S., Sandow, B., Veeck, L., and Mantzavinos, T.H., 1983, Correlation of HMG/HCG stimulation and oocyte quality in an in vitro fertilization program, Fertil. Steril., 39:438.

Ben-Rafael, Z., Dor, J., Mashiach, S., Blankstein, J., Lunenfeld, B., and Serr, D.M., 1983, Abortion rate in pregnancies following ovulation induced by human menopausal gonadotropin/human chorionic gonadotropin, Fertil. Steril., 39:157.

Bergquist, C., Nillius, S.J., and Wide, L., 1983a, Human gonadotropin therapy. I. Serum estradiol and progesterone patterns during conceptual cycles, Fertil. Steril., 39:761.

Bergquist, C., Nillius, S.J., and Wide, L., 1983b, Human gonadotropin therapy. II. Serum estradiol and progesterone

patterns during nonconceptual cycles, Fertil. Steril., 39:766.
Buttery, B., Trounson, A., McMaster, R., and Wood, C., 1983, Evaluation of diagnostic ultrasound as a parameter of follicular development in an in vitro fertilization program, Fertil. Steril., 39:458.
Buxton, C.L., 1953, The pitfalls of clinical research, J. Clin. Endocrinol. Metab., 13:231.
Edwards, R.G., and Steptoe, P.C., 1975, Induction of follicular growth, ovulation and luteinization in the human ovary, J. Reprod. Fert., 22:121.
Edwards, R.G., Steptoe, P.C., and Purdy, J.M., 1980, Establishing full-term human pregnancies using cleaving embryos grown in vitro, Br. J. Obstet. Gynecol., 87:737.
Fritz, M.A., and Speroff, L., 1982, The endocrinology of the menstrual cycle: The interaction of folliculogenesis and neuroendocrine mechanisms, Fertil. Steril., 38:509.
Garcia, J.E., Jones, G.S., Acosta, A.A., and Wright, G., 1983a, Human menopausal gonadotropin/human chorionic gonadotropin follicular maturation for oocyte aspiration: Phase I, 1981. Fertil. Steril., 39:167.
Garcia, J.E., Jones, G.S., Acosta, A.A., and Wright, G., 1983b, Human menopausal gonadotropin/human chorionic gonadotropin follicular maturation for oocyte aspiration: Phase II, 1981. Fertil. Steril., 39:174.
Garcia, J.E., Acosta, A., and Jones, H.W., 1983c, Advanced endometrial maturation after ovulation induction with HMG/HCG for in vitro fertilization, Fertil. Steril., 39: 426.
Gemzell, C.A., Diczfalusy, E., and Tillinger, K.G., 1958, Clinical effect of human pituitary follicle stimulating hormone, J. Clin. Endocrinol. Metab., 18:1333.
Haning, R., Austin, C.W., Kuzma, D.L., Shapiro, S.S., and Zweibel, W.J., 1982, Ultrasound evaluation of estrogen monitoring for induction of ovulation with menotropins, Fertil. Steril., 37:627.
Hodgen, G.D., 1982, The dominant ovarian follicle, Fertil. Steril., 38:281.
Insler, V., and Potashnik, G., 1983, Monitoring of follicular development in gonadotropin-stimulated cycles, in: "Fertilization of the Human Egg In Vitro". H.M. Beier and H.R. Lindner, eds., Springer-Verlag Publishers, Berlin.
Jones, H.W., Jones, G.S., Andrews, M.C., Acosta, A., Bundren, C., Garcia, J., Sandow, B., Veeck, L., Wilkes, C., Witmyer, J., Wortham, J.E., and Wright, G., 1982, The program for In vitro fertilization at Norfolk, Fertil. Steril., 38:14.
Jones, H.W., Acosta, A.A., Garcia, J.E., Sandow, B.A., and Veeck, L., 1983a, On the transfer of conceptuses from oocytes fertilized in vitro, Fertil. Steril., 39:241.
Jones, H.W., Acosta, A., Andrews, M.C., Garcia, J.E., Jones, G.S., Mantzavinos, T.H., McDowell, J., Sandow, B., Veeck, L., Whibley, T., Wilkes, C., and Wright, G., 1983b, The importance

of the follicular phase to success and failure in in vitro fertilization, Fertil. Steril., 40:317.
Johnston, I., Lopata, A., Spiers, A., Hoult, I., Kellow, G., and Du Plessis, Y., 1981, In vitro fertilization: The challenge of the eighties, Fertil. Steril., 36:699.
Johnston, I.W.H., 1983, Discussion of Vargyas, J.M., Saito, H., Gibbons, W.E., Sueldo, C., Yee, W., and Marrs, R.P., Effects of different methods of ovarian stimulation on the human in vitro fertilization and embryo transfer procedure, presented at 39th Annual Meeting of the American Fertility Society, April 16-20, 1983, San Francisco, CA.
Kerin, J.F., Warnes, G.M., Quinn, P.J., Jeffrey, R., Kirby, C., Matthews, C.D., Seamark, R.F., and Cox, L.W., 1983, Incidence of multiple pregnancy following human in vitro fertilization and embryo transfer, Lancet, 2:537.
Lopata, A., Johnston, I.W.H., Hoult, I.J., and Speirs, A.L., 1980, Pregnancy following intrauterine implantation of an embryo obtained by in vitro fertilization of a preovulatory egg, Fertil. Steril., 33:117.
Lopata, A., 1983, Concepts in human in vitro fertilization and embryo transfer, Fertil. Steril., 40:289.
Lunenfeld, B., Menzi, A., and Valet, B., 1960, Clinical effects of a human post menopausal gonadotropin, Ross. Clin. Ter. Sci. Affini., 59:213.
Mantzavinos, T.H., Garcia, J.E., and Jones, H.W., 1983, Follicular ultrasound measurement in human gonadotropin ovulation induction patients for in vitro fertilization, Fertil. Steril., 39:415.
Olson, J.L., Rebar, R.W., Schreiber, J.R., and Vaitukaitis, J.L., 1983, Shortened luteal phase after ovulation induction with human menopausal gonadotropin and human chorionic gonadotropin, Fertil. Steril., 39:284.
Quigley, M.M., Schmidt, C.L., Beauchamp, P.J., Pace-Owens, S., and Wolf, D.P., 1984, Menopausal gonadotropins compared to clomiphene citrate for enhanced follicular recruitment in an in vitro fertilization program, Fertil. Steril., (in press).
Renaud, R., Macler, J., Ehret, M.C., Aron, C., Plas-Roser, S., Spira, A., and Pollack, H., 1983, Echographic study of follicular maturation and ovulation during the normal menstrual cycle, Fertil. Steril., 33:272.
Schenker, J.G., and Weinstein, D., 1978, Ovarian hyperstimulation syndrome: a current survey, Fertil. Steril., 30:255.
Schenker, J.G., Yarkoni, S., and Granat, M., 1981, Multiple pregnancies following induction of ovulation, Fertil. Steril., 35:105.
Schwartz, M., and Jewelewicz, R., 1981, The use of gonadotropins for induction of ovulation, Fertil. Steril., 35:3.
Spiers, A.L., Lopata, A., Gronow, M.J., Kellow, G.N., and Johnston, I.W.H., 1983, Analysis of benefits and risks of

multiple embryo transfer, Fertil. Steril., 39:468.
Steptoe, P.C., Edwards, R.G., and Purdy, J.M., 1980, Clinical aspects of pregnancies established with cleaving embryos grown in vitro, Br. J. Obstet. Gynecol., 87:757.
Vargyas, J.M., Saito, H., Gibbons, W.E., Sueldo, C., Yee, W., and Marrs, R.P., 1983, Effect of different methods of ovarian stimulation on the human in vitro fertilization and embryo transfer procedure, Fertil. Steril., 39:438.
Wood, C., Trounson A., Leeton, J., Talbot, J. McK., Buttery, B., Webb, J., Wood, J., and Jessup, D., 1981, A clinical assessment of nine pregnancies obtained by in vitro fertilization and embryo transfer, Fertil. Steril., 35:502.
Wortham, J.W.E., Veeck, L.L., Witmyer, J., and Jones, H.W., 1983, Vital initiation of pregnancy (VIP) using human menopausal gonadotropin and human chorionic gonadotropin ovulation induction: Phase I, 1981, Fertil. Steril., 39:785.
Yuen, B.J., Sy, L., and Cannon, W., 1981, Regulation of ovarian follicular and luteal function during treatment with exogenous gonadotropins in anovulatory infertility, Am. J. Obstet. Gynecol., 140:629.

8

MONITORING FOLLICULAR DEVELOPMENT WITH ULTRASOUND

Nabil F. Maklad

Ultrasound scanning of the pelvis to demonstrate the ovaries and to directly visualize the presence, size, and number of developing follicles has significantly increased over the past few years as a safe and reliable noninvasive method and has become an integral part of most in vitro fertilization and embryo transfer (IVF-ET) programs throughout the world. Ultrasound has been used to assess human follicular development in spontaneous cycles (Queenan et al., 1980), and in stimulated cycles during which patients were given either clomiphene citrate (O'Herlihy et al., 1980a), human menopausal gonadotropin (Ylostalo et al., 1981), or a combination of both (Hoult et al., 1981). Although many centers treating human infertility by IVF-ET utilize primarily measurements of serum or urinary estrogen to monitor follicular maturation (see Chapter 9), essentially all centers also rely upon ultrasonographic scanning to determine follicular size, location, and number.

FOLLICULAR SIZE AND NUMBER DEMONSTRATED BY ULTRASONOGRAPHIC EXAMINATION

Queenan et al., (1980) were able to detect ovulation in more than 80% of the spontaneous cycles studied by serial measurements of the follicular diameter and by the morphologic changes occurring with follicular rupture and corpus luteum formation. Moreover, a good correlation has been established between ultrasound measurements of follicular diameter in the spontaneous cycle and measurements of peripheral plasma hormone levels (Hackeloer et al., 1979).

A close correlation in follicular size and number between ultrasonographic observations and direct visualization at laparoscopy has been established by various groups of investigators (O'Herlihy et al., 1980b; Quigley et al., 1982). Ultrasonographic measurements of follicular size and determination of number of follicles are, in many cases, more accurate than the laparoscopic observations. Direct measurements of follicular diameter at laparoscopy can be unreliable when only a portion of the follicular surface is visible. Also, estimation of the follicular diameter by calculation from the aspirated fluid volume may be inaccurate if follicular fluid is lost at the time of aspiration or if the follicle is not spherical in shape.

ULTRASOUND VERSUS ESTIMATION OF SERUM ESTRADIOL FOR FOLLICULAR MONITORING

Most IVF-ET programs utilize frequent measurements of serum estradiol levels to determine when sufficient follicular maturation has been achieved to induce oocyte maturation with human chorionic gonadotropin (hCG). Few centers rely exclusively on ultrasonographic measurements as the determinate for hCG administration (Hoult et al., 1981; Quigley et al., 1983). Many studies have established an excellent correlation between mean follicular diameter measured by ultrasonography and mean estradiol levels during both spontaneous (Hackeloer et al., 1979) and clomiphene stimulated cycles (Vargyas et al., 1982). Ultrasonography has the advantage of monitoring individual follicular development as opposed to monitoring a composite or average of all ovarian follicular units. The combination and integration of both ultrasonographic follicular imaging and measurement of serum estradiol may prove to be superior to either monitoring technique alone. However, practical considerations often result in only one modality being available 7 days per week.

TECHNIQUES OF ULTRASOUND SCANNING

A full urinary bladder is a prerequisite for visualization of the female pelvic structures. This can usually be achieved by asking the patient to drink approximately 1200 cc of fluid (6 to 8 cups) one to two hours prior to the scan. Overdistension of the urinary bladder is unnecessary, tends to compress and distort the pelvic structures, and is an ordeal for the patient. In cases where overdistension occurs, most patients can void partially to achieve relief and minimize compression of the pelvic structures.

Adequate visualization of the uterus and ovaries can be achieved with either static or sector real time scanners. Linear array real time scanners, on the other hand, rarely produce adequate visualization of the ovaries in a cross sectional plane and their use for follicular monitoring is generally unsatisfactory. The static scanner (General Electric Datason), in our experience, produces the most accurate results (Figure 1). In cases where the ovaries cannot be identified easily, static scanning can be combined with a sector real time scanner (Advanced Diagnostic Research) for accurate follicular measurement. The major disadvantage of sector real time scanning is the larger degree of error in measurement.

We begin scanning patients with sagittal and parasagittal views of the pelvis. Identification of the uterus is an important initial step to provide orientation to the pelvic anatomy. Once the uterus is located and identified, scanning continues in the parasagittal planes along both sides of the uterus. The ovaries are usually visualized as oval shaped structures with well defined margins (Figure 2). Identification of the ovaries is facilitated by demonstration of the iliac vessels and the ureter as tubular

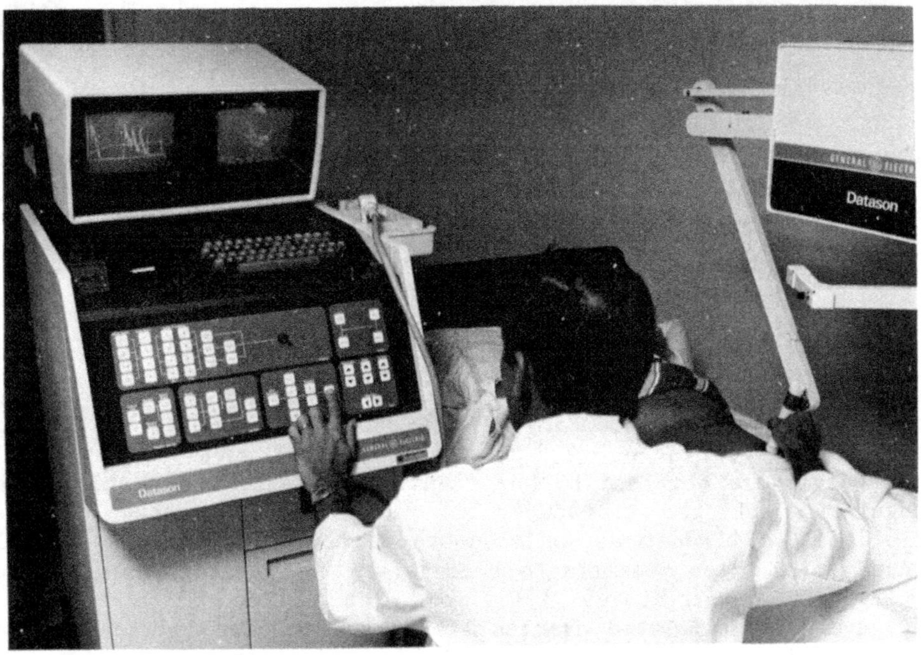

Figure 1

Ultrasonographic scanning of ovarian follicles using static mode scanner

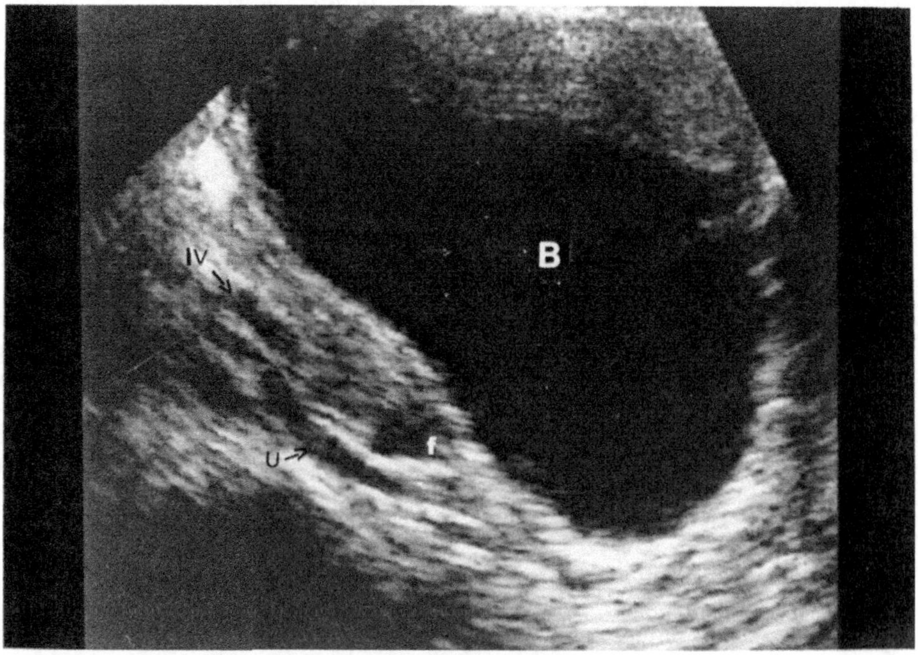

Figure 2

Parasagittal scan to the right of the uterus. The right ovary is the oval homogenously echogenic structure posterior to the urinary bladder (B). A small developing follicle (f) is seen in the inferior part of the ovary. The ureter (U) and iliac vein (IV) are seen coursing along the posterior boundary of the ovary.

structures with central echolucency and echogenic walls, coursing along the posterior boundary of the ovary (Figure 3). Following the parasagittal scans of both ovaries, cross sectional scans of the pelvis are obtained in the transverse plane, with appropriate angulation of the transducer to take full advantage of the fluid-filled bladder as an acoustic window. On cross sectional scans it is often possible to demonstrate both ovaries as rounded, well defined structures lying on either side of the uterus (Figure 4). Stimulated ovaries are larger in size and tend to be better defined allowing for easier identification (Figure 5). In most cases, multiple follicles are demonstrated in the ovaries in varying stages of development, spatially distributed within the cortical region of each ovary at random. Follicles are usually oval in outline, indicating unequal compression by stroma and adjacent follicles. Occasionally only one large follicle is seen

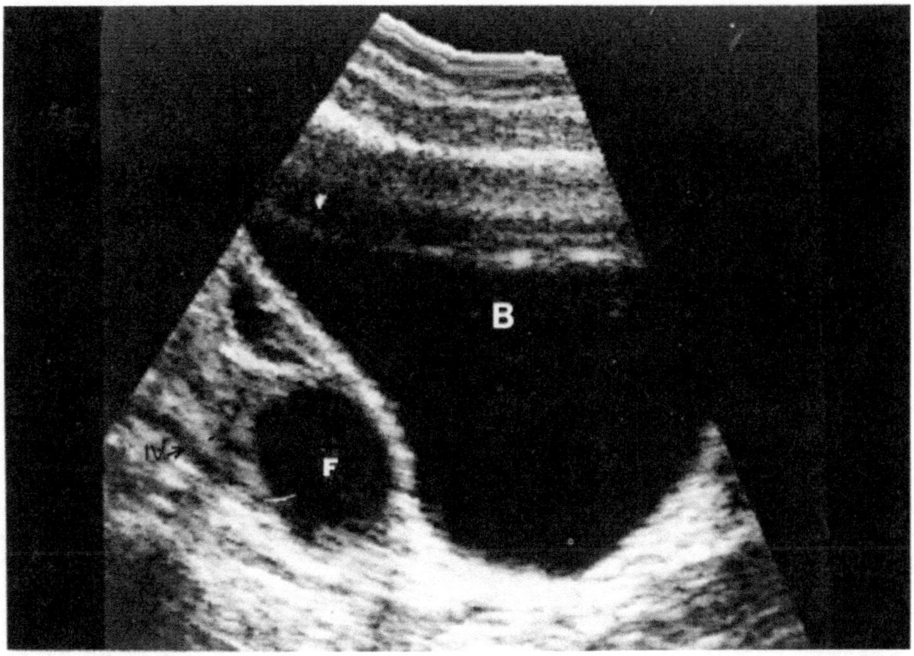

Figure 3

Parasagittal scan showing a dominant follicle (F) in the ovary. The iliac vein (IV) courses along the posterior aspect of the ovary.

in an ovary and this tends to be spherical in shape with equal diameters in all three planes.

Every follicle $\geq$ 10 mm within each ovary is measured daily using electronic calipers. Follicular diameters should be measured in three planes and the average diameter then calculated for each follicle. Although some investigators (Queenan et al., 1980) advocate measurement of the longest diameter of the follicle as an identification of its size, relying on this measurement for oval shaped follicles is not an accurate assessment of size in all cases.

In approximately one-third of the large follicles examined, an echogenic area can be demonstrated attached to one of the follicular walls, representing the cumulus oophorus (Figure 6). Attempts at correlating the presence or absence of this observation with oocyte recovery at follicular aspiration have been unsuccessful to date.

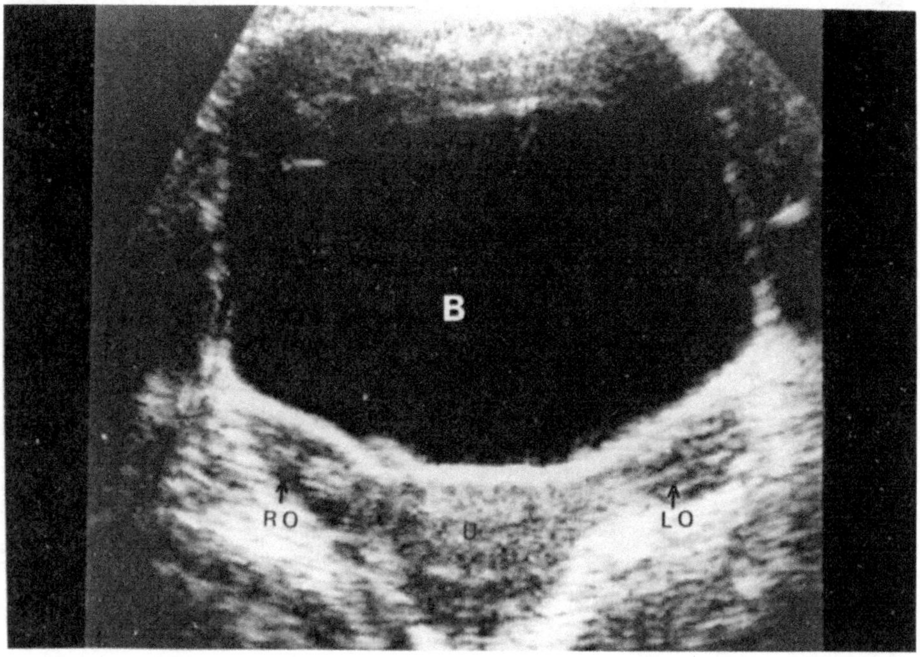

Figure 4

Cross sectional scan of the pelvis. The uterus (U), the right ovary (RO) and the left ovary (LO) are seen posterior to the distended urinary bladder (B).

FOLLICULAR MONITORING

Physiologic Cycles

In monitoring follicular development by daily sonographic examination during spontaneous cycles, typically only one follicle developed progressively (dominant follicle), while other smaller follicles did not change appreciably in size. The maximum size of the dominant follicle was found to vary between 18 and 24 mm (unpublished observations). This is a narrower range of diameters for preovulatory follicles than the range of 14 to 28 mm reported by Queenan et al. (1980). Following ovulation, the follicle disappeared and no distinguishable corpus luteum could be seen. In some cases, an irregular fluid filled area was seen in the place of the dominant follicle and only rarely did the follicle fill in with ultrasonographic echoes that gradually disappeared on subsequent scans. Replacement of the follicle by a corpus luteum cyst was very rarely seen.

Clomiphene Citrate Induced Cycles

Clomiphene citrate is the most commonly used ovulation induction agent in IVF-ET programs and is given to increase the number of preovulatory follicles, and thus, the number of recoverable oocytes. Ultrasonographic examination of the pelvis is started on day 10 and continued daily until one or more dominant follicles reach 20 mm in mean diameter. Each day all follicles greater than or equal to 10 mm in mean diameter are imaged in two planes with the three diameter measurements being averaged to give the mean follicular diameter for that day. Clomiphene citrate stimulated ovaries are larger and better defined than the ovaries in a spontaneous cycle, and usually contain multiple follicles (Figure 7). These findings agree with O'Herlihy et al. (1980a) who reported that in clomiphene stimulated cycles, the follicles were similar both in ultrasound appearance and size at ovulation to those developing in spontaneous

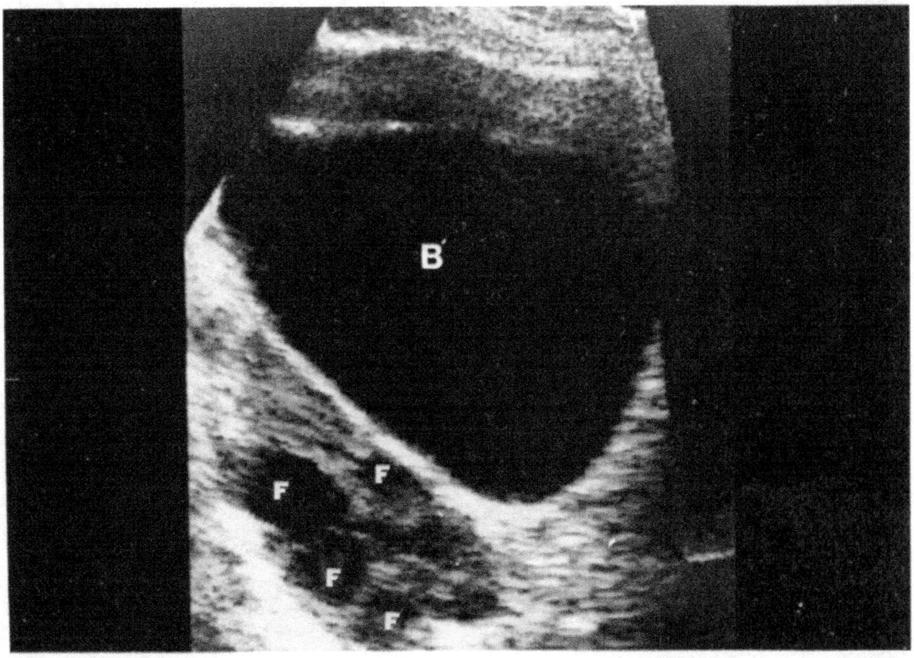

Figure 5

Parasagittal scan to the left of the uterus. Stimulated ovary is larger in size and is better defined allowing for its easy identification. Multiple follicles (F) at various stages of development are noted within the ovary.

cycles, although the rate of follicular growth was faster in clomiphene stimulated cycles.

Human Menopausal Gonadotropin Induced Cycles

Human menopausal gonadotropins in varying regimens are also used in IVF-ET programs. A comparative study using either human menopausal gonadotropins (4 ampules per day, beginning cycle day 3) or clomiphene citrate (50 mg per day, cycle days 5-9) for follicular recruitment was performed on two groups of patients. Ultrasound scanning in the HMG group began on cycle day 8 with the clomiphene group scans beginning on day 10. The ovaries stimulated by human menopausal gonadotropins were usually larger in size and contained a larger number of follicles (Figure 8), however, individual follicles were usually smaller in size, and showed a slower rate of growth (Figure 9). Preovulatory follicular diameters of 15 to 22 mm were reported by Ylostalo et al. (1981) during induction of ovulation with human menopausal gonadotropin. Generally, smaller follicles were found in cycles induced with

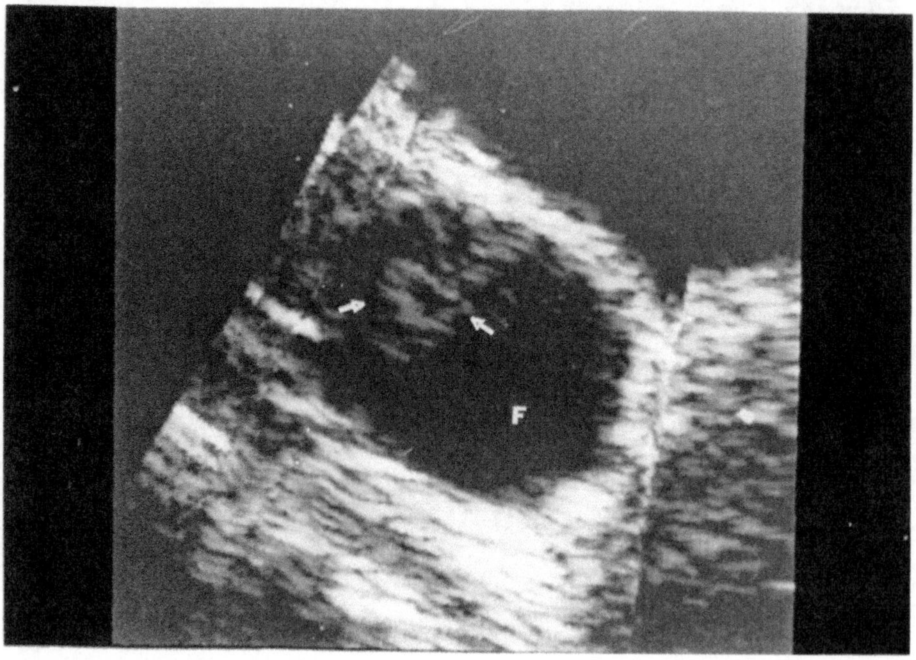

Figure 6

A large follicle (F) with an echogenic area attached to the superior wall (arrows) representing the cumulus oophorus.

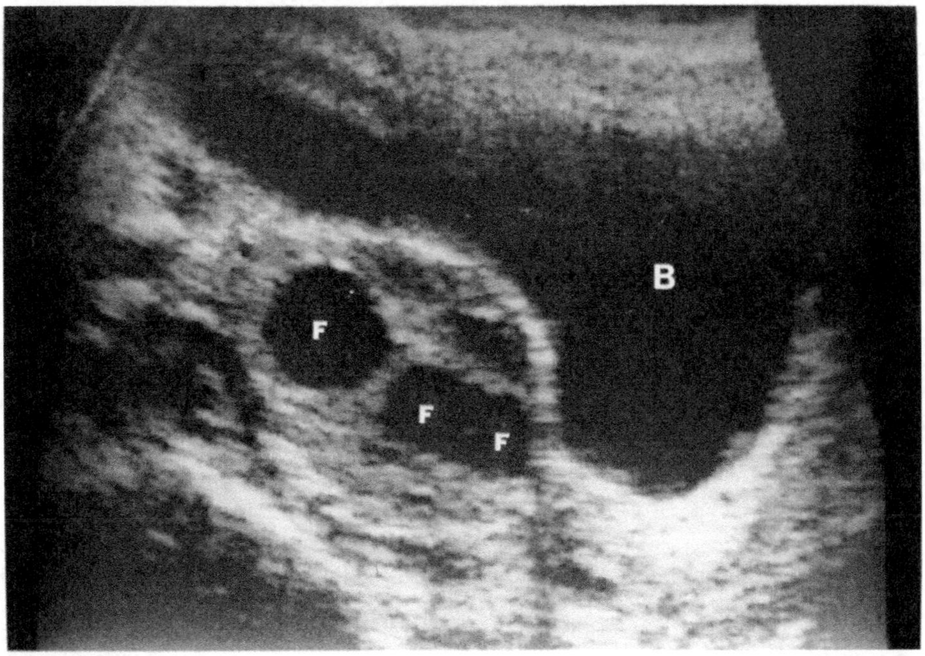

Figure 7

Parasagittal scan of the right ovary following clomiphene citrate stimulation. The right ovary is enlarged and very well defined. The ovarian stroma is echogenic. Multiple follicles (F) at various stages of development are seen within the ovary.

human menopausal gonadotropins compared with normal cycles or clomiphene stimulated cycles (Figure 10).

Clomiphene and hMG Induced Cycles

A combination of the two most commonly used follicular recruitment agents (clomiphene citrate; 50 mg per day, cycle days 5-9 plus human menopausal gonadotropin (Pergonal) 2 ampules per day, cycle days 6, 8 and 10) was used in a group of 17 patients. This group of patients was compared with a similar group receiving only 50 mg of clomiphene citrate per day, cycle days 5-9. All patients were monitored with daily follicular ultrasound measurements beginning on day 10. The total number of follicles available for aspiration was increased in the combination group, 5.1 follicles per patient as compared with 3.7 follicles per patient in the clomiphene alone group. The increase in follicle number in the combination group was primarily in follicles 10 to 14 mm in diameter (Figure 11). At laparoscopy, the number of oocytes recovered per patient was greater in the combination group (2.8 oocytes per patient) as compared with the clomiphene alone group (1.9 oocytes per patient) ($p < .05$). The increased number of oocytes obtained in the combination group resulted in an increased (not statistically significant) number of embryos transferred.

ADVANTAGES AND DISADVANTAGES OF ULTRASOUND FOLLICULAR MONITORING

A major advantage of ultrasonographic monitoring is the ability to determine early in the cycle the side on which the follicle or follicles are developing. This information is important in those patients in whom only one ovary is accessible for laparoscopic follicular aspiration. A second major advantage of ultrasonographic monitoring is to avoid unnecessary laparoscopy

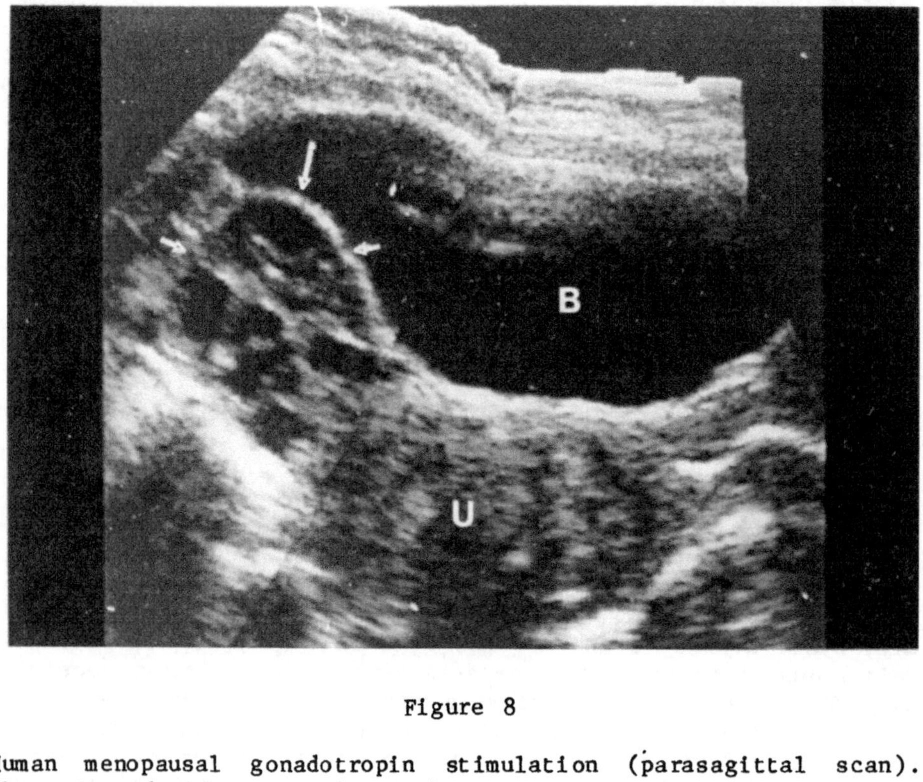

Figure 8

Human menopausal gonadotropin stimulation (parasagittal scan). The enlarged left ovary (arrows) contains a large number of small follicles and is seen posterior to the urinary bladder (B) and superior to the retroflexed uterus (U).

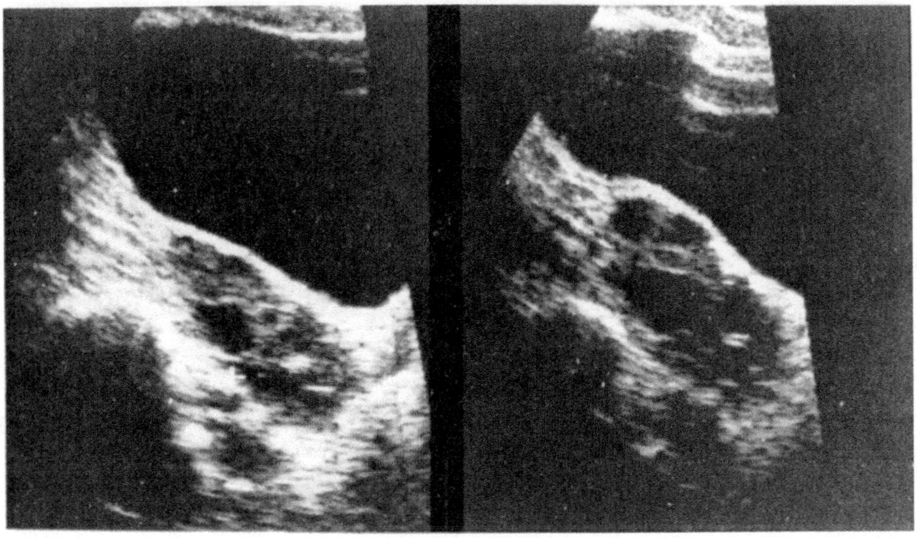

Figure 9

Parasagittal scans of right ovary on cycle days 8 and 10 following human menopausal gonadotropin stimulation demonstrating growth of multiple follicles.

in patients in whom abnormal follicular development is occurring (non-growing or shrinking follicles) or in whom premature ovulation has occurred. Additionally, in selected cases, when the mid-cycle LH surge has occurred prior to hCG administration, ultrasonographic demonstration of preovulatory follicles still within the ovary at the time of laparoscopy can be used to support the clinical decision to proceed with the scheduled laparoscopic follicular aspiration. Finally, a recent report (Quigley et al., 1982) has shown a reduced chance that a patient will undergo embryo transfer if there is only one preovulatory follicle developing. Ultrasound imaging can therefore play a role in the clinical management of the patient.

There are few disadvantages of follicular monitoring by ultrasound. One is that ultrasonographic examination of the ovaries is operator dependent and should be undertaken only by experienced personnel. In a few cases, it is difficult to differentiate between other fluid filled structures in the adnexa (such as a hydrosalpinx), and ovarian follicles. An important differentiating point between other cystic structures and ovarian follicles is the steady rate of growth of the latter on

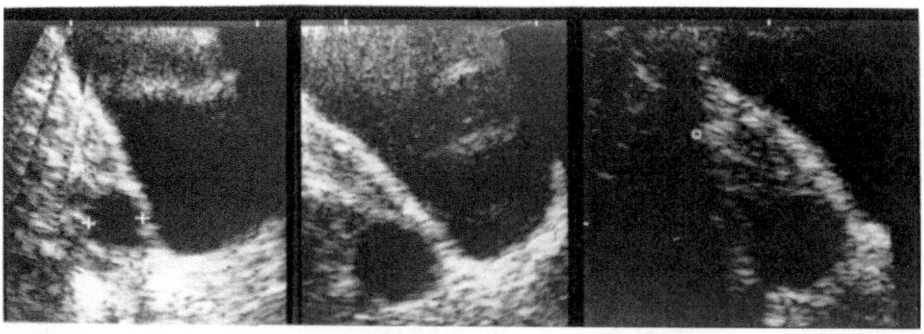

Figure 10

Clomiphene citrate stimulation. Parasagittal scan of right ovary on cycle days 10, 11 and 12 demonstrating rapid growth of a single follicle.

ultrasonographic examinations. The possible toxic effects of ultrasound on the ovary and on subsequent offspring is of theoretical concern. Studies in animals have shown that there is no increase in the percentage of offspring with anomalies following ultrasonographic exposure (Erdmann et al., 1977). There have been no reported adverse biologic effects of ultrasound when used at the lower frequency levels currently employed for diagnostic purposes.

SUMMARY AND CONCLUSIONS

Ultrasonography offers a rapid, noninvasive technique for monitoring follicular growth and development during IVF-ET treatment cycles where enhanced follicular recruitment protocols usually result in the development of multiple follicles. In general, the development of these follicles is asynchronous (see Chapter 6) and ultrasonographic imaging, by monitoring the development of individual follicles, aids significantly in determining the ideal time for administration of the pre-ovulatory dose of hCG.

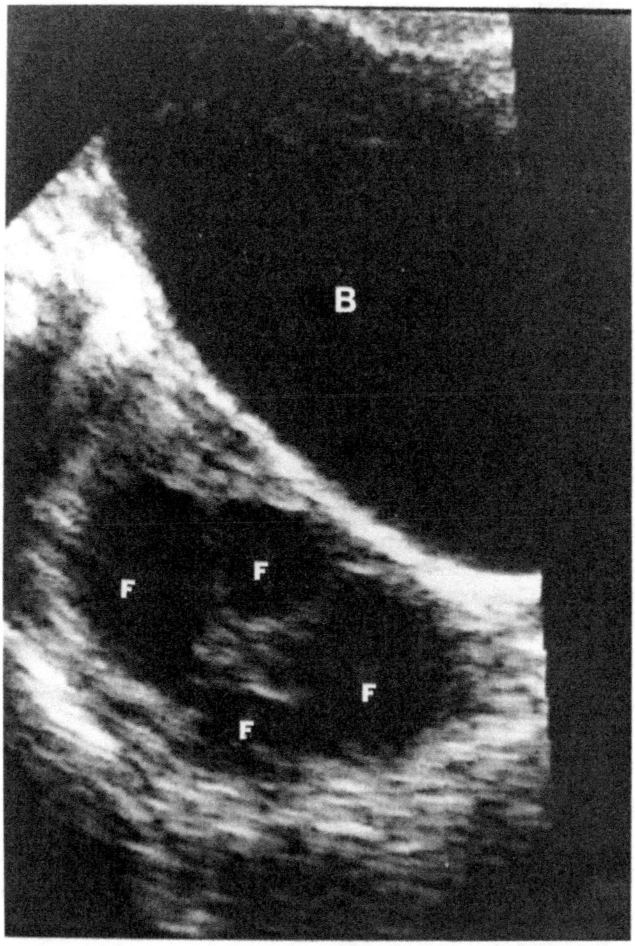

Figure 11

Ovarian stimulation by combination of clomiphene and human menopausal gonadotropin. This parasagittal scan shows the enlarged ovary containing 4 well-defined follicles (F) ranging in size from 10 to 22 mm in diameter (B = urinary bladder).

REFERENCES

Erdmann, W.A., Johnson, L.K. and Baird, A.I., 1977, Ultrasound toxicity study, Ultrasound Med. Biol., 3:351.

Hackeloer, B.J., Fleming, R., Robinson, H.P., Adam, A.H., and Coutts, J.R.T., 1979, Correlation of ultrasonic and endocrinologic assessment of human follicular development, Am.J. Obstet. Gynecol., 135:122.

Hoult, I.J., deCrespigny, L. Ch., O'Herlihy, C., Speirs, A.L., Lopata, A., Kellow, G., Johnston, I., and Robinson, H.P., 1981, Ultrasound control of clomiphene/human chorionic gonadotropin stimulated cycles for oocyte recovery and in vitro fertilization, Fertil. Steril., 36:316.

O'Herlihy, C., deCrespigny, L. Ch., and Lopata, A., 1980(b), Preovulatory follicular size: A comparison of ultrasound and laparoscopic measurements. Fertil. Steril., 34:24.

Queenan, J.T., O'Brien, G.D., Bains, L.M., Simpson, J., Collins, W.P., and Campbell, S., 1980, Ultrasound scanning of ovaries to detect ovulation in women, Fertil. Steril., 34:99.

Quigley, M.M., Maklad, N.F., and Wolf, D.P., 1983, Comparison of two clomiphene citrate dosage regimens for follicular recruitment in an in vitro fertilization program, Fertil. Steril., 40:53.

Quigley, M.M., Wolf, D.P., Maklad, N.F., Dandekar, P.V., and Sokoloski, J.E., 1982, Follicular size and number in human in vitro fertilization, Fertil. Steril., 38:678.

Quigley, M.M., Kendall, J.Z., Maklad, N.F., Wolf, D.P., 1983, Monitoring follicular development in an IVF-ET program: Serum estrogen versus ultrasonography, Fertil. Steril., 39:416.

Sallam, H.N., Marinho, A.O., Collins, W.P. , Rodeck, C.H., Campbell, S., 1982, Monitoring gonadotropin therapy by real time ultrasonic scanning of ovarian follicles, Br. J. Obstet. Gynaecol., 89:155.

Vargyas, J.M., Marrs, R.P., Kletzky, O.A., and Mishell, D.R., 1982, Correlation of ultrasonic measurement of ovarian follicle size and serum estradiol levels in ovulatory patients following clomiphene citrate for in vitro fertilization, Am. J. Obstet. Gynecol., 144:569.

Ylostalo, P., Lindgren, P.C., and Nillius, S.F., 1981, Ultrasonic measurement of the ovarian follicles, ovaries and uterine size during induction of ovulation with human gonadotropins, Acta Endocrin., 98:592.

9

MONITORING FOLLICULAR DEVELOPMENT WITH ESTROGENS

Pedro J. Beauchamp

Daily measurements of serum or urinary estrogen(s) concentrations have been used to monitor follicular development in patients undergoing ovulation induction with human menopausal gonadotropins (hMG). In these patients, biochemical (estrogen) monitoring of the follicular response to hMG is necessary to determine the optimal time to administer the ovulatory dose of human chorionic gonadotropin (hCG) or to withhold hCG in cases of ovarian overstimulation. The goals of such monitoring in anovulatory ovulation induction are: 1) to achieve pregnancy; 2) to minimize ovarian hyperstimulation syndrome; and 3) to minimize the rate of multiple gestation. Similarly, measurements of estrogens have been used in monitoring follicular development for in vitro fertilization and embryo transfer (IVF-ET) in order to: 1) predict the exact time of ovulation; 2) determine the appropriate time for hCG administration; 3) assess follicular functional well being; 4) avoid biochemical hyperstimulation; and 5) terminate the treatment cycle in the face of abnormal estrogen secretory patterns. The object of this chapter is to discuss estrogen monitoring, and to review the experience with it in the context of IVF-ET.

ESTRADIOL DURING THE NORMAL AND STIMULATED MENSTRUAL CYCLE

Spontaneous Cycles

The preovulatory follicle(s) is responsible for over 90% of the estradiol (E_2) production during the preovulatory period (Baird and Fraser, 1974). The E_2 results from direct secretion by the theca cells plus aromatization of androgen precursors by the granulosa cells. Increasing E_2 levels during the first half of the cycle reflect increasing follicular size, number and/or aromatase activity (Fritz and Speroff, 1982; Chapters 4 and 5). After ovulation, the corpus luteum is the main source of circulating estradiol.

The preovulatory E_2 peak (E_2 level over 200 pg/ml sustained for up to 50 hours) triggers the onset of the LH surge (Fritz and Speroff, 1982). The timing of the preovulatory E_2 peak is not a reliable predictor of ovulation as ovulation occurs 24-72 hours (mean interval 34 $\pm$ 3 hours) after the peak E_2 value (Pauerstein et al., 1978; García et al., 1981). Such a wide fluctuation makes E_2 monitoring too imprecise for the timing of ovulation. Follicular size (as determined by ultrasound) likewise varies from 17mm to 25mm at the time of ovulation during a natural cycle (O'Herlihy et al., 1980) and 15 to 23mm during clomiphene citrate stimulation (Buttery et al., 1983). The onset of the LH surge is a more accurate predictor of ovulation than either the time of the estrogen peak or follicular size by ultrasound (Pauerstein et al., 1978; Garcia et al., 1981; Bryce et al., 1982; Lemay et al., 1982).

During a normal spontaneous cycle, estradiol levels rise linearly to maximum levels of 300-600 pg/ml 1-3 days prior to ovulation (Garcia et al., 1981; Fritz and Speroff, 1982; Pauerstein et al., 1983; Polan et al., 1983). With the onset of the LH surge, E_2 levels decrease to lower levels (100-200 pg/ml) 2-3 days after ovulation. During the midluteal phase, there is a secondary E_2 rise to about half the preovulatory E_2 level. This cyclic E_2 pattern is reproduced in stimulated, conception cycles (Figure 1).

Clomiphene Stimulated Cycles

Most groups treating patients by IVF-ET use stimulated cycles with timed administration of hCG for preovulatory maturation prior to laparoscopic follicular aspiration. A few groups allow the endogenous LH surge to occur instead of administering hCG (Frydman et al., 1982; Lopata, 1983; Kerin et al., 1983). Their rationale for this practice is to allow completion of the normal physiologic events leading to ovum maturation and ovulation, thereby potentially improving fertilization and pregnancy rates.

The number of follicles and their growth rate are best monitored with ultrasound. E_2 monitoring is utilized by most groups to assess the functional development of preovulatory follicles (See chapter 7). Plasma E_2 levels have been shown to

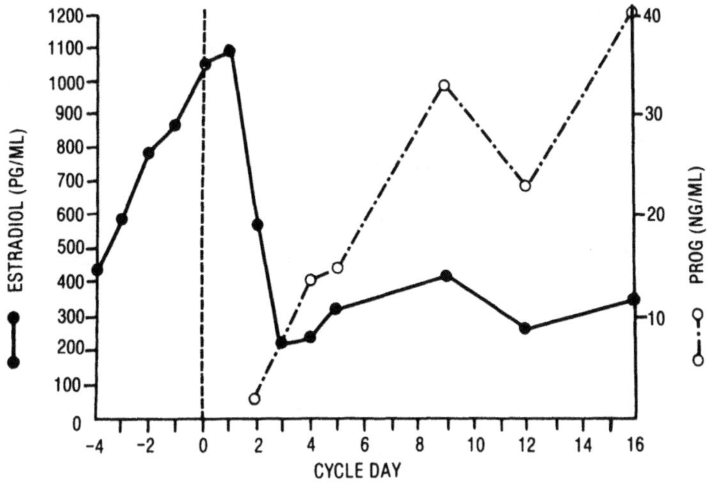

Figure 1

Serum estradiol and progesterone values during a conceptual cycle. Follicular recruitment was enhanced with clomiphene citate 50 mg/day cycle days 5-9. HCG (2500 IU) was administered on Day 0. Laparoscopic follicular aspiration was performed on Day 2 and one embryo was transferred on Day 4. Progesterone in oil 12.5 mg intramuscular was administered daily from Day 4 to 8.

correlate with total ovarian follicular volume (Haning et al., 1982). Thus the E_2 level is proportional to the size and number of follicular units. A good correlation between follicular growth (as determined by ultrasound) and E_2 production has been demonstrated during natural cycles (Hackeloer et al., 1979; Kerin et al., 1981), and in cycles stimulated with clomiphene citrate (Vargyas et al., 1982) or hMG (Marrs et al., 1983). The limitation of monitoring follicular number and development with E_2 is that multiple small follicles can produce the same amount of E_2 as a single large follicle, if the total follicular volume is the same (Haning et al., 1982). An average value of E_2 per follicle can, of course, be calculated. However, in doing this, the assumption is made that each follicle contributes equally to the total E_2 level, which may not always be true. In either case, peripheral E_2 monitoring measures the total steroidogenic capacity of the developing follicles.

Ovulatory cycles stimulated with clomiphene citrate (150 mg/day for 5 days) have average peak E_2 levels of 1150 $\pm$ 65 pg/ml (mean ± SEM), probably reflecting multiple follicular recruitment (Vargyas et al., 1982). The mean E_2 value per large (≥18mm) follicle was 459 ± 19 pg/ml (range 275-670 pg/ml) in that report. Recent studies at our institution have demonstrated that IVF-ET patients taking 150 mg of clomiphene citrate from days 5 through 9 of the cycle have significantly higher total peak E_2 levels of 973 ± 100 pg/ml (mean ± SEM) compared to 614 ± 63 pg/ml for those receiving 50 mg clomiphene citrate on the same schedule ($p < .01$; Figure 2; unpublished observations). The mean number of follicles per patient were similar for both groups, 2.3 ± 0.1 follicles versus 2.4 ± 0.2 follicles per patient for 50 and 150 mg clomiphene citrate, respectively (Quigley et al., 1983). The mean peak E_2 levels per follicle were 477 ± 49 pg/ml and 262 ± 31 pg/ml for 150 and 50 mg clomiphene citrate, respectively ($p < .01$; Figure 3). The higher LH levels produced by the 150 mg dose of clomiphene citrate are probably responsible for the higher E_2 levels relative to the 50 mg dose of clomiphene citrate seen in spite of a similar number of developing follicles (unpublished observations).

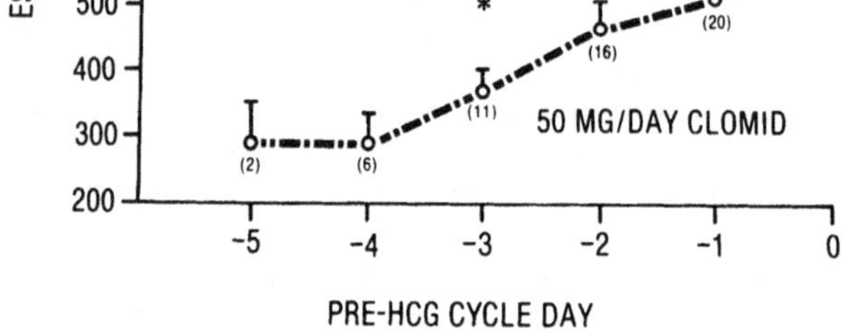

Figure 2

Total serum estradiol measured in patients receiving either 50 or 150 mg/day clomiphene citrate, cycle days 5-9. The day of hCG administration is cycle Day 0. The number of patients is in parentheses (* $p < 0.05$; ** $p < .01$).

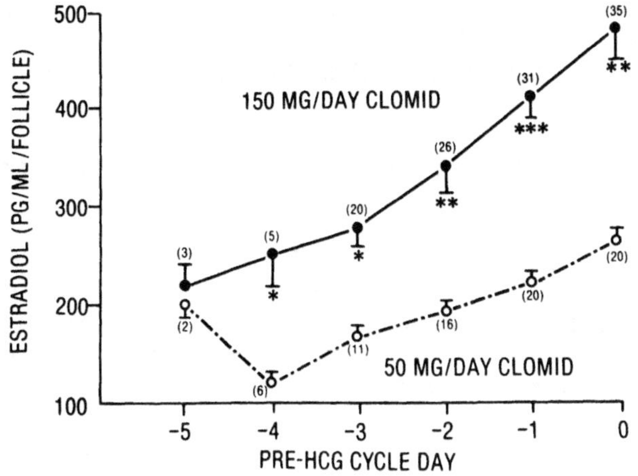

Figure 3

Serum estradiol expressed per follicle $\geq$ 15mm diameter in patients receiving 50 and 150 mg clomiphene citrate cycle day 5-9. Day of hCG administeration is cycle Day 0. The number of patients is in parentheses. (* $p < .05$; ** $p < .01$; *** $p < .001$).

Gonadotropin Stimulated Cycles

The E_2 response to hMG depends on dosage, duration of treatment, and state of the follicles at the beginning of therapy. During hMG administration to anovulatory women, there is an initial latent phase, analogous to the first 5-7 days of the menstrual cycle, when E_2 levels are low in spite of relatively high FSH and LH levels. The duration of the latent phase will depend on the state of the follicles at the beginning of therapy and ranges from 3-9 days in anovulatory women. Once a certain level of gonadotropins is reached (referred to as the effective daily dose and marking the beginning of the active phase of E_2 production), follicular growth is enhanced, as reflected in increasing serum E_2 levels. Thereafter, a progressive logarithmic increase in E_2 level occurs, dependant on the dose of hMG and the ovarian sensitivity to that dose (Insler and Potashnik, 1983).

Timing of blood sampling in relation to the previous hMG

injection is important. Even though the 24 hour post-injection E_2 values are indicative of ovarian stimulation, peak E_2 levels are observed 8 to 10 hours post-hMG injection (Klopper et al., 1974). Groups that use hMG for follicular recruitment in an IVF-ET program should draw blood samples at a constant interval post-hMG injection for their data analysis to be meaningful. This consideration is probably not necessary in clomiphene citrate stimulated cycles due to clomiphene's long half life.

E_2 MONITORING FOR ASSESSMENT OF FOLLICULAR MATURITY AND FUNCTIONAL WELL-BEING

Obtaining mature, fertilizable oocytes is essential for successful _in vitro_ fertilization. In cycles stimulated with clomiphene citrate and/or hMG, determination of optimal follicular maturation is critical for proper timing of hCG administration. The goal of such monitoring is to maximize the recovery rate of fertilizable oocytes.

The Eastern Virginia Medical School group relies on E_2 monitoring and clinical parameters for hMG-stimulated IVF cycles (Garcia et al., 1983a, b). Ultrasound is utilized in patients that cannot be followed by clinical parameters, and to confirm the presence of adequate number and size of follicles. They have divided patients into low, normal or high E_2 responders corresponding to $E_2 < 300$, 300-600, or > 600 pg/ml, respectively, at the time of the "clinical estrogen shift." For further details and significance of such monitoring, the reader is referred to Chapter 7.

Determination of follicular maturation is important for optimal timing of hCG administration. Premature injection of hCG can result in recovery of small immature oocytes, with lower fertilizing capacity. Likewise, post mature, fragmented oocytes with luteinized granulosa cells can result from overmaturation (Chapter 7). Establishment that a follicle contains an oocyte with a high probability of subsequent fertilization may be accomplished by integration of ultrasound measurements and serum E_2 levels (Trounson and Leeton, 1982; Lopata, 1983; Garcia et al., 1983a, b). In addition, it may be possible to identify patients with diminished chances of establishing a pregnancy and in whom laparoscopy should be discouraged.

E_2 MONITORING FOR PREVENTION OF BIOCHEMICAL HYPERSTIMULATION

As previously indicated in Chapter 7, very high pre-ovulatory E_2 levels frequently result in disruption of the luteal phase.

Data reported by Edwards et al. (1980) demonstrated that high preovulatory E_2 levels were associated with lower progesterone levels during the luteal phase. Biochemical ovarian hyperstimulation has been shown to decrease pregnancy rates and increase spontaneous abortion rates (Edwards et al., 1980; Olson et al., 1983; Ben-Rafael et al., 1983). E_2 monitoring may, thus, also pre-select patients with excessively high E_2 response, in whom pregnancy rates may be lower and in whom laparoscopy may be discouraged (See also Chapter 7).

ESTRADIOL MONITORING AT THE UNIVERSITY OF TEXAS AT HOUSTON

Our data from clomiphene citrate stimulated cycles has shown that preovulatory peak E_2 levels ranged between 468 and 1100 pg/ml in the first 9 patients who achieved pregnancy. Timing of injection of the pre-ovulatory dose of hCG was determined by ultrasound findings of at least one follicle measuring 20mm in diameter. It appears that during clomiphene citrate stimulated follicular recruitment, the optimal pre-ovulatory E_2 range is between 400-1200 pg/ml in the presence of at least one preovulatory follicle $\geq$ 20mm diameter.

Data from our IVF-ET program has detected several abnormal E_2 patterns (Beauchamp et al., 1984). Follicular recruitment was enhanced with clomiphene citrate, 50 mg or 150 mg daily from days 5 through 9; timing of hCG was determined by ultrasound monitoring as described elsewhere or in Chapter 8. Daily serum E_2 determinations were used for retrospective evaluation of these cycles.

Follicular Phase Hyperstimulation

Figure 4 depicts a cycle in which administration of clomiphene citrate, 150 mg/day, resulted in pre-hCG E_2 values $\geq$ 2,000 pg/ml. Four follicles $\geq$ 15mm developed in this patient, five oocytes were recovered and 2 embryos were transferred. Pregnancy was not established. Progesterone values were 17.2 ng/ml on the day of transfer and rose to peak levels of 51.1 ng/ml. The luteal phase (interval from follicular aspiration to onset of menses) lasted 14 days. The overall E_2 pattern of a normal cycle was reproduced but at a much higher level.

Follicular Phase Hypostimulation

Inadequate preovulatory E_2 rise in one patient is shown in Figure 5. She received clomiphene citrate, 50 mg/day for 5 days, and developed two follicles $\geq$ 15mm; one oocyte was obtained and one embryo was transferred. Pregnancy was not established.

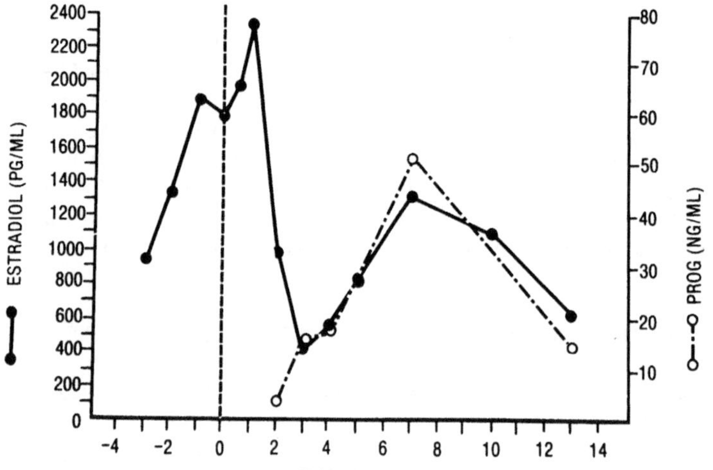

Figure 4

Serum estradiol and progesterone values during a hyperstimulated cycle. Patient received 150 mg clomiphene citrate/day, cycle days 5 to 9. 2500 IU of hCG were administered on cycle Day 0 when four follicles ≥ 15mm in diameter were present. Please note that the scale of the ordinate is twice the scale of figures 1, 5, 6 and 7. The overall hormonal pattern of a normal cycle was reproduced but at a much higher level.

Luteal phase progesterone values were 7.8 ng/ml on the day of embryo transfer and rose to a maximum of 10.7 ng/ml even with progesterone supplementation (12.5 mg/day X 5 days starting on the day of the transfer). The luteal phase lasted 15 days. In this case, the overall E_2 pattern of a normal cycle was reproduced but at a much lower level.

Persistent elevation of E_2 during the early luteal phase

As previously indicated, E_2 decreases to lower levels 2-3 days after ovulation and rises later in the midluteal phase. Figure 6 shows a case in which E_2 levels remained elevated early in the luteal phase. This patient had received 150 mg clomiphene citrate per day for 5 days. She developed one follicle 22mm in diameter which was aspirated. No secondary follicles developed. One oocyte was obtained and one embryo was transferred. Implantation did not occur. The midluteal progesterone value was

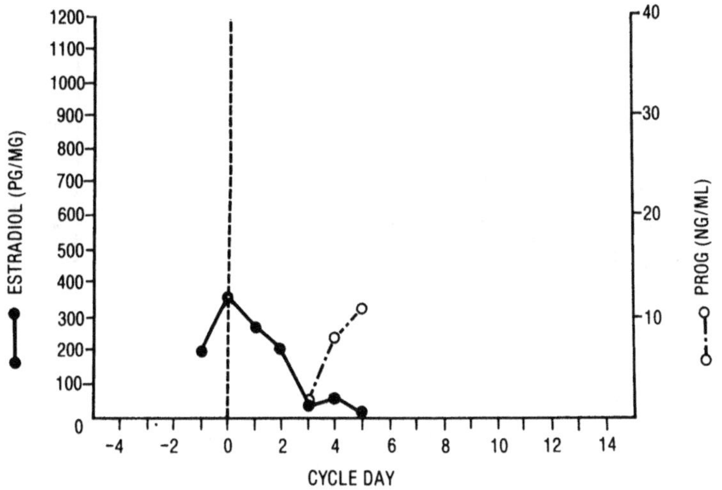

Figure 5

Serum estradiol and progesterone values during a hypostimulated cycle. Patient received 50 mg clomiphene citrate cycle day 5-9. 2500 IU of hCG were administered on cycle Day 0 when two follicles $\geq$ 15mm in diameter were present. The overall hormonal pattern of a normal cycle was reproduced but at a much lower level.

17 ng/ml on the day of embryo transfer which increased to a peak of 38.1 ng/ml. The duration of the luteal phase was 12 days.

Elevated E_2 levels for several days after ovulation inhibits implantation; this observation is the principle behind post-coital contraception (interception; Morris and Van Waganer, 1973; Yuzpe and Percival-Smith, 1983). It is possible that high E_2 levels during the early luteal phase may interfere with endometrial maturation causing an out-of-phase endometrium and implantation failure (Edwards et al., 1980).

Failure of midluteal E_2 rise

Peak E_2 levels coincide with peak progesterone levels during the luteal phase. This secondary E_2 rise is thought to be responsible for initiation of the mechanism eventually resulting in luteolysis (Fritz and Speroff, 1982). In certain animal species e.g., rodents, estrogens are necessary for implantation to occur. In animals oophorectomized within 3 days after ovulation,

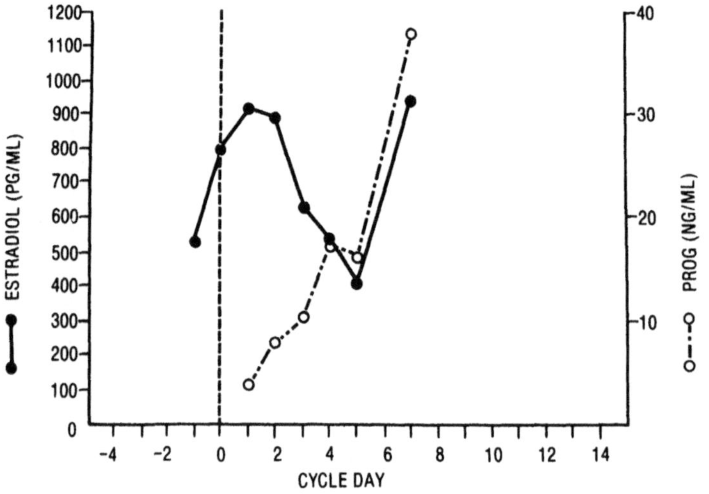

Figure 6

Serum estradiol and progesterone values in a cycle with persistent elevation of E_2 during the luteal phase. Patient received 150 mg clomiphene citrate per day cycle days 5-9. The hCG (2500 IU) was administered on cycle Day 0. One follicle $\geq$ 15mm in diameter (22mm) was present and aspirated on Day 2. The lowest early luteal phase E_2 value (400 pg/ml) was observed on Day 5 (3 days after laparoscopic aspiration).

implantation can be delayed for up to 2-3 weeks if they are given adequate progesterone supplementation. Implantation can be induced during this period of "delayed implantation" within 48 hours after an injection of estradiol benzoate (Perry, 1971; Psychoyos, 1973). It is not known what role, if any, E_2 plays in the process of human implantation.

Figure 7 shows the E_2 curve of a patient receiving 50 mg clomiphene citrate per day for 5 days during an IVF-ET cycle. She developed 3 follicles $\geq$ 15mm from which 2 oocytes were obtained and one embryo was transferred. Implantation did not occur. The progesterone value was 13.2 ng/ml on the day of embryo transfer and rose to 22.1 ng/ml with progesterone supplementation. The duration of the luteal phase was 14 days. The overall E_2 pattern was normal except for a flat luteal phase (luteal phase E_2 rise was only 30 pg/ml over baseline).

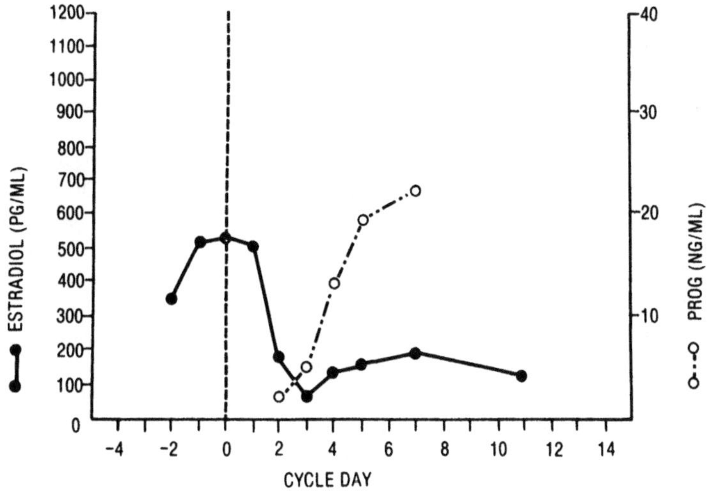

Figure 7

Serum estradiol and progesterone values in a cycle with failure of midluteal E_2 rise. The patient received 50 mg clomiphene citrate per day, days 5-9. The hCG (2500 IU) was administered on cycle Day 0 when three follicles $\geq$ 15mm in diameter were present. The overall progesterone and E_2 pattern was normal except for minimal rise in midluteal E_2 level (30 pg/ml over baseline).

THE USE OF PROSPECTIVE ESTRADIOL MONITORING IN IVF-ET.

This section will give practical advise on the use of estradiol and ultrasound for monitoring follicular development. Such prospective monitoring requires the availability of ultrasound measurements and estradiol determinations on a daily basis.

Irrespective of the protocol utilized for follicular recruitment, estradiol and ultrasound monitoring should be started about 4 days prior to the expected day of hCG administration. Several parameters should be taken into consideration in order to determine the optimal timing of hCG administration: 1) the number and size of follicles developing in both ovaries (even if only one is accessible); 2) the absolute total E_2 value; and 3) the shape of the preovulatory E_2 curve. All three parameters are of equal importance.

The total E_2 value can be utilized prospectively to modify the follicular recruitment protocol, as is done by the Eastern Virginia Medical School group with their hMG regime (See Chapter 7). An optimal E_2 level range (window) should be attained at the time of hCG administration. Our data indicate that an E_2 level between 400 and 1200 pg/ml appears to be ideal in cycles stimulated with clomiphene citrate alone. During cycles stimulated with hMG alone, the Eastern Virginia Medical School group has obtained the highest pregnancy rates with the "normal" E_2 responders (E_2 level 300-600 pg/ml), followed by the "high" E_2 responders ($E_2 \geq 600$ pg/ml; See Chapter 7). Even though the highest E_2 level that they observed during a conceptual cycle was not mentioned, it is reasonable to assume that an E_2 window between 300 and 1200 pg/ml is adequate for cycles stimulated with hMG alone. The peak E_2 levels in our pregnancies established during combination clomiphene citrate-hMG stimulated cycles have been in this same range.

By the time that adequate serum E_2 levels have been reached, ultrasound results should allow further evaluation of follicular growth rate and indicate the number and size of follicles. During cycles stimulated with hMG alone, it is desirable to have at least two preovulatory follicles $\geq$ 16mm in mean diameter when the E_2 window is reached. Since larger follicles develop with clomiphene citrate stimulation, at least two preovulatory follicles $\geq$ 18mm in mean diameter (preferably $\geq$ 20mm) should be present when the E_2 window is reached during clomiphene citrate alone or clomiphene citrate-hMG follicular recruitment protocols. Conversely, ultrasound monitoring could also be utilized prospectively to modify the follicular recruitment protocol, as is done by Lopata and coworkers (1983). In their clomiphene citrate-hMG protocol, the dosage of hMG varies depending on follicular size, number and growth rate. In this case, E_2 monitoring could then be utilized to assure attainment of an appropriate E_2 window.

Lastly, the shape of the preovulatory E_2 curve should be evaluated for further assessment of follicular well-being. Jones and coworkers (1983) have described several preovulatory E_2 patterns in response to hMG stimulation. Their data indicate that the highest pregnancy rates were obtained in cycles in which E_2 levels progressively increased each day and reached peak levels either on the day of hCG administration or the next day. A plateau in E_2 levels or decreasing E_2 levels were associated with very low pregnancy rates. Similar results from clomiphene stimulated cycles have been reported recently by Lopata (1983).

The optimum timing of hCG administration in IVF-ET should be on the day when at least 2 preovulatory follicles reach a critical size (depending on the follicular recruitment protocol used), the serum E_2 levels have been progressively increasing and the total E_2 value falls within a certain window (approximately 300 to 1200 pg/ml). Patients not meeting these criteria may be discouraged from undergoing laparoscopy and the cycle terminated. Measurement of the LH levels at the time of hCG administration is a wise precaution to ensure that LH levels are basal and the endogenous LH surge had not started.

SUMMARY AND CONCLUSIONS

The functional development of the preovulatory follicle can be evaluated by biochemical (E_2) monitoring. A good correlation between E_2 levels and ultrasound measurement of total follicular volume has been demonstrated during natural cycles and in cycles stimulated with clomiphene citrate and hMG. Monitoring the E_2 response to follicular stimulation may be useful to assess the steroidogenic capacity of the developing follicles. By this monitoring, cases of ovarian hyper- or hypostimulation (in which pregnancy rates are lower) can be identified prior to laparoscopy. Analysis of the E_2 cycle pattern may be used to evaluate the individual's response to ovarian stimulation and possibly, to alter the stimulation protocol in the current or subsequent cycles.

Monitoring follicular development with E_2 in conjunction with ultrasound is a valuable clinical and research tool in IVF. Its principal clinical application lies in determining the time of optimal follicular maturation, and in assessing the normalcy of the follicular response. Establishment that a follicle contains an oocyte with a high probability of subsequent fertilization and implantation may be accomplished by integration of ultrasound measurement and serum E_2 levels. Accordingly, it should become possible to pre-select patients with diminished chances of establishing a pregnancy and in whom laparoscopy should be discouraged.

REFERENCES

Baird, D.T. and Fraser, I.S., 1974, Blood production and ovarian secretion rates of estradiol and estrone in women throughout the menstrual cycle, J. Clin. Endocrinol. Metab., 38:1009.

Beauchamp, P.J., Quigley, M.M., Schmidt, C.L., Gilbert, S., Pace-Owens, S., and Wolf, D.P., 1984, Abnormal serum estradiol patterns in patients receiving clomiphene citrate for enhanced follicular recruitment in *in vitro* fertilization, Fertil. Steril., (in press).

Ben-Rafael, Z., Dor, J., Mashiach, S., Blankstein, J., Lunenfeld, B. and Serr, D.M., 1983, Abortion rate in pregnancies following ovulation induced by human menopausal gonadotropin/human chorionic gonadotropin, Fertil. Steril., 39:157.

Bryce, R.L., Shuter, B., Sinosich, M.J., Stiel, J.N., Picker, R.H. and Saunders, D.M., 1982, value of ultrasound, gonadotropin, and estradiol measurements for precise ovulation prediction, Fertil. Steril., 37:42.

Buttery, B., Trounson, A., McMaster, R. and Wood, C., 1983, Evaluation of diagnostic ultrasound as a parameter of follicular development in an in vitro fertilization program, Fertil. Steril., 39:458.

Edwards, R.G., Steptoe, P.C. and Purdy, J.M., 1980, Establishing full-term human pregnancies using cleaving embryos grown in vitro, Brit. J. Obstet. Gynecol., 87:737.

Frydman, R., Testart, J., Giacomini, P., Imbert, M.C., Martin, E. and Nahoul, K., 1982, Hormonal and histological study of the luteal phase in women following aspiration of the preovulatory follicle, Fertil. Steril., 38:312.

Fritz, M.A. and Speroff, L., 1982, The endocrinology of the menstrual cycle: the interaction of folliculogenesis and neuroendocrine mechanisms, Fertil. Steril., 38:509.

Garcia, J.E., Jones, G.S. and Wright, G.L., 1981, Prediction of the time of ovulation, Fertil. Steril., 36:308.

Garcia, J.E., Jones, G.S., Acosta, A.A. and Wright, G., 1983a, Human menopausal gonadotropin/human chorionic gonadotropin follicular maturation for oocyte aspiration: Phase I, 1981, Fertil. Steril., 39:167.

Garcia, J.E., Jones, G.S., Acosta, A.A. and Wright, G., 1983b, Human menopausal gonadotropin/human chorionic gonadotropin follicular maturation for oocyte aspiration: Phase II, 1981, Fertil. Steril., 39:174.

Haning, R.V., Austin, C.W., Kuzma, D.L., Shapiro, S.S. and Zweibel, W.J., 1982, Ultrasound evaluation of estrogen monitoring for induction of ovulation with menotropins, Fertil. Steril., 37:627.

Hackeloer, B.J., Fleming, R., Robinson, H.P., Adam, A.H. and Coults, J.R.T., 1979, Correlation of ultrasonic and endocrinologic assessment of human follicular development, Am. J. Obstet. Gynecol., 135:122.

Insler, V. and Potashnik, G., 1983, Monitoring of follicular development in gonadotropin-stimulated cycles, in: "Fertilization of the Human Egg In Vitro", H.M. Beier and H.R. Lindner, eds., Springer-Verlag, Berlin.

Jones, H.W., Acosta, A., Andrews, M.C., Garcia, J., Jones, G.S., Mantzavinos, T.H., McDowell, J., Sandow, B., Veeck, L., Whibley, T., Wilkes, C., and Wright, G., 1983, The importance of the follicular phase to success and failure in in vitro fertilization, Fertil. Steril., 40:317.

Kerin, J.F., Edmonds, E.K., Warnes, G.M., Cox, C.W., Seamark, R.F., Matthews, C.D., Young, G.B. and Baird, D.T., 1981,

Morphological and functional relations of graafian follicle growth to ovulation in women using ultrasonic, laparoscopic and biochemical measurements, Brit. J. Obstet. Gynecol., 88:81.
Kerin, J.F., Warners, G.M., Quinn, P.J., Jeffrey, R., Kirby, C., Matthews, C.D., Seamark, R.F. and Cox, L.W., 1983, Incidence of multiple pregnancy following human in vitro fertilization and embryo transfer, Lancet, 2:537.
Klopper, A., Aiman, J. and Besser, M., 1974, Ovarian steroidogenesis resulting from treatment with menopausal gonadotropin, Eur. J. Obstet. Gynecol. Reprod. Biol., 4:25.
Lemay, A., Bastide, A., Lambert, R. and Rioux, J.C., 1982, Prediction of human ovulation by rapid luteinizing hormone (LH) radioimmunoassay and ovarian ultrasonography, Fertil. Steril., 38:194.
Lopata, A., 1983, Concepts of human in vitro fertilization and embryo transfer, Fertil. Steril., 40:289.
Marrs, R.P., Vargyas, J.M. and March, C.M., 1983, Correlation of ultrasonic and endocrinologic measurements in human menopausal gonadotropin therapy, Am. J. Obstet. Gynecol., 145:417.
Morris, J.M. and Van Waganen, G., 1973, Interception: The use of postovulatory estrogens to prevent implantation, Am. J. Obstet. Gynecol., 115:101.
O'Herlihy, C., DeCrespigny, L., Lopata, A., Johnston, I., Hoult, I., and Robinson, H., 1980, Preovulatory follicular size: A comparision of ultrasound and laparoscopic measurements, Fertil. Steril., 34:24.
Olson, J., Rebar, R.W., Schreiber, J.R. and Vaitukaitis, J.L., 1983, Shortened luteal phase after ovulation induction with human menopausal gonadotropin and huma chorionic gonadotropin, Fertil. Steril., 39:284.
Pauerstein, C.J., Eddy, C.A., Croxatto, H.D., Hess, R., Siler-Khodr, T.M. and Croxatto, H.B., 1978, Temporal relationships of estrogens, progesterone and luteinizing hormone levels to ovulation in women and infrahuman primates, Am. J. Obstet. Gynecol., 130:876.
Perry, J.S., 1971, Ovarian periodicity, in: "The ovarian cycle of mammals", J.S. Perry, ed., Oliver and Boyd, Edinburgh.
Psychoyos, A., 1973, Endocrine control of egg implantation, in: "Handbook of Physiology", (Section 7, Endocrinology, Volume II, Part 2), R.O. Greep and E.B Astwood, eds. American Physiological Society, Washington, DC.
Polan, M.L., Totora, M., Caldwell, B.V., DeCherney, A.H., Haseltine, F.P., and Kase, N., 1982, Abnormal ovarian cycles as diagnosed by ultrasound and serum estradiol levels, Fertil. Steril., 37:342
Quigley, M.M., Maklad, N. and Wolf, D.P., 1983, Comparison of two clomiphene citrate dosage regimens for follicular recruitment in an in vitro fertilization program, Fertil. Steril., 40:178.
Trounson, A.O. and Leeton, J.F., 1982, The endocrinology of

clomiphene citrate stimulation, in: "Human Conception in Vitro", R.G. Edwards and J.M. Purdy, eds., Academic Press, London.

Vargyas, J.M., Marrs, R.P., Kletzky, O.A. and Mishell, D.R., 1982, Correlation of ultrasonic measurement of ovarian follicle size and serum estradiol levels in ovulatory patients following clomiphene citrate for in vitro fertilization, Am. J. Obstet. Gynecol., 144:569.

Yuzpe, A.A. and Percival-Smith, R., 1983, Use of hormonal steroids for pregnancy interception, Volume 6, in: "Gynecology and Obstetrics", J.J. Sciarra, ed., Harper and Row, Philadelphia.

10

LAPAROSCOPIC FOLLICULAR ASPIRATION

Pedro J. Beauchamp

The collection of mature, fertilizable oocytes is crucial for successful IVF-ET. Human oocytes are usually recovered by aspirating the pre-ovulatory follicle(s) using a needle introduced into the pelvic cavity at the time of laparoscopy. The object of this chapter is to review laparoscopy in general, and to describe step by step the technique and equipment used by our team at The University of Texas at Houston.

HISTORICAL BACKGROUND

Visual inspection of the abdominal cavity without laparotomy was introduced by Ott (1901). He performed a culdotomy through which, with the use of vaginal retractors and mirror-directed incandescent light, he was able to visualize the pelvic and abdominal organs.

The first "laparoscopic" abdominal endoscopy was performed by Kelling (1902) on a dog and by Jacobaeus (1910) on a human. Since then, there have been many reports of this method and technique.

In America, Decker and Cherry (1944) described and popularized culdoscopy in the 1940's and 1950's. However, due to the cumbersome knee-chest positioning of the patient during culdoscopy and the limited view of the pelvis and abdomen obtained by this technique, laparoscopy was reintroduced in the 1960's. Since then, laparoscopy has gained increasing popularity as a diagnostic and therapeutic tool, initially, for female sterilization and now adapted for follicular aspiration in IVF-ET. The first attempts of human laparoscopic follicular aspiration for IVF-ET were reported by Steptoe and Edwards (1970), Morgenstern and Soupart (1972) and Lopata et al. (1974).

CONTRAINDICATIONS TO LAPAROSCOPY

Laparoscopy is a relatively safe, low risk procedure. Nonetheless, the procedure is contraindicated in the following circumstances: 1) Patients for whom anesthesia would be contraindicated. Patients with chronic medical problems in whom laparoscopy and pregnancy are contraindicated or unsafe are not candidates for IVF-ET. Patients with acute medical conditions when general anesthesia is unsafe (e.g., acute upper respiratory infections, bronchitis, pneumonia or asthma) should have the laparoscopy postponed to a later date when the acute process has resolved; 2) Patients with intestinal obstruction or peritonitis, since they are at higher risk for injury to the abdominal viscera; and 3) Patients with a large hiatal hernia where establishing a pneunoperitoneum is associated with the potential risk of pneumothorax and cardiopulmonary complications.

Laparoscopy may be more difficult, and at slightly higher risk to the patient, when there is a previous history of peritonitis, prior laparotomies and known abdominal and pelvic adhesions. Obviously, most of the infertility patients undergoing IVF-ET have had one or more of the above, making the risk of inadvertent bowel or bladder damage somewhat greater. Accordingly, laparoscopy should be done with utmost care in order to minimize the risk to the patient. In addition, IVF-ET should not be attempted whenever there is evidence of acute or chronic genital tract infection or inflammation. Since the chances of a successful implantation and pregnancy are lower in patients with acute pelvic infections, it is wiser to delay laparoscopy until appropriate therapy is instituted, the erythrocyte sedimentation rate is normal and there is no evidence of endometritis on endometrial biopsy.

ANESTHESIA

Laparoscopy is a minor surgical procedure requiring major anesthesia (Cohen, 1983). Although technically feasible, local anesthesia for follicular aspiration is not recommended due to patient discomfort from the multiple puncture sites and intraperitoneal manipulation of abdominal and pelvic organs. Regional anesthesia (spinal, epidural) is also not recommended due to the respiratory compromise induced by the pneumoperitoneum and steep Trendelenburg position required. For these reasons, laparoscopic follicular aspiration is best performed under general, endotracheal anesthesia.

The majority of our patients have the laparoscopy performed on an ambulatory basis. Even in instances when the day surgery unit is closed (weekends) and the patient has to be admitted to the hospital the evening prior to laparoscopy, they are usually discharged from the hospital once fully recovered from the anesthesia. This practice requires the use of minimal or no premedication, and selection of anesthetic agents that will allow a deep enough anesthesia to carry out the procedure comfortably, yet be short acting enough to permit rapid recovery with minimal post operative nausea.

In general, at our institution, patients are not premedicated with narcotics or hypnotics, anesthesia is induced with intravenous pentothal, muscle relaxation is accomplished with succinylcholine, and inhalation of nitrous oxide, O_2 and isoflurane or enflurane is used for maintenance.

The influence of midcycle general anesthesia and different anesthetic agents on the hormonal profile of the ensuing luteal phase has been a matter of debate. Soules et al. (1980) reported endocrine data from three patients undergoing midcycle general anesthesia. They noted a statistically significant decrease in serum progesterone levels and an increase in prolactin when compared with the control group. However, there were no significant changes in LH or 17 β estradiol levels.

In a well conducted study by Szalay et al. (1982), the effect of different anesthetic agents were evaluated in 35 patients undergoing laparoscopy for oocyte retrieval during spontaneous cycles. They found no significant changes in the values of FSH, progesterone, estradiol or testosterone during and up to 12 hours after anesthesia. There was a slight but significant elevation of LH 10-40 minutes after onset of anesthesia. In addition, prolactin levels showed a highly significant rise 20-60 minutes after the onset of anesthesia. The lowest prolactin elevation occurred with the combination of thiopental and halothane, but even with these agents prolactin levels approached 100 ng/ml. In spite of the supraphysiologic increase in prolactin and the removal of follicular contents by aspiration, they did not find evidence of luteal phase insufficiency (as judged by progesterone levels and the onset of the following menses). Therefore, it appears that midcycle general anesthesia does not usually have a detrimental effect on circulating steroid hormones during the luteal phase of the menstrual cycle.

INSTRUMENTATION AND SET UP

Laparoscopy is performed with the patient in the supine position. Lithotomy position is not necessary since adequate exposure of the ovaries is usually achieved by placing the patients in Trendelenberg position. No instruments are placed in the vagina or cervix; only on rare occasion is it necessary to have an assistant elevate the cervix and uterus by digital intravaginal manipulation.

Our laparoscopic equipment for oocyte retrieval begins with the basic laparoscopy set (Figure 1). A Verres needle (R. Wolf, Rosemont, IL, Model E8302.08) is utilized for insufflation of the peritoneal cavity. The needle is 80mm long and consists of a movable, inner blunt stylet within an outer sharp tip cannula. The hub of the needle contains a spring which allows the inner blunt stylet to retract as resistance is met through the abdominal wall layers. Upon entry into the peritoneal cavity, a decrease in resistance springs the blunt stylet beyond the sharper tip, reducing the chances of laceration or puncture of the abdominal viscera. The Verres needle is connected to the insufflator by flexible rubber tubing.

The gas insufflator we use is also manufactured by R. Wolf, Model 2043.50. The insufflator should contain a regulator to control pressure and flow rate of gas, an insufflating pressure meter with automatic high pressure shut-off valve, a meter to monitor the amount of gas insufflated, a flow rate indicator, and a tank pressure gauge.

For the first (transumbilical) puncture site, we use a 10mm laparoscopic trocar with triangular tip (Olympus Corporation, Hyde Park, NY, Model A 5224) and sleeve (Olympus Corporation, Model A 5205). We use a 10 mm wide, 37 cm long laparoscope (Olympus Corporation, Model A 5214) with a 180° forward-directed objective. The additional light transmitted with a 10 mm laparoscope is desirable when video cameras or teaching attachments are employed. We use the laparoscope for visualization only, therefore extra channels for operating instruments are not necessary.

Good illumination is essential for adequate visualization. Our light source (Olympus Corporation, Model ILK-3) consists of a light projector with a 150 watt, 15 volt light bulb connected to the laparoscope by a fiberoptic cable with a focusing lens (Olympus Corporation, Model A 3045).

The second puncture trocar and sleeve is introduced in the suprapubic area. A 5mm self seal insulated trocar and sleeve (KLI

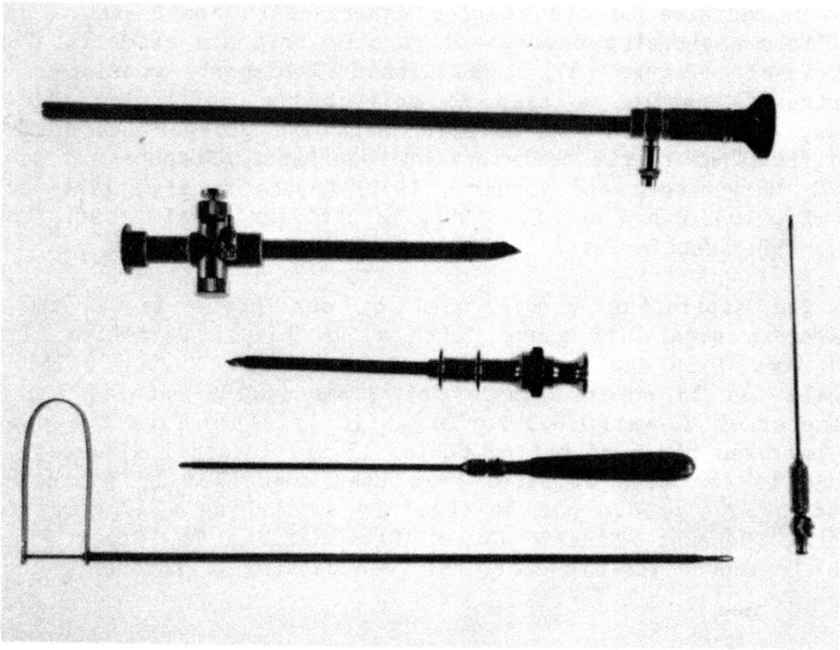

Figure 1

Basic laparoscopy equipment including: Verres needle; laparoscope; laparoscope trocar and sleeve; second puncture trocar and sleeve; sleeve and trocar for aspiration needle; and grasping forceps.

Inc. Newtown, PA, Model SS51235) is used for insertion of the grasping forceps. The forceps (WISAP, Reznik Instruments, Inc. Skokie IL, Model 7655) is 5 mm wide, 37 cm long and has two atraumatic jaws. It is designed so that when the handle is released, the jaws are closed, grasping tissue. Pressure has to be applied to open the jaws.

A needle sleeve and trocar (custom made by American V. Mueller, Chicago, IL, Model CD 10289) is used for the third puncture. The sleeve is 16 cm long and has an inner diameter of 2.9 mm, through which the aspirating needle is passed.

In addition to the regular laparoscopic equipment, a special follicle aspirating device and an ovum trap are essential for egg retrieval (Figure 2). The basic equipment consists of an aspirating needle, a trap to collect the follicular fluid and ovum, and a suctioning device. Many IVF groups have introduced modifications to the technique and equipment (Steptoe and Edwards, 1970; Morgenstern and Soupart, 1972; Lopata et al., 1974; Frydman et al., 1981;Renou et al., 1981; Feichtinger et al., 1981; Wood et al., 1981; Mettler et al., 1982; Jones et al., 1982).

The aspirating needle used by our group is 23 cm long, stainless steel, 12 gauge, with a 30° bevel (Perfektum, Propper and Sons Inc, New Hyde Park, NY, Catalogue Number 7421). The needle has an outer diameter of 2.8mm (0.109 inches) and inner diameter of 2.2mm (0.085 inches). It is lined from the tip with an unbroken piece of teflon tubing (1.3mm internal diameter) which leads to the trap modified from that described by Renou et al. (1981). The needle can be lined by stretching a 17 gauge teflon tubing (Penntube Plastic Co. Clifton Height, PA, Stock # 17 S/W FEP) to reduce its diameter, and then passing it through the

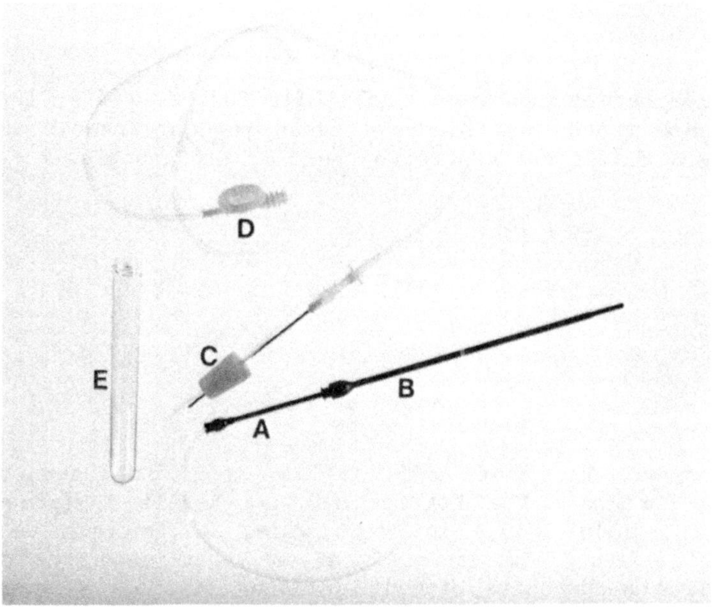

Figure 2

Aspirating device consisting of (A) aspirating needle (B) needle sleeve (C) silicone stopper (D) thumb suction control regulator (E) Follicular fluid collection device.

needle from the hub end and pulling it into the needle so that the unstretched teflon tubing snugly fits inside the needle. The teflon tube is then cut off flush with the bevel of the needle. The overall length of the teflon tubing, from tip of needle to ovum trap is 50-60 cm long and holds 1 to 1.5 ml of fluid volume. At the opposite end of the needle, the teflon tubing passes through a silicone stopper (A.H. Thomas Co. Philadelphia PA, Catalog No. 8747-E23, Size 0) and projects 2-3 cm into the ovum trap. Similar needles are commercially available from Rocket, USA (Branford, CT). The aspirating needle is introduced into the peritoneal cavity through the needle sleeve. The sleeve, once in place, will protect the needle and will allow clear entry into the peritoneal cavity without picking up foreign material from the abdominal wall.

Trauma to the oocyte can occur during aspiration. To prevent this, low suctioning pressures and larger bore size needles have been tested. Since the expanded cumulus containing the oocyte can be 1.0 - 1.5 mm in diameter or larger, narrow needles could potentially distort or tear off fragments of cumulus, fracture the zona pellucida or fragment the oocyte. However, large bore size needles (2.2 mm internal diameter) are not as efficient as medium sized (1.4 mm internal diameter) needles with regard to oocyte recovery rates (Renou et al., 1981). Medium size needles increase the velocity of fluid flow and reduce fluid dead space and turbulence inside the needle, thereby improving oocyte recovery rates. Furthermore, teflon lining reduces surface friction and eliminates connectors in which the cumulus could get stuck or traumatized. For these reasons, we prefer the device described above and have experienced little evident trauma to the cumulus and oocyte with its use.

The ovum trap consists of a polystyrene plastic tissue culture tube (Falcon, Oxnard, CA, Catalog Number 3033) which measures 16 X 125 mm, has a capacity of 15 ml, and a screw cap. The silicone stopper (Size 0) fits snugly into the culture tube to prevent any suction vacuum leaks.

The tubing leading away from the tissue culture tube is designed for thumb controlled suctioning. The silicone stopper is traversed by an 18 gauge, 3 1/2 inch long spinal needle (Becton Dickinson Co., Rutherford, NJ). The spinal needle is connected by plastic extension tubing (Pharmaseal Extension Tube, Toa Alta, PR, Model K50L, 33 inches long, capacity 3.3 ml) to a thumb controlled, Regu Vac Suction catheter with regulator (Bard Parker). This is in turn connected by regular suction tubing to wall suction (Figure 2).

A pressure regulator is used to adjust the vacuum pressure to 100-120 mm Hg. Vacuum pressures in this range have been suitable for follicular aspiration. Higher vacuum pressures (>200 mm Hg) are undesirable since they may traumatize the oocyte, cause early collapse of the follicular wall and impair its aspiration, and/or lead to follicular bleeding and excessive granulosa cell removal.

FOLLICULAR ASPIRATION TECHNIQUE

When adequate follicular development has been achieved, the pre-ovulatory dose of human chorionic gonadotropin (hCG) is administered and the laparoscopy is scheduled 36 hours later. For convenience, laparoscopies are scheduled for 9:00 AM, 10:00 AM or 11:00 AM; therefore, hCG is administered at 9:00 PM, 10:00 PM or 11:00 PM respectively 36 hours earlier. Laparoscopies are performed in a designated operating room in close proximity to the in vitro fertilization laboratory.

The patient is placed on the operating table in the supine position after the bladder is emptied. General endotracheal anesthesia is administered and the patient prepped and draped in routine fashion. The pneumoperitoneum is established by placing the Verres needle transumbilically into the peritoneal cavity. The method preferred by the author (Special gratitude is expressed to Drs. Celso-Ramon Garcia, and Luigi Mastroianni, Jr. who taught me this technique) consists of everting the umbilicus with an Allis clamp and holding the intraumbilical skin with towel clips, one on each side. A small stab incision is made through the umbilical scar. A Verres needle is attached to the gas tubing and the insufflating pressure is checked with the needle valve in the open and closed position. The needle valve is then opened and the needle is inserted vertically through the abdominal wall layers (held by towel clips) while insufflating. Normally, the insufflating pressure reading increases as gas outflow is obstructed by the abdominal wall tissues. As soon as the needle enters the peritoneal cavity, the insufflating pressure drops to the level previously seen when the needle valve was open and there was no resistance. This indicates to the surgeon that the needle is in the peritoneal cavity and that further advancement of the needle is not necessary, minimizing trauma to abdominal organs. The transumbilical route is the shortest distance between the skin and the peritoneum. In addition, at the umbilicus, the peritoneum is usually firmly adherent to the abdominal wall, decreasing the chances of preperitoneal insufflation.

Another technique frequently used involves insertion of the Verres needle through a vertical incision in the lower edge of the umbilicus or through a semicircular, transverse infraumbilical incision. Once the needle is inserted into the peritoneal cavity, a drop of sterile saline is placed in the hub of the needle. The abdominal wall is grasped and elevated. If the needle has been correctly placed in the peritoneal cavity, the negative intraperitoneal pressure will suction the drop of saline inwards. The gas tubing is then connected and insufflating pressure is checked.

The abdomen is insufflated with sufficient carbon dioxide to adequately distend the abdomen (generally 2-3 liters). Early investigators used the same gas mixture employed in the incubator (5% CO_2, 5% O_2, 90% N_2) for establishment of the pneumoperitoneum, but lack of evidence for improved fertilization or cleavage rates, and the risk of potentially fatal gas embolism with this mixture (Johnston, 1982) have led most groups to utilize pure CO_2.

The effect of pure CO_2 on follicular fluid pH has been a matter of debate. The pH of follicular fluid measured within one minute of collection is 7.4 (Trounson, 1982). When follicular fluid is exposed to ambient air, its pH begins to rise to a level of 7.8 or more. It appears that a 5% CO_2 environment results in optimal buffering capacity; mixing follicular fluid and 100% CO_2 results in a major drop in pH. However, no significant difference in fertilization and cleavage rates have been observed with pure CO_2 pneumoperitoneum when compared to the three-gas mixture. Nonetheless, in the technique of follicular aspiration (described below), it is important to prevent bubbling of follicular fluid with CO_2. We have established pregnancies in patients whose intact follicles were aspirated after 45 minutes of 100% CO_2 pneumoperitoneum. Follicular fluid pH does not change when intact follicles are exposed to 100% CO_2 peritoneum for up to one hour (Trounson, 1982). Thus, it appears that intact follicles can buffer any CO_2 that could have diffused through the follicle wall.

While the abdomen is insufflating, the aspirating device is assembled, tested, and the pressure is adjusted to 100-120mm Hg if necessary. Following insufflation, the laparoscope's trocar and sleeve are introduced bluntly through the transumbilical incision. The laparoscope is inserted, light source and gas tubing are attached and the patient is placed in Trendelenburg position. In the midline suprapubic area (1-2 fingerbreadths above the pubic symphisis) a small (5 mm) incision is made, and the second puncture trocar and sleeve is inserted under direct visualization (to avoid trauma to bladder, bowel or blood vessels). The grasping forcep is introduced through the second puncture sleeve and the pelvic organs are manipulated gently in order to expose the ovaries.

Depending on the position and accessibility of the ovaries, the site for the third puncture is determined by estimating the best line of approach. Most commonly, an area in the right or left quadrant is used although a midline infra-umbilical area a few centimeters above the second puncture site may occasionally be preferred. A small (3 mm) incision is made after transillumination of the abdominal wall with the laparoscope's light to avoid puncturing a large vessel. The third puncture trocar and needle sleeve is introduced under direct visualization.

In cases where the ovaries are 100% accessible and no pelvic adhesions are present, the ovaries are brought into view by grasping the utero-ovarian ligament. Both ovaries are quickly inspected and the larger ($\geq$15mm) follicles are identified. The most accessible ovary containing the largest follicles (as determined by visual inspection and/or prior ultrasound) is aspirated first. Manipulation of the ovaries should be minimized prior to aspiration to prevent follicular rupture. The aspirating needle should be inserted immediately after the grasping forceps so that everything is ready to aspirate in case a follicle ruptures during ovarian manipulation.

If any follicles have ovulated, the cul de sac and any peri-ovarian fluid is promptly aspirated, labeled and sent to the laboratory for microscopic examination. The needle is then introduced into the ovulated follicle and suction is applied in an effort to recover an oocyte-containing cumulus that may have been trapped and was not extruded. If no oocyte is obtained, the follicle is then flushed (see below). We, as well as others, have successfully recovered oocytes which have fertilized and cleaved from peritoneal fluid and ovulated follicles.

If all follicles are intact, the ovary is stabilized against the pelvic side wall by grasping the utero-ovarian ligament with the grasping forceps (See Figure 3). The assistant is asked to hold the grasping forceps with one hand. The surgeon advances the aspirating needle to the surface of the follicle and estimates its size. After the needle tip is in contact with the follicular wall, and immediately prior to puncture of the follicle, the assistant is asked to occlude the thumb control to create the negative pressure necessary for aspiration. This will minimize the introduction of CO_2 into the follicular aspirate. The follicle is promptly punctured under visualization in an avascular area. If possible, the needle is introduced at the most superior surface of the follicle to minimize fluid leakage around the needle. We prefer to puncture the follicle through the stigma since the increased pressure needed to puncture the thicker part of the follicular wall may cause spontaneous rupture through the weaker stigma. Others prefer to puncture the follicle away from

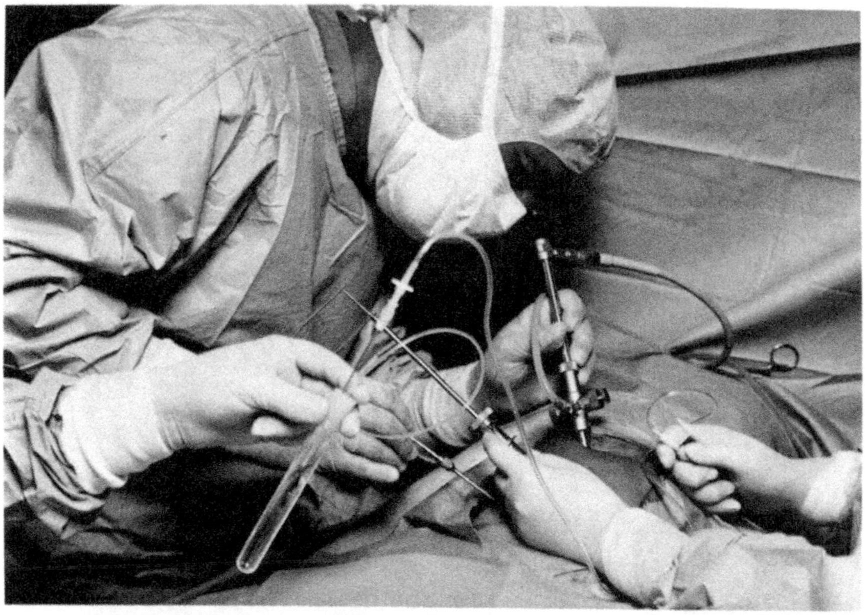

Figure 3

Laparoscopic follicular aspiration. The assistant holds the second puncture sleeve and grasping forceps with the left hand, and thumb controlled suction regulator with the right hand. The surgeon is advancing the aspirating needle to the surface of the follicle under direct visualization. The scrub nurse holds the collection device and reports on the aspirated follicular contents.

the very thin stigma because the hole in the follicular wall frequently extends and leakage of follicular fluid may occur. Once most of the follicular fluid is aspirated, the needle is moved in a circular fashion inside the follicle to assist in the dislodgement of the cumulus and to allow all parts of the follicle to be aspirated (See Figure 4). After aspiration is complete, suction is discontinued (by releasing the thumb control) to prevent aspiration of CO_2, and the needle is removed from the abdomen. Once the needle is outside the peritoneal cavity, suction is reapplied to empty the fluid contained within the teflon tubing into the ovum trap. The ovum trap is then changed and heparinized culture medium (See Chapter 13) is aspirated into a second tube to rinse the needle and to insure that the oocyte is

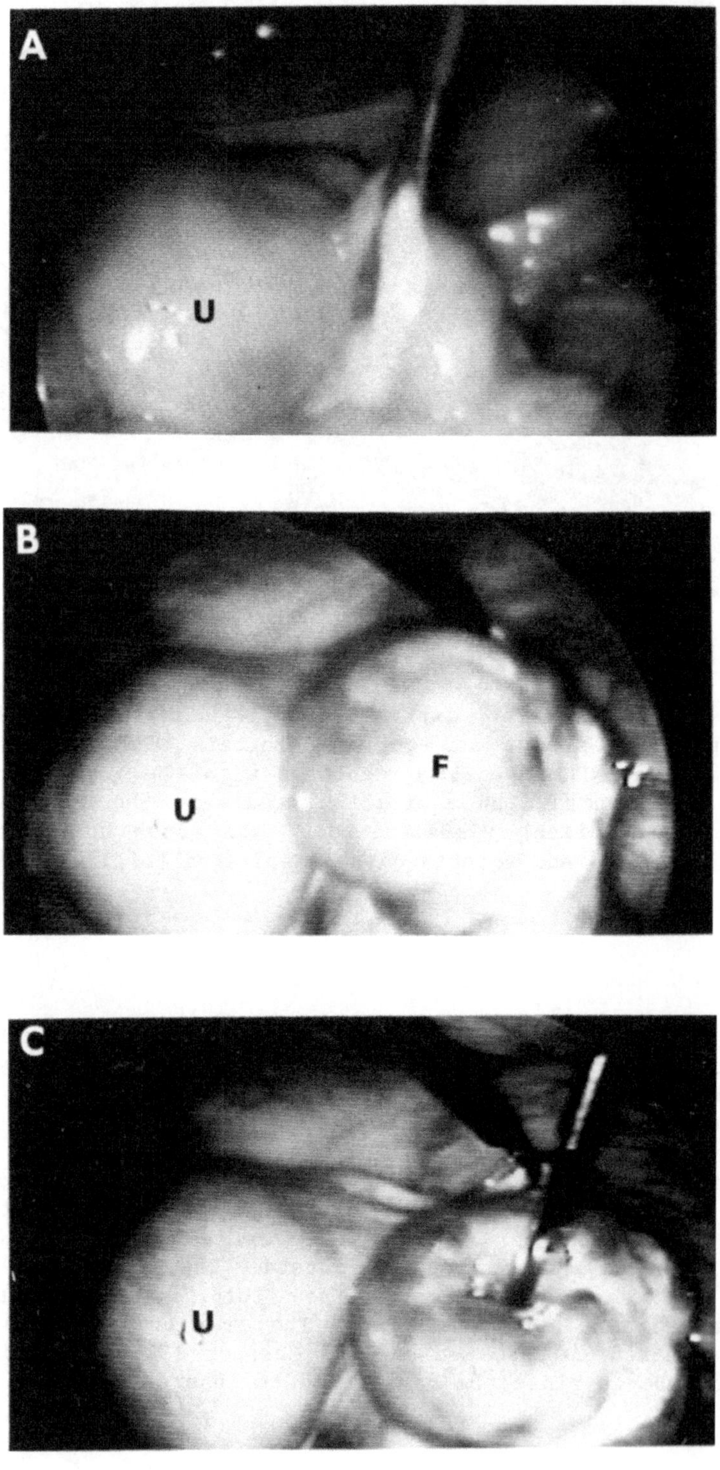
A
U
B
U
F
C
U

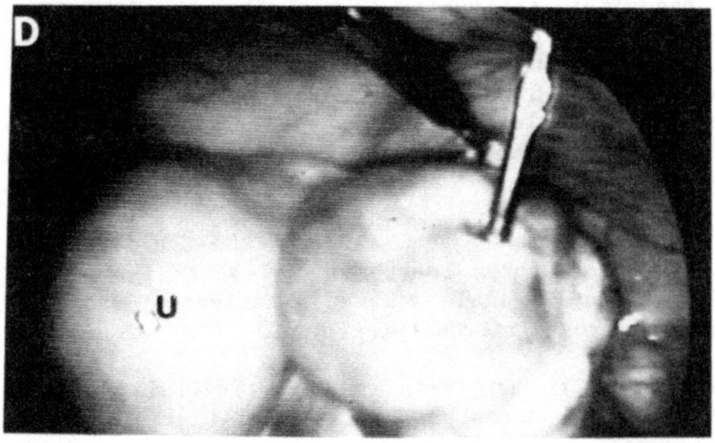

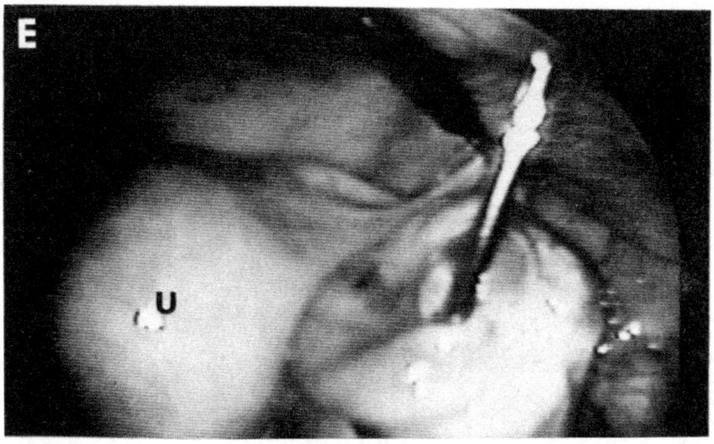

Figure 4

Technique of follicular aspiration

A) Grasping the right utero ovarian ligament (U=uterus)
B) Exposing and stabilizing the follicle (F) which measured 25mm on the right ovary
C) Puncturing the follicle at the most superior surface (suction is applied prior to follicular puncture)
D) Entry of the aspiration needle into the follicle
E) Collapse of the follicular wall after aspirating its contents.

not retained within the tubing (Figure 5). The flushing medium is kept at 37°C in a portable incubator (Lab Line Instrument Inc., Melrose Park, IL, Catalogue Number 150). The follicular aspirate is identified as L1 or R1, representing the first follicle aspirated from the left or right ovary respectively. Numbering sequence is done on the basis of order of aspiration and not on follicle size.

The circulating nurse hand carriers the fluid to the in vitro fertilization laboratory, located a few steps from the operating room. The follicular fluid volume is estimated, and the fluid is inspected grossly and microscopically.

If an oocyte is obtained, the next follicle is aspirated in the same fashion. Occasionally, the follicular fluid or needle rinse may contain only granulosa cells or a piece of cumulus but no oocyte. The follicle is then irrigated in the following fashion: flushing medium is introduced in a retrograde manner into the teflon tubing at the silicone stopper end using a 6 cc syringe with a 18 gauge blunt needle (Becton-Dickinson #8208) and

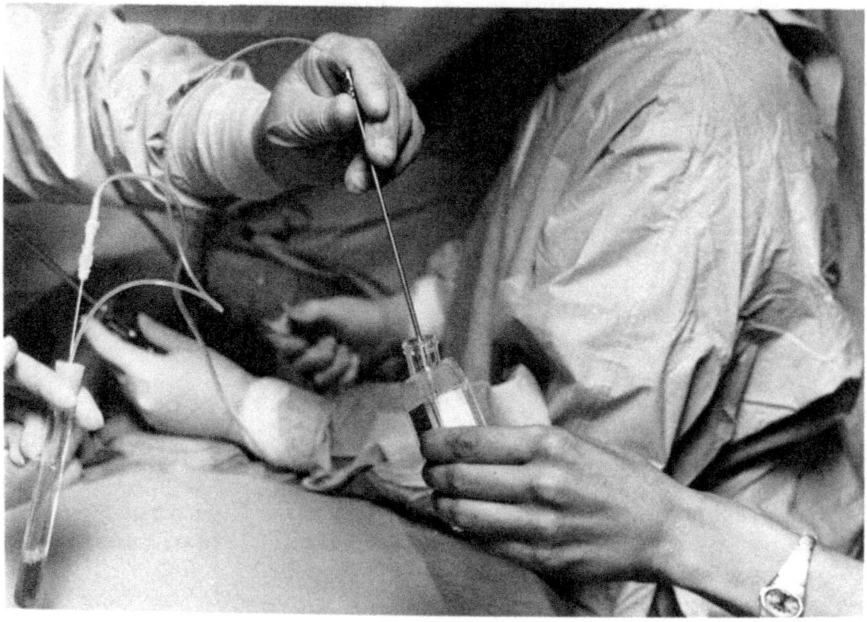

Figure 5

Rinsing the needle. The needle and tubing are rinsed by aspirating heparinized culture medium after attaching a second culture tube.

the tubing is purged to expel the air. The aspirating needle is then re-introduced into the follicle through the previously made puncture hole. A volume of flushing media calculated to be 0.5 to 1.0 cc less than the volume of the aspirated follicular fluid is instilled, redistending the follicle (Figure 6). A new ovum trap is attached, suction is reapplied and the follicle is reaspirated as the needle is manipulated inside the follicle in an effort to dislodge any adherent cumulus. When all the fluid is recovered, suction is discontinued, the needle removed and rinsed by aspirating flushing medium.

Follicles are aspirated one at a time and subsequent follicles are not aspirated until an oocyte is identified microscopically or the follicle is irrigated. This practice prevents follicular fluid from "backing up" in the laboratory before the personnel have a chance to examine it.

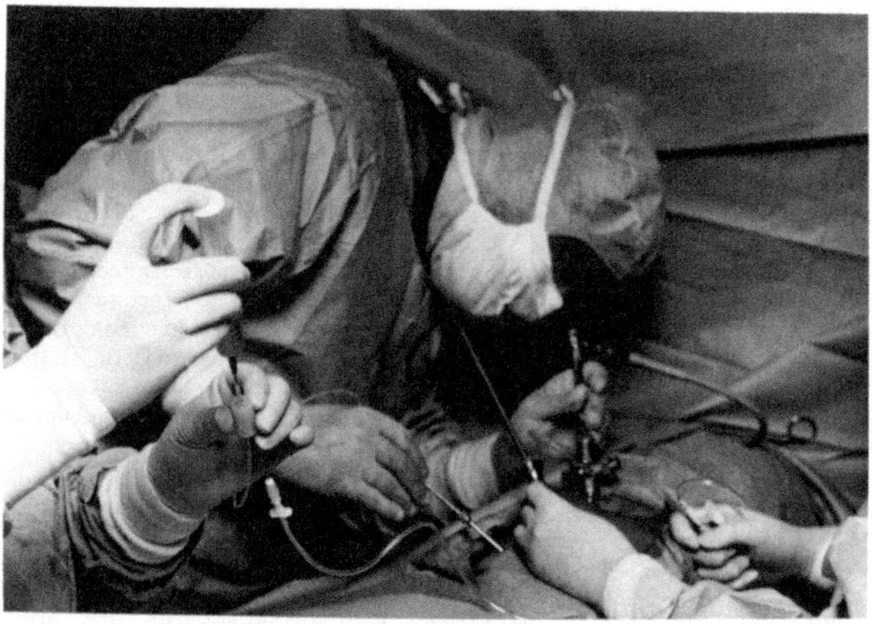

Figure 6

Irrigating the follicle. The scrub nurse injects heparinized culture medium into the teflon tubing at the silicone stopper end until the tubing is purged of air. The aspirating needle is then reintroduced into the follicle, medium is injected and the follicle is redistended. The culture tube is attached and suction applied until the follicle collapses. The needle is then rinsed as above.

In many patients, accessibility to one or both ovaries is compromised by pelvic adhesions. In these cases, follicles are aspirated in the most accessible ovary first since it requires less ovarian manipulation and lesser chance of iatrogenically rupturing a follicle. If an ovary is partly accessible but one follicle (not necessarily the dominant one) can be identified without manipulation, it is aspirated prior to ovarian manipulation. Once all visible follicles are aspirated, an attempt is made to lyse adhesions (bluntly or with electrocautery) to visualize additional ovarian surface. Often, the introduction of additional operating instruments through a fourth puncture may be useful.

Frequently, in cases of partly accessible ovaries, ultrasound may have shown one or more pre-ovulatory follicles that cannot be seen at the time of laparoscopy. In those cases, the aspirating needle is inserted into the ovary and different areas are probed while aspirating. In this way, we have reached follicles developing deep in the ovary and those developing, for example, near the ovarian surface attached to the pelvic sidewall by adhesions.

Ovaries that have been stimulated by clomiphene citrate usually contain a limited number of distinct, large follicles, whose domes protrude from the ovarian surface. Human menopausal gonadotropin (hMG) stimulated ovaries differ in that they usually contain several medium sized follicles next to each other with less distinct domes. On occasion, in the hMG stimulated patient, more then one egg is obtained from aspiration of presumably one follicle. Even though polyovular follicles are present in most ovaries (Gougeon, 1981), the most likely explanation is that the contents of more than one follicle have been aspirated. The presence of more than one oocyte within the same cumulus mass suggests that a true polyovular follicle has been aspirated.

On two occasions (both following clomiphene citrate stimulation) we have found large (4-5 cm) follicles containing abnormal granulosa cells, a large volume of thick follicular fluid (15-25 ml) and no oocyte. These were probably large atretic, degenerated follicles. Sometimes, cystic structures are present on the ovarian surface (such as inclusion cysts or adherent hydatids of Morgagni) and should be distinguished from follicles. They may be aspirated to improve access to or visualization of the ovarian surface.

The laparoscopic procedure is terminated once all available follicles are aspirated (irrigated if necessary) or the maximum number of oocytes (five) is obtained. The carbon dioxide is vented and the instruments are removed. The umbilicus is sutured with 3-0 absorbable suture in a subcuticular, purse-string manner.

The second puncture site is sutured with a horizontal mattress subcuticular stitch. Adhesive strips are applied to the third puncture site. The patient is awakened and taken to the recovery room, where routine post operative care is instituted. The patient is discharged from the day surgery unit when fully awake and stable.

CLEANING AND STERILIZING THE EQUIPMENT

Most of the laparoscopic equipment is cleaned with tap water and autoclaved unless it contains plastic or rubber. The laparoscope, trocars, sleeves and grasping forceps are sterilized in Cidex (Surgikos, Arlington, TX, Catalogue Number 2250) immediately prior to use, and well rinsed with sterile saline solution. The aspirating needle and tubing are gas sterilized with ethylene oxide after special processing (See Appendix A).

POTENTIAL COMPLICATIONS

Laparoscopy carries a small risk of bleeding, intraperitoneal or abdominal wall infection, trauma to abdominal viscera, or anesthesia complications. Bleeding as a result of follicular aspiration is minimal. A few minutes after follicular aspiration, the empty, collapsed follicle distends with blood, forming a corpus hemorrhagicum. Depending on the size of the puncture hole and the extent of follicular trauma, a few drops to several milliliters of blood will accumulate in the pouch of Douglas. In no case has a laparotomy been needed as a result of continued or perfuse ovarian bleeding.

Oophoritis is a potential complication even though no cases have been reported or have occurred in our experience. Superficial wound infection or drainage have occurred infrequently and have promptly responded to oral antibiotics and/or local care.

The effect of follicular aspiration and removal of granulosa cells on corpus luteum function has been a matter of concern (Garcia et al., 1981; Kreitmann et al., 1981; Feichtinger et al., 1982; Frydman et al., 1982). Pre-ovulatory follicles contain an average of 50-60 million granulosa cells (McNatty et al., 1979; Gougeon, 1982). An average of 3 million granulosa cells are removed by follicular aspiration (range: 6,000 to 12 million; Garcia et al., 1981). It is reasonable to assume that the larger the numbers of granulosa cells removed, the greater are the chances of subnormal progesterone production and luteal phase disruption.

In monkeys, removal of increasing numbers of granulosa cells by midcycle follicular aspiration during a spontaneous cycle is highly correlated with decreasing progesterone production by the corpus luteum (Kreitmann et al., 1981). These observations were confirmed in humans undergoing follicular aspiration during a natural cycle (Garcia et al., 1981). Luteal progesterone levels were lowest in patients requiring vigorous aspiration and repeated follicular irrigations. In spite of progesterone deficiency, the duration of the luteal phase was not significantly different between aspirated natural and stimulated cycles (Garcia et al., 1981; Frydman et al., 1982).

Luteal phases following aspirations during clomiphene citrate stimulated cycles appear to be different. Progesterone levels in clomiphene citrate stimulated cycles were significantly higher than in natural cycles 3 days after aspiration and were similar to or higher than levels seen in natural, non-aspirated, control cycles. It appears that the multiple follicles developing in response to clomiphene form multiple corpora lutea which prevent subnormal progesterone production.

RESULTS

The oocyte recovery rate will depend on the following variables: the instruments and aspirating device used, experience of the surgeon, number and size of the follicles present, ovarian accessibility, quality of the fluid sent to the laboratory and experience of the laboratory personnel. For these reasons, oocyte recovery rates have ranged from 20% in the earlier reports to 90% in recent series.

Results can be reported as recovery rates per aspirated follicle or per patients undergoing laparoscopy. Experience from our institution (Quigley et al., 1982) show that, from July 1981 to September 1982, during ultrasound monitored cycles, in patients receiving either 50 or 150 mg clomiphene daily for 5 days, at least one oocyte was obtained in 49 of 56 patients (88%). In seven patients, no oocytes were recovered due to: inaccessible ovaries (one), ovulation prior to laparoscopy (two), no oocyte identified in aspirated fluid (four). The overall recovery rate per follicle aspirated was 89/142 or 63%, with a significantly higher rate associated with follicles $\geq$ 20mm diameter (67%) compared to smaller follicles (33%).

During a 12 month period between May 1982 and April 1983, at least one oocyte was recovered in 84 of 95 patients undergoing laparoscopy (88%). Reasons for failed oocyte retrieval were: Follicle aspirated but no oocyte recovered (eight patients), all follicles ovulated prior to laparoscopy (two) and no follicles identified at laparoscopy (one patient) (Quigley and Wolf, 1984).

SUMMARY AND CONCLUSIONS

Collection of mature, fertilizable oocytes is crucial for successful IVF-ET. In this chapter, laparoscopy in general has been reviewed, with special emphasis on follicular aspiration. Pure carbon dioxide is used to establish the pneumoperitoneum. Follicular aspiration is accomplished by means of a three puncture technique that has been described in detail. The aspirating needle used for follicular aspiration is hand made, 12 gauge, lined by an unbroken piece of teflon tubing, with an internal diameter of 1.3 mm. Wall suction, adjusted to 100-120mm Hg and regulated by a thumb-controlled device, is used for aspiration.

Midcycle general anesthesia does not seem to affect the ensuing luteal phase. Follicular aspiration during natural, unstimulated cycles has been associated with lowered progesterone production during the luteal phase, probably correlated with the amount of granulosa cells removed. However, in clomiphene citrate stimulated cycles, normal or supra-normal progesterone levels are seen.

Using our technique at least one oocyte has been recovered from 88% of patients undergoing laparoscopic follicular aspiration during clomiphene citrate stimulated cycles, with 63% of aspirated follicles yielding an oocyte.

REFERENCES

Cohen, M.R., 1983, Gynecologic Laparoscopy, in: "Gynecology and Obstetrics", J.J. Sciarra, ed., Harper and Row, Philadelphia.

Decker, A., and Cherry, T., 1944, Culdoscopy, a new method in the diagnosis of pelvic disease, Am. J. Surg., 64:40.

Feichtinger, W., Szalay, S., Beck, A., Kemeter, P., and Janisch, H., 1981, Die gewinnung reifer menschlicher Eizellen mittels laparoskopie zum Zwecke der In Vitro Fertilisierung, Geburtsh Frauenheilk, 41:400.

Feichtinger, W., Kemeter, P., Szalay, S., Beck, A., and Janisch, H., 1982, Could aspiration of the graafian follicle cause luteal phase deficiency? Fertil. Steril., 37:205.

Frydman, R., Feinstein, M.C., Testart, J., Thebault, A., Labbe, A., Grenier, J., Roger, M., and Scholler, R., 1981, Receuil d' ovocytes humains en phase preovulatoire. Interet du dosage radioimmunologuique rapide de la LH Plasmatique, J. Gynecol. Obstet. Biol. Reprod. (Paris), 10:127.

Frydman, R., Testart, J., Giacomini, P., Imbert, M.C., Martin, E., and Nahoul, K., 1982, Hormonal and histological study of the luteal phase in women following aspiration of the preovulatory follicle, Fertil. Steril., 38:312.

Garcia, J., Jones, G.S., Acosta, A.A., and Wright, G.L., 1981, Corpus luteum function after follicle aspiration for oocyte retrieval, Fertil. Steril., 36:565.

Gougeon, A., 1981, Frequent occurrence of multiovular follicles and multinuclear oocytes in the adult human ovary, Fertil. Steril., 35:417.

Gougeon, A., 1982, Rate of follicular growth in the human ovary, in: "Follicular Maturation and Ovulation", R. Rolland, E.V. Van Hall, S.G. Hillier, K.P. McNatty and J. Schoemaker, eds., Excerpta Medica, Amsterdam.

Jacobaeus, H.C., 1910, Uber die Moglichkeit die Zystoskope bei Untersuchungseroser Hohlung anzuwenden, Munch. Med. Wochenschr., 57:2090.

Johnston, I.W.H., 1982, Discussion on the laparoscopic recovery of oocytes, in: "Human Conception In Vitro". R.G. Edwards and J.M. Purdy, eds., Academic Press, New York.

Jones, H.W., Acosta, A.A., and Garcia, J., 1982, A technique for the aspiration of oocytes from human ovarian follicles, Fertil. Steril., 37:26.

Kelling, G., 1902, Uber Oesophagoskopie, gastroskopie und Colioskopie, Munch. Med. Wochenschr., 49:21.

Kreitmann, O., Nixon, W.E., and Hodgen, G.D., 1981, Induced corpus luteum dysfunction after aspiration of the preovulatory follicle in monkeys, Fertil. Steril., 35:671.

Lopata, A., Johnston, I.W.H., Leeton, J.F., Muchniki, D., Talbot, J.M., and Wood, C., 1974, Collection of human oocytes at laparoscopy and laparotomy, Fertil. Steril., 25:1030.

McNatty, K.P., Smith, D.M., Makris, A., Sathanond, R., and Ryan, K.J., 1979, The microenvironment of the human graafian follicle: Interrelationship among the steroid levels in antral fluid, the population of granulosa cells and the status of the oocyte in vivo and in vitro, J. Clin. Endocrinol. Metab., 49:851.

Mettler, L., Seki, M., Baukloh, V., and Semm, K., 1982, Human ovum recovery via operative laparoscopy and in vitro fertilization, Fertil. Steril., 38:30.

Morgenstern, L.L., and Soupart, P., 1972, Oocyte recovery from the human ovary, Fertil. Steril., 23:751.

Ott, D.O., 1901, Ventroscopic illumination of the abdominal cavity in pregnancy, Zakus i Zhensk, 15:7.

Quigley, M.M., Wolf, D.P., Maklad, N., Dandekar, P., and Sokoloski, J., 1982, Follicular size and number in human in vitro fertilization, Fertil. Steril., 38:678.

Quigley, M.M., and Wolf, D.P., 1984, Human in vitro fertilization and embryo transfer at The University of Texas, Houston, J. In Vitro Fert., 1: (in press)

Renou, P., Trounson, A.O., Wood, C., and Leeton, J.F., 1981, The collection of human oocytes for in vitro fertilization. I. An instrument for maximizing oocyte recovery rate, Fertil. Steril., 35:409.

Soules, M.R., Sutton, G.P., Hammond, C.B., and Haney, A.F., 1980, Endocrine changes at operation under general anesthesia: reproductive hormone fluctuations in young women, Fertil. Steril., 33:364.

Steptoe, P.C., and Edwards, R.G., 1970, Laparoscopic recovery of preovulatory human oocytes after priming of ovaries with gonadotropins, Lancet, 1:683.

Steptoe, P.C., and Webster, J., 1981, Laparoscopy of the normal and disordered ovary, in: " Human Conception In Vitro". R.G. Edwards & J.M. Purdy, eds., Academic Press, New York.

Szalay, S., Feichtinger, W., Kemeter, P., Beck, A., Janisch, H., and Neumark, J., 1982, Changes in Hormonal parameters under different kinds of general anesthetics during laparoscopic oocyte recovery, in: "Human Conception In Vitro", R.G. Edwards and J.M. Purdy, eds., Academic Press, New York.

Trounson, A.O., 1982, Discussion on the laparoscopic recovery of oocytes, in: "Human Conception In Vitro", R.G. Edwards and J.M. Purdy, eds., Academic Press, New York.

Wood, C., Leeton, J., McTalbot, J., and Trounson, A.O., 1981, Technique for collecting mature human oocytes for in vitro fertilization, Br. J. Obstet. Gynecol., 88:756.

11

SPERM CAPACITATION

Jeffrey Boldt and Don P. Wolf

In 1951, C. R. Austin and M. C. Chang published what have become classic papers in the field of mammalian reproduction. In their studies, rabbits induced to ovulate at prescribed times were artificially inseminated via the fallopian tube at various time intervals before and after ovulation. After some 30-40 hours, the eggs were recovered and examined for evidence of fertilization. An interesting pattern emerged as only eggs recovered from animals inseminated several hours before ovulation were fertilized; those inseminated either just prior to or after ovulation yielded only a few fertilized ova. The conclusion reached by both investigators was that sperm must reside within the oviduct for some time prior to ovulation to acquire fertilizing ability. The acquisition of fertilizing ability, termed capacitation by Austin (1952), is now recognized as an essential feature of mammalian fertilization.

Since its discovery, capacitation has been the subject of intensive investigation, an endeavor facilitated greatly by the development of _in vitro_ fertilization techniques in a variety of animal models (see Rogers, 1978 for review). Despite the advances made in defining various biochemical and physiological changes attending this process, our knowledge concerning basic mechanisms remains limited. The study of human sperm capacitation specifically has been neglected for several reasons. The lack of suitable bioassays for human sperm function has been a major contributing factor; obviously major limitations are associated with the use of human eggs. Another consideration is that comparative information derived from capacitation studies in lower mammals has involved largely epididymal sperm, perhaps a poor paradigm for a cell exposed to seminal plasma. The recent development of bioassays for human sperm function, together with the advent of human IVF-ET programs, has focused increased attention on human sperm capacitation. In this chapter, we review current methods used to study human sperm capacitation in vitro, and discuss parameters that may impact upon this process. Where relevant and instructive, aspects of capacitation in other animal model systems are discussed.

"DEFINITION" OF CAPACITATION

Capacitation is a complex process involving an interplay of biochemical, metabolic, and physiological alterations (see review by Yanagimachi, 1981). Due to this complexity, it has been impossible to designate one factor as "the" critical event. Capacitation, therefore, is commonly "defined" in an operational sense, i.e., sperm that have penetrated an egg are considered capacitated. Conceptually, however, it is important to recognize that capacitation represents the initial steps in a continuum of events that culminate in the ability of the sperm to fuse with and penetrate the ovum. The consensus in the field is that capacitation is a necessary pre-requisite to the acrosome reaction which, in turn, is required for sperm-egg fusion and subsequent penetration (see discussions by Yanagimachi, 1981; Bedford, 1983). Based on these considerations capacitation can best be "defined" in a functional sense as a process that provides sperm with the ability to undergo appropriate modification (i.e., the acrosome reaction) such that sperm-egg fusion can occur. Using this definition, sperm are considered capacitated if they have undergone an acrosome reaction, penetrated eggs, or both. Since capacitation is defined in functional terms, it follows that dead or inactive sperm, regardless of the status of their acrosomes, cannot be considered capacitated.

An increase in flagellar activity known as hyperactivation is a characteristic feature of capacitation in several species (Yanagimachi, 1981). For example, mouse (Fraser, 1982), guinea pig (Yanagimachi and Usui, 1974), and hamster (Katz and Yanagimachi, 1980) sperm all display vigorous flagellar beat patterns when incubated under capacitating conditions. Functionally, hyperactivation is thought to facilitate penetration of the egg investments, i.e., cumulus oophorous and/or zona pellucida (Yanagimachi, 1981; Bedford, 1983). However, it is not yet established whether hyperactivation is a universal phenomenon in mammals (Yanagimachi, 1981) and, in fact, it has not been described in the human.

ASSAYS FOR HUMAN SPERM CAPACITATION *IN VITRO*

Many investigations in animal model systems rely on fertilization to assess whether or not sperm are capacitated, an approach that is impractical in the human. The establishment of human IVF-ET programs opens the possibility of the direct study of human sperm capacitation *in vitro*. However, the fact that only laboratories connected with IVF-ET programs could conduct such research, together with the small number of eggs available and the attendant ethical considerations, limits the usefulness of this approach. Thus, we are left with the need for a convenient model system that mimics the conditions of normal human fertilization.

Several bioassays for human sperm capacitation have been described. At present, the most widely used is the zona-free hamster egg test (see Chapter 14). Hanada and Chang (1972) and Yanagimachi (1972a) first established that the hamster egg, when stripped of its zona pellucida, was capable of incorporating heterologous sperm. In a landmark paper, Yanagimachi et al. (1976) extended these observations to human sperm. Since then, the test has been employed extensively for evaluation of male fertility potential and in studies of capacitation (Table 1; Chapter 14). The usefulness of the assay is dependant upon the fact that only acrosome-reacted sperm can bind to the egg, and that a true fusion of sperm and egg plasma membranes occurs during penetration, as opposed to a non-specific phagocytic-like incorporation (Yanagimachi et al., 1976; Koehler et al., 1982; Talbot and Chacon, 1982).

A second bioassay involves the use of non-living human oocytes collected from cadavers or from ovaries surgically removed for gynecological considerations (Overstreet and Hembree, 1976; Yanagimachi et al., 1979; Overstreet et al., 1980a; Gould et al., 1983). The eggs can be frozen (Overstreet et al., 1980a) or stored in hypertonic salt solution (Yanagimachi et al., 1979), allowing accumulation of suitable numbers for study. When placed in fresh culture medium and inseminated, sperm will readily bind to and penetrate the zona pellucida although binding to the vitellus proper does not occur. This assay purports to measure important features of human sperm fertilizing ability, the binding to and subsequent penetration of the zona pellucida, which require that sperm be capacitated and/or acrosome reacted (Bedford, 1983). An additional advantage is that interaction of sperm with its homologous egg is measured, an important point since sperm binding to the human zona pellucida is highly species specific (Bedford, 1977; Yanagimachi, 1977).

A combination bioassay utilizes both the non-living human oocyte and the zona-free hamster egg (Overstreet et al., 1980a;

Gould et al., 1983). In this case, the two egg types are combined and inseminated, the advantage being that two aspects of sperm fertilizing ability are tested simultaneously; zona penetration with the human oocyte and sperm-egg fusion with the hamster egg.

These bioassays may not adequately represent the physiologic events of fertilization. In the case of the non-living human oocyte, zona penetration may not be completely analagous to that occurring with a viable, mature oocyte. With the zona-free hamster egg bioassay, a heterologous egg is involved and then only after exposure to hydrolytic enzymes for cumulus and zona removal. Additionally, these bioassays are usually conducted at sperm concentrations 1 to 2 orders of magnitude higher than those used successfully in human IVF-ET. The most limiting feature of these bioassays is that they provide information about only a very small fraction of sperm in a given population, those which have penetrated the zona and/or ovum. While it is safe to conclude that penetrating sperm have undergone capacitation and the acrosome reaction, such techniques provide no direct information about the physiological state of the remainder of the population. This dilemma is by no means restricted to studies of human sperm but applies to capacitation in other model systems and, in fact, to any experimental system where the performance of a few is used to assess the status of an entire population.

As an alternative to the bioassays discussed above, quantitation of acrosome reactions can be used as a measure of capacitation. The acrosome is a membrane-limited secretory organelle located within the anterior portion of the sperm head (Figure 1). The acrosomal membrane can be subdivided into the outer membrane situated just beneath the plasma membrane, and the inner membrane closely apposed to the nucleus. Posterior to the acrosomal cap proper is the equatorial segment and the post-acrosomal region of the sperm head. Under appropriate physiological conditions, which can be mimicked chemically with the Ca^{2+} ionophore A23187, sperm undergo an acrosome reaction. The typical pattern for the mammalian sperm acrosome reaction has been described by a number of authors (Barros et al., 1967; Bedford and Cooper, 1978; Meizel, 1978; Yanagimachi, 1981) and is shown schematically in Figure 2A. The reaction is characterized by fusion between the outer acrosomal and plasma membranes, resulting in the formation of a vesiculated structure through which the acrosomal contents may pass. As the reaction progresses, the vesicles are lost and the sperm with its intact inner acrosomal membrane and equatorial segment remains. In the human, acrosome reactions induced during insemination of human oocytes (Soupart and Strong, 1974; McMaster et al., 1978), zona-free hamster ova (Yanagimachi et al., 1976), and upon ionophore treatment (Russell et al., 1979) show a membrane

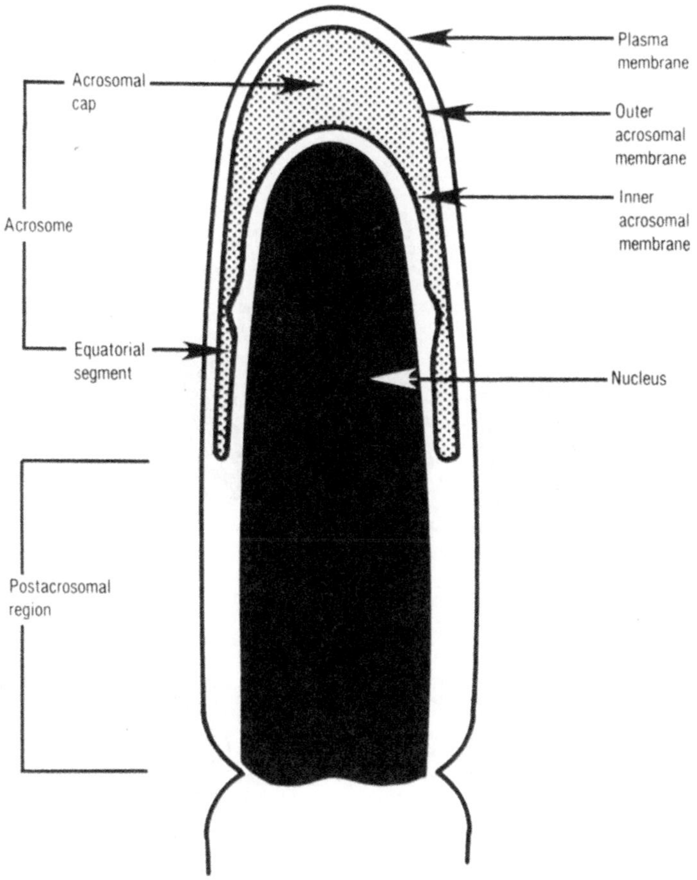

Figure 1

Schematic representation of the acrosomal region of the mammalian sperm. Redrawn from Yanagimachi (1981).

vesiculation pattern similar to other species, i.e., as seen in Figure 2A. However, based on recent observations by Jamil and White (1981) and ourselves, the chemically induced acrosome reaction may be different mechanistically. As shown in Figure 2B, the outer acrosomal membrane alone, at least in some cells, begins vesiculation independent of the plasma membrane. The intact plasma membrane is shed, followed by loss of the outer acrosomal membrane vesicles, leaving behind the intact inner acrosomal membrane and equatorial segment. It is unclear at this time why a different vesiculation pattern might exist; perhaps there is a

A

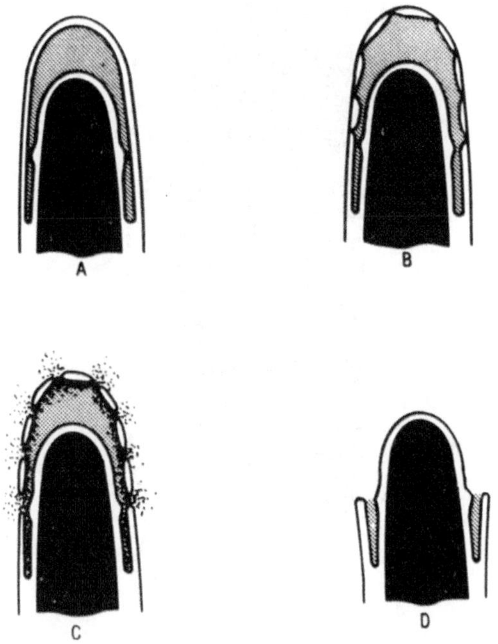

Figure 2A

Schematic representation of the mammalian acrosome reaction. Before initiation of the reaction the plasma and outer acrosomal membranes are intact (A). Initiation of reaction involves fusion of the plasma and outer acrosomal membranes (B) resulting in the formation of vesicles and release of the acrosomal contents (C). Completion of the reaction leaves the sperm with an intact inner acrosomal membrane (D).

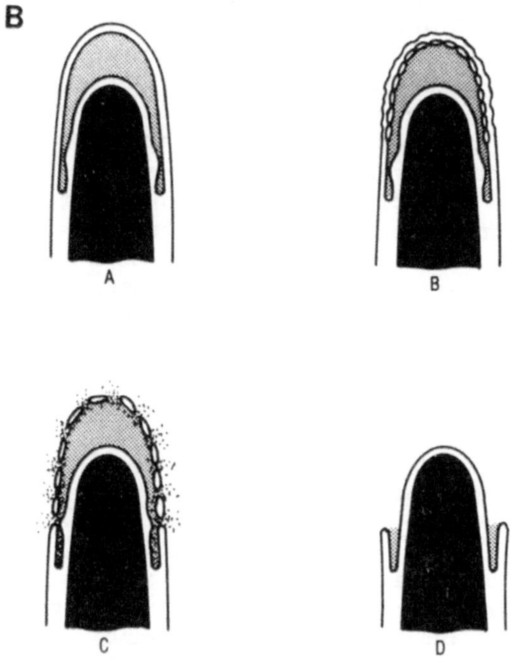

Figure 2B

Proposed model for the chemically induced acrosome reaction in human sperm. Before induction of the reaction both the plasma and outer acrosomal membranes are intact (A). Upon exposure to ionophore A23187 the outer acrosomal membrane alone vesiculates; the plasma membrane may deform somewhat but remains intact (B). As the reaction proceeds, the plasma membrane is lost (C). The outer acrosomal membrane components and acrosomal contents are finally dispersed, leaving the sperm with an intact inner acrosomal membrane (D).

unique mechanism for the human sperm acrosome reaction, although artifacts associated with fixation technique or ionophore treatment cannot be completely discounted.

Quantitation of acrosome reactions as a means to assay capacitation offers the obvious advantage that large numbers of sperm can be scored easily, as opposed to the few sperm scored in penetration assays. This is especially true in species such as the guinea pig and hamster, where the acrosome is large and can be readily observed with the light microscope (Yanagimachi, 1969; Yanagimachi and Usui, 1974; Lui and Meizel, 1977; Hyne and Garbers, 1981). In the human, where the acrosome is too small to be visualized directly, specific staining techniques are available. Talbot and Chacon (1980) used a fluorescent lectin probe and, more recently, a triple stain method (Talbot and Chacon, 1981) for the evaluation of normal acrosome reactions. The advantage of the triple stain technique is that it differentiates between physiological acrosome reactions and abnormal reactions associated with degenerating or dead sperm. The disadvantages of the technique, however, is that it requires the use of fixed cells, is somewhat time consuming, and is, at least in our hands, somewhat capricious.

Our laboratory is currently pursuing the use of monoclonal antibodies (MAb) as markers for human sperm capacitation and/or the acrosome reaction. In theory this approach can be applied directly to the living cell. MAb's have been generated in the mouse against ejaculated human sperm preparations in collaboration with Dr. Kathleen Bechtol at the Wistar Institute (Wolf et al., 1983). Hybridoma supernatants are screened by radioimmunoassay and indirect immunofluorescence, using immobilized intact sperm as the antigen source. One MAb, designated HS-21, is of particular interest since it binds exclusively to the acrosomal cap region (Figure 3). The intense, uniform staining pattern is observed in both fresh sperm and sperm incubated under capacitating conditions. Upon addition of ionophore A23187, a decrease (~30%) in the number of stained caps is observed. This approach is promising and at present we are defining conditions under which acrosome reactions can be induced in the entire sperm population, with the intent of correlating HS-21 staining patterns with transmission electron microscopic observations.

The MAb approach not only provides a method for detecting acrosome reactions, but also for quantitating specific sperm surface changes associated with capacitation _per se_. This requires the use of MAb's directed against surface antigens that are altered during capacitation, an accomplishment that has not yet been realized with human sperm. In the guinea pig, Myles and

Primakoff (1983) have used MAb's to detect an antigen localized on the surface of the posterior sperm tail that migrates to the anterior tail during capacitation. The challenge ahead lies in developing MAb's that recognize antigens localized to the sperm head that are altered during capacitation, since this is where events of capacitation preliminary to the acrosome reaction take place.

METHODOLOGY FOR HUMAN SPERM CAPACITATION IN VITRO

In the following sections culture conditions are described that support human sperm capacitation and IVF.

Culture Media and Media Supplements

Culture Media. Several types of culture media have been utilized for human sperm capacitation *in vitro* (Table 1). These can, for convenience, be grouped into two categories: simple and complex. Simple media, such as BWW and Tyrode's, are in general bicarbonate-buffered balanced salt solutions with ionic compositions similar to human serum (Bavister, 1981a). Complex media include Ham's F-10 and Menezo's B-2, which are supplemented with various vitamins, amino acids, and monosaccharides. For comparative purposes, the chemical composition of several simple and complex media are listed in Table 1 of Chapter 13.

Media Supplements: a) Protein sources. The use of protein sources, specifically serum albumin, to support capacitation and IVF stems from findings in several mammalian systems (see Rogers, 1978 for review). A number of years ago, Yanagimachi (1969, 1970) described a heat stable, non-dialyzable fraction from blood serum or follicular fluid that could induce capacitation of hamster spermatozoa, and he showed that some albumin preparations could effectively replace this fraction. Subsequently, albumin was identified as the active non-dialyzable fraction of follicular fluid by Lui et al. (1977). In more recent experiments, albumin in the culture media used for *in vitro* fertilization was replaced with a synthetic polymer, polyvinyl alcohol (PVA); hamster sperm motility was normal but PVA did not support the occurrence of acrosome reactions or fertilization (Bavister, 1981b). In the mouse, fertilization rates *in vitro* are greatly reduced in the absence of albumin (Miyamoto and Chang, 1973a; Hoppe and Whitten, 1974; Quinn et al., 1982) and in the rat, Davis (1976) implicated serum albumin for *in vitro* fertilization since other exogenous proteins (ovalbumin, globulins) were ineffective. In contrast to the above species, capacitation in the guinea pig apparently does not depend absolutely upon the presence of serum albumin, since acrosome reactions can be induced in minimal culture medium devoid

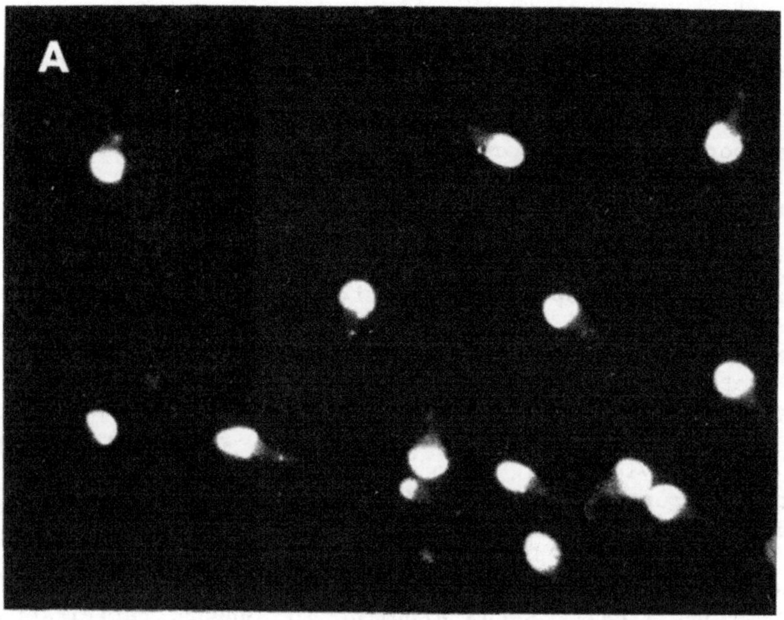

Figure 3A

Epifluorescence image of human sperm labelled with monoclonal antibody HS-21. Fresh ejaculates were washed 3x with PBS, fixed briefly (15 min.) with 1% paraformaldehyde, washed 2x with 0.2M glycine, and air-dried onto glass slides. Indirect immunofluorescence was performed using affinity-purified HS-21 as first antibody, followed by affinity-purified FITC-goat anti-mouse IgG (Kirkegaard and Perry; Gaithersburg, MD). Excess antibody was removed by washing with 0.01% NP-40, 0.1% β-mercaptoethanol, 1% albumin in PBS. Slides were mounted with n-propyl gallate in glycerol and examined under oil at 500x. Note the intense, uniform staining of the acrosomal cap region.

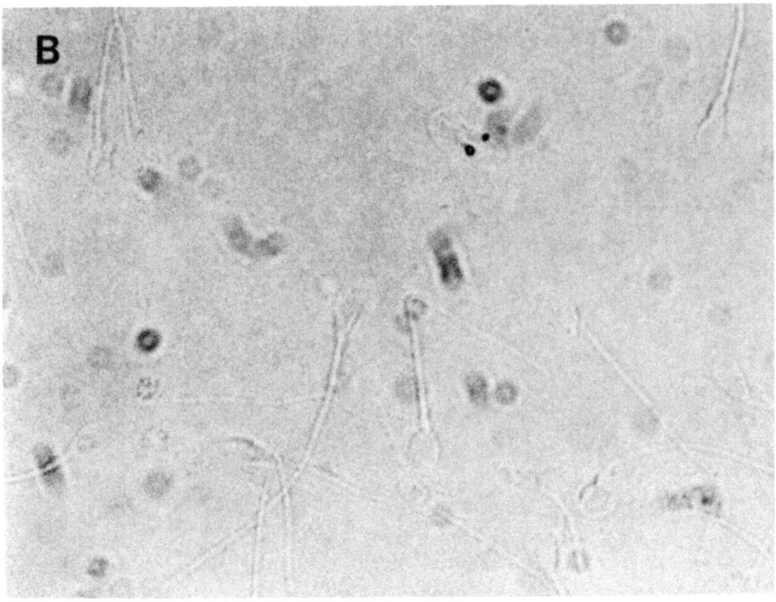

Figure 3B

Corresponding bright field image (see facing page).

of any macromolecular substances (Yanagimachi, 1972b; Barros et al., 1973).

The precise mechanism by which serum albumin influences capacitation and/or IVF is not clearly understood. Albumin is notorious for its ability to bind or chelate ions, fatty acids, or other physiologically active substances. Several suggestions have been offered concerning specific effects of albumin. One possibility is that albumin directly induces alterations in lipid constituents of the sperm plasma membrane. Albumin pre-saturated with cholesterol does not support capacitation of rat or mouse sperm (Davis, 1976; Go and Wolf, 1983) and sperm from these species pre-incubated in albumin-containing media display decreased cholesterol: phospholipid ratios (Davis et al., 1980; Go and Wolf, 1983). In the hamster, fatty acid-free BSA is more effective at stimulating acrosome reactions than BSA of high fatty acid content (Lui and Meizel, 1977). Quinn et al. (1982) have

Table 1. Culture conditions for human sperm capacitation and fertilization *in vitro*

Author	Test System	Culture Media	Protein Source	Energy Sources	Osmolarity (mOsm)	pH	Gas Phase
Yanagimachi et al., (1976)	ZFHE[1]	BWW[2]	0.3% HSA[1]	G,P,L[1]	-	7.5–7.6[3] 8.1–8.3[4]	5%CO_2 in air; air only
Rogers et al., (1979b & 1983)	ZFHE	BWW	0.3% HSA	G,P,L	-	7.5	Air
Overstreet et al., (1980a)	ZFHE and non-living human oocyte	BWW	3.5% HSA	G,P,L	-	-	Air
Binor et al., (1980)	ZFHE	BWW	0.3% HSA	G,P,L	-	7.5	5%CO_2 in air
Dor et al., (1981)	ZFHE	BWW	1.8% HSA	G,P,L	-	-	5%CO_2 in air
Bronson et al., (1981)	ZFHE	BWW w/7mM Caffeine	3.0% HSA	G,P,L	-	-	5%CO_2 in air
Tyler et al., (1981)	ZFHE	BWW w/ Hepes[1]	0.3% HSA	G,P,L	-	7.2[3]–8.2[4]	5%CO_2 in air; air only
Karp et al., (1981)	ZFHE	BWW w/ Hepes	0.4% HSA	G,P,L	-	7.4	1%CO_2 in air
Wolf and Sokoloski (1982)	ZFHE	BWW	0.3–3.5% HSA	G,P,L	-	7.4–7.6	5%CO_2 in air

Hall (1981)	ZFHE	Tyrode's	1.0% BSA[1]	G,P, L?[5]	290	7.5	5% CO_2 in air
Aitken et al., (1982a)	ZFHE	BWW w/Hepes	1.8% HSA	G,P,L	305	7.4–7.5	5% CO_2 in air
Perreault and Rogers (1982)	ZFHE	BWW	0.3% HSA	G,P,L	-	7.5	air
Berger et al., (1983)	ZFHE	Ham's F-10	0.5% HSA or 10% Serum	G,P,L	280	7.4	5% CO_2 in air
Soupart and Strong (1974)	Human Oocyte	Tyrode's ± Steroid Hormones	0.25% BSA	G,P	327	7.6	5% CO_2 in air
Overstreet and Hembree (1976)	Non-Living Human Oocyte	Tyrode's	0.25% BSA	G,P	-	-	5% CO_2 in air
McMaster et al., (1978)	Human Oocyte	BWW	15% Serum	G,P,L	-	-	5% CO_2 in air
Yanagimachi et al., (1979)	Non-Living Human Oocyte	BWW	0.3% HSA	G,P,L	308	7.4–7.5	5% CO_2 in air
Overstreet et al., (1980b)	Non-Living Human Oocyte	BWW	15% Serum	G,P,L	-	-	5% CO_2 in air
Lopata et al., (1978)	Human Oocyte	Medium S	0.5% HSA	G,P,L	285–295	7.45–7.55	5% CO_2 in air

(continued)

Table 1. (Continued)

Lopata et al., (1980)	Human IVF-ET	Ham's F-10	0.5% HSA	G,P,L	280	7.30–7.35	5%CO_2, 5%O_2, 90%N_2
Trounson et al., (1980)	Human IVF-ET	Hoppe-Pitts	0.3% BSA	G,P,L	-	-	5%CO_2, 5%O_2, 90%N_2
Trounson et al., (1982)	Human IVF-ET	Ham's F-10 Hoppe-Pitts	0.5% HSA	G,P,$\pm$L	280	7.4	5%CO_2, 5%O_2, 90% N_2
Edwards et al., (1981)	Human IVF-ET	Earle's, Tyrode's, Hanks	0.36% BSA w/5–7.5% Serum	G,P	280–285	7.2–7.3	5%CO_2, 5%O_2, 90%N_2
Purdy (1982)	Human IVF-ET	Earle's	8% Serum	G,P	282–286	7.3	5%CO_2, 5%O_2, 90%N_2
Plachot et al., (1982)	Human IVF-ET	Menezo's B_2	0.5% HSA	G,P,L	-	-	5%CO_2, 5%O_2, 90%N_2
Wortham et al., (1983a)	Human IVF-ET	Ham's F-10	0.5% BSA	G,P,L	285–295	7.4–7.45	5%CO_2 in air
Testart et al., (1982)	Human IVF-ET	Menezo's B_2	HSA, BSA	G,P,L	-	-	5%CO_2, 5%O_2, 90%N_2

Testart et al., (1983)	Human IVF-ET	Menezo's B_2	HSA, BSA (%-)	G,P,L	-	-	$5\%CO_2$, $5\%O_2$, $90\%N_2$
Wortham et al., (1983b)	Human IVF-ET	Ham's F-10	7.5% Fetal Cord Serum	G,P,L	280	7.4	$5\%CO_2$ in air
Feichtinger et al., (1983)	Human IVF-ET	Ham's F-10 Menezo's B_2	15% serum; 1% BSA	G,P,L	280	7.4	$5\%CO_2$ in air, $5\%CO_2$, $5\%O_2$, $90\%N_2$
University of Texas-Houston	Human IVF-ET	Ham's F-10	7.5% Serum	G,P,L	280	7.4-7.6	$5\%CO_2$, $5\%O_2$, $90\%N_2$

1. Abbreviations: ZFHE - zona free hamster egg test; BWW - Biggers, Whitten, Whittingham's media(Biggers et al., 1971); HSA, BSA - human serum albumin, bovine serum albumin; G,P,L - glucose, pyruvate, lactate; Hepes - N-2-Hydroxyethylpiperazine-N -2-ethanesulfonic acid.

2. The original formulation of BWW media includes 5.56 glucose, 21.58 mM sodium lactate, and 0.25mM sodium pyruvate at 308 mOsm.

3 pH when incubated under 5% CO_2 in air.

4. pH when incubated under air only

5. Tyrode's medium is generally based on the formulation of Bavister (1969), which includes glucose and pyruvate. It is not clear in most cases whether lactate is included.

suggested an alternative role for albumin in IVF. In their study, untreated BSA supported fertilization of both zona-intact and zona-free mouse ova. Trichloroacetic acid-precipitated BSA, which stimulates hamster sperm acrosome reactions in vitro (Lui et al., 1977), supported penetration of zona-free but not zona-intact eggs. Based on these observations, it was suggested that acrosomal enzymes necessary for zona penetration are regulated by BSA.

Serum albumin is used routinely for human sperm capacitation and IVF (Table 1). Albumin is added to the medium in several forms: either as crystalline protein, Cohn's Fraction V, or as heat inactivated preovulatory or fetal cord serum. The albumin requirement for human sperm capacitation has not been rigorously investigated. Gould et al. (1983) compared sperm pre-incubated in 3.5% HSA for 18-24 hours versus fresh, non-preincubated sperm. After a 4 hour insemination period, penetration of zona-free hamster ova was enhanced with the 18-24 hour sperm. In contrast, however, zona penetration of non-living human oocytes was not supported by this treatment, despite the fact that the percentage of acrosome reacted cells was increased. This effect was specific for HSA; BSA at equivalent concentrations did not influence zona penetration. The authors suggested that senescent changes, involving alterations of the acrosomal region and/or motility, occurred in the sperm during the prolonged exposure to the high HSA concentration, limiting their ability to penetrate the zona.

Some evidence suggests that there may not be an absolute albumin requirement for capacitation in the human. Perreault and Rogers (1982a) demonstrated that sperm from some donors effect penetration in the zona-free hamster egg test without preincubation, i.e., without prolonged pre-exposure to albumin. However, inseminations were conducted in albumin-containing media so capacitation most likely took place in this time period. Recent studies in our laboratory indicate that sperm pre-incubated in albumin-free media, then used for insemination of zona-free hamster eggs also in albumin-free media, still support penetration albeit at decreased levels compared to controls (Figure 4). In these experiments, the only source of albumin was that carried over with the zona-free eggs; egg processing was conducted in albumin containing media although eggs were rinsed in test media before insemination.

b) Energy Sources. The energy sources pyruvate, lactate, and glucose are usually present in culture media supporting mammalian sperm capacitation and IVF (Rogers, 1978). Requirements are species specific. In the mouse, in vitro fertilization occurs with glucose alone (Hoppe, 1976) and glucose is required for induction of the acrosome reaction in both mouse (Fraser and Quinn, 1981) and hamster (Dravland and Meizel, 1981) sperm. In contrast, the acrosome reaction in guinea pig sperm is retarded in the presence of glucose (Rogers and Yanagimachi, 1975; Rogers et al., 1979a). Despite the lack of an absolute dependence on pyruvate and lactate, these compounds are beneficial for capacitation in the mouse (Miyamoto and Chang, 1973a), rat (Toyoda and Chang, 1974), guinea pig (Rogers and Yanagimachi, 1975) and hamster (Bavister and Yanagimachi, 1977). In the human, energy sources are included routinely in capacitating media (Table 1) despite the lack of unequivocal evidence that they are required. Purdy (1982) has reported successful fertilization _in vitro_ using media containing low pyruvate and no lactate. Human sperm capacitation, as measured by the zona-free hamster egg test, is stimulated by glucose more so than fructose or pyruvate and

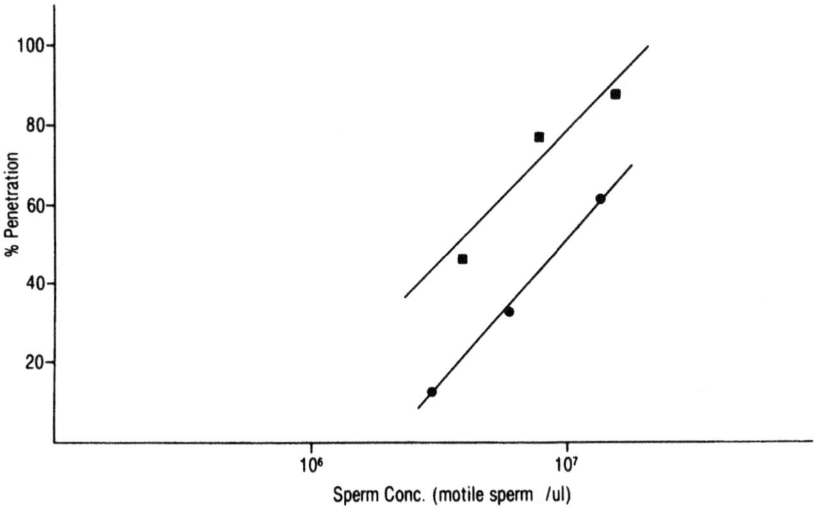

Figure 4

Albumin and human sperm capacitation _in vitro_. Ejaculates were washed 3x with BWW containing either _0.3%_ (-■-) or zero (-●-) HSA, then preincubated for 3 hours in BWW with 3.5% (-■-) or zero (-●-) HSA. Zona-free hamster eggs were inseminated at the indicated concentrations, and scored for penetration after 3 hours. Inseminations were in the same media used for pre-incubation.

lactate alone (Perreault and Rogers, 1981) and the stimulatory effect of glucose is concentration dependent over a 0.1-1% range (Munemasa et al., 1983).

Other Media Conditions: a) Osmolarity. Osmotic pressures from 280-330 mOsm have been used for human sperm capacitation and/or IVF (Table 1); an optimum osmotic pressure has not been defined. In the mouse and hamster, Miyamoto and Chang (1973b) defined optimum osmotic pressure ranges of 270-400 and 300-365 mOsm, respectively. In the rabbit and bovine, a brief exposure to hyperosmotic (∿ 390 mOsm) conditions enhances capacitation *in vitro* (Brackett and Oliphant, 1975, Triana et al., 1980; Oliphant and Eng, 1981; Brackett et al., 1982). The effect of hyperosmotic treatment on human sperm capacitation has not yet been reported.

b) pH. A pH range of 7.2-8.2 is compatible with human sperm capacitation and IVF (Table 1); however a precise pH optimum has not been established. In other systems a somewhat basic pH is ideal. Miyamoto et al. (1974) defined optimal pH ranges of 7.3-7.7, 6.8-8.2 and 7.8 for fertilization *in vitro* in the mouse, hamster and rat, respectively, and Mahi and Yanagimachi (1978) showed that the percentage of acrosome-reacted canine sperm increased with increasing pH (from 7.4-8.0). In the latter investigation zona penetration actually decreased at pH 8.0, perhaps reflecting an adverse effect on motility. The pH requirement for capacitation and/or acrosome reactions in the guinea pig has been studied by Hyne and Garbers (1981). Acrosome reactions were observed in minimal culture medium (devoid of macromolecular components) at pH values above 7.8. At more physiologic pH levels (∿ 7.4) serum factors were required to initiate acrosome reactions.

c) Gas atmosphere. Either 5% CO_2 in air, or 5% CO_2, 5% O_2, 90% N_2 are used routinely for human sperm capacitation and for IVF (Table 2). A CO_2 environment is essential for pH maintenance since the media used are bicarbonate buffered. In some cases, media are supplemented with HEPES to insure adequate buffering capacity, or are overlaid with oil to minimize gas exchange (Purdy, 1982). The particular gas phase used is probably not critical to results so long as some bicarbonate is present and adequate pH control is maintained.

d) Temperature. All studies of human sperm capacitation and IVF have been conducted at $37 \pm 1^{o}C$. A critical evaluation of temperature effects on capacitation has not been undertaken although elevated temperatures are no doubt detrimental. In other species such as hamster (Mahi and Yanagimachi, 1973) and bovine (Lenz et al., 1983), temperatures between 35-40°C appear optimal.

Sperm Preparation

Washing Procedures. Sperm used for zona-free hamster egg bioassays or IVF are routinely washed free of seminal plasma following liquifaction. This step is necessary as seminal plasma has a significant inhibitory effect on these processes (Rogers et al., 1983; see discussion below). Two methods for washing are commonly employed (see Chapters 13 and 14). Semen can be cycled through several centrifugation-resuspension steps. Alternatively a "swim-up" procedure can be used (Overstreet et al., 1980a). In this procedure, semen is layered underneath culture medium and motile sperm are allowed to "swim-up" into medium for approximately 1 hour. The highly motile sperm are then collected by centrifugation and used for insemination.

Preincubation Time. Sperm used for mammalian fertilization *in vitro* are generally pre-incubated for a given time period to effect capacitation. Optimal preincubation times vary between and within species (Bedford, 1970; Chang and Hunter, 1975; Rogers, 1978). Human sperm capacitation times in an IVF-ET setting have not been defined precisely since sperm are either preincubated for several hours or used immediately after washing (Table 2). Sperm and eggs are then cultured, usually for about 14-18 hours, and examined for evidence of fertilization. This approach yields little information as to when fertilization, and hence capacitation, actually occurred.

Several investigators have addressed the question of capacitation kinetics in human sperm. Lopata et al. (1978) pre-incubated sperm for 1.5 hrs. before insemination; the insemination period lasting 3 hours. In 3 of 4 ova examined after this time, morphological evidence of fertilization was observed, suggesting that at least some sperm had undergone capacitation within the 4 1/2 hour time period. McMaster et al. (1978) provided evidence that capacitation can take place within a shorter time interval. Human oocytes matured *in vitro* and inseminated with non-preincubated sperm had sperm within the perivitelline space within 2 hours of insemination, indicating that capacitation was completed at some point during this period. Overstreet et al. (1980b) showed that capacitation could occur within an even shorter time period. Their method involved washing sperm through a column of cervical mucus into droplets containing non-viable human oocytes. In some cases, sperm attached to and penetrated the zona within 1 hour.

Defining the kinetics of human sperm capacitation becomes more complex if results from zona-free hamster egg bioassays are considered. Here, preincubation times for capacitation range from

Table 2. Sperm parameters for capacitation and fertilization *in vitro*

Author	Test System	Pre-Incubation Time (Hrs)	Sperm-Egg Contact (Insemination) Time (Hrs)	Insemination Concentration
Yanagimachi et al., (1976)	ZFHE	4; 7-7.5	0.5-3	$3\text{-}6 \times 10^5$/ml
Rogers et al., (1979 & 1983)	ZFHE	18-20	2-4	$0.5\text{-}2.0 \times 10^7$/ml
Overstreet et al., (1980a)	ZFHE & non-human oocyte	Zero	1-20	$1\text{-}20 \times 10^6$/ml
Binor et al., (1980)	ZFHE	7.5	4-5.5	$5 \times 10^2\text{-}5 \times 10^6$/ml
Dor et al., (1981)	ZFHE	6	3	1×10^7/ml
Bronson et al., (1981)	ZFHE	2-3	4	5×10^6/ml
Tyler et al., (1981)	ZFHE	18	2.5	$10^6\text{-}10^7$/ml
Karp et al., (1981)	ZFHE	7	3	2×10^7/ml

Wolf and Sokoloski (1982)	ZFHE	2-22	3-5	$5x10^6$motile/ml
Hall (1982)	ZFHE	15-18	3	$0.5-1.5x10^6$/ml
Aitken et al., (1982)	ZFHE	7	3	$5.4x10^6$motile/ml
Perreault and Rogers (1982)	ZFHE	0-22	2-3	$1x10^7$/ml
Berger et al.,(1983)	ZFHE	3	5	10^6-10^7motile/ml
Soupart and Strong (1974)	Human Oocyte	Zero	24	$2x10^7$/ml
Overstreet and Hembree (1976)	Non-Living Human Oocyte	Zero	8-24	$2x10^4-1.5x10^7$
McMaster et al., (1978)	Human Oocyte	Zero	2-7	$5x10^6$/ml
Yanagimachi et al., (1979a)	Non-Living Human Oocyte	Zero	7-9	$1x10^6$/ml
Overstreet et al., (1980b)	Non-Living Human Oocyte	Zero	1-20	$1x10^4-4x10^6$/ml
Lopata et al., (1978)	Human Oocyte	1.5	3-6	$1.5-2.5x10^6$/ml

(continued)

Table 2 (Cont'd)

Mettler et al., (1982)	Human IVF-ET	2-3	12	$1x10^6$motile/ml
Lopata et al., (1980)	Human IVF-ET	47 min.	15.5	$1x10^6$motile/ml
Trounson et al., (1980)	Human IVF-ET	1	8-15	$1-18x10^5$/ml
Trounson et al., (1982)	Human IVF-ET	Zero	12-23	$3-8x10^5$/ml
Edwards et al., (1981)	Human IVF-ET	Zero	16	$4x10^5-4x10^6$/ml
Purdy (1982)	Human IVF-ET	Zero	4-24	-
Plachot et al., (1982)	Human IVF-ET	Zero	12-18	$0.5-1.0x10^6$/ml
Wortham et al., (1983a)	Human IVF-ET	Zero	7-9	$8x10^5$/ml
Testart et al., (1982)	Human IVF-ET	Zero	20	$5x10^4-1.5x10^6$/ml
Testart et al., (1983)	Human IVF-ET	Zero	20	$1.5x10^5$motile/ml

Table 2 (Cont'd)

Wortham et al., (1983b)	Zero	14	0.5-1.5x10^6 motile/ml
University of Texas-Houston	6	16	5x10^4 motile/ml

1. Pre incubation times do not include the time required for washing. Zero pre-incubation time refers to inseminations conducted immediately after washing.

0-22 hours (Table 2), and results are donor specific, i.e., individual donors show marked differences in pre-incubation times required for maximal penetration (Perreault and Rogers, 1982a; Wolf and Sokoloski, 1982). In the former case, one donor gave approximately 30% penetration levels with no pre-incubation, i.e., insemination immediately after washing. Not only are there differences in capacitation rates between donors, but also between specimens from the same donors (Wolf and Sokoloski, 1982). Thus, interdonor as well as intradonor variability must be considered when attempting to define optimal capacitation times.

Considering the above findings, it is difficult to assign an optimal pre-incubation time for capacitation of human sperm *in vitro*. Some pre-incubation time undoubtedly increases the likelihood of obtaining greater numbers of capacitated sperm, and factors such as specific washing and/or culturing conditions undoubtedly influence the kinetics of the process. One should recall that only a small subpopulation of sperm can actually be assessed using penetration assays and it is likely that in a given population subsets of sperm undergo capacitation at differing rates.

Other Factors. Other variables associated with sperm preparation include sperm concentration and sperm-egg interaction times. Regarding sperm concentration, lower sperm numbers can be used successfully for human IVF-ET as compared to zona-free hamster egg bioassays (Table 2). Penetration in human IVF-ET programs has been reported at concentrations as low as 1-5 x 10^4 sperm/ml (Craft et al., 1981; Testart et al., 1982; Wortham, Jr. et al., 1983b; see Chapter 12). In contrast, inseminations in the zona-free hamster egg bioassay are normally conducted at concentrations in excess of 1 x 10^6 sperm/ml (Table 2), with optimal concentrations within the 5-10 x 10^6 sperm/ml range (Berger et al., 1983; Rogers et al., 1983).

Sperm-egg interaction or insemination times also vary (Table 2) most notably in zona-free hamster egg studies. Insemination times may affect interpretation of results if insufficient to allow completion of penetration and pronuclear development. Rogers et al. (1983) have indicated that a 2-3 hr. insemination period is optimal for the hamster egg bioassay.

To summarize, human sperm capacitation and/or IVF can take place under a variety of experimental conditions. Many, if not all, of the potential variables such as media, media supplements, pH, osmolarity, etc. have not been systematically investigated. By and large, culture conditions used to support human sperm capacitation and IVF have been extrapolated from other mammalian systems, and confirmation of success has relied almost exclusively on empirical observation.

MOLECULAR CORRELATES OF HUMAN SPERM CAPACITATION

Defining the molecular correlates of human sperm capacitation or, in fact capacitation in general, is problematic. It would be ideal, of course, if the molecular events of capacitation were identical in all species, such that direct inferences to the human could be drawn. Whether this is in fact true, however, remains uncertain. Several factors contribute to the dilemma. The divergent, often non-specific conditions that support capacitation *in vitro* hampers comparison of capacitation mechanisms between species. Another variable involves the source of sperm. In the common laboratory rodents (hamster, mouse, guinea pig, rat) epididymal sperm are routinely used whereas studies of human sperm have necessarily relied on ejaculated cells. In the rabbit and bovine, where both cell types have been investigated, there is evidence to suggest that epididymal and ejaculated sperm behave somewhat differently with regard to capacitation mechanisms (Babcock et al., 1979; Oliphant and Eng, 1981).

Clearly a major aspect of capacitation, in both epididymal and ejaculated sperm, involves cell surface alterations. Changes in both extrinsic and intrinsic properties of the sperm plasma membrane occur concomitant with capacitation (Clegg, 1983). During transit within the male reproductive tract, the sperm surface is coated by a variety of macromolecular substances, and the removal or alteration of these coating materials is of critical importance to capacitation (Bedford, 1970; Johnson, 1975; Yanagimachi, 1981; Clegg, 1983). Certainly some coating of the sperm surface occurs prior to or during epididymal transit. A number of lectin and antibody-labelling studies have demonstrated a loss or redistribution of extrinsic surface components upon capacitation of epididymal sperm (reviewed by Koehler, 1978, 1981). Upon ejaculation, the sperm surface is further modified. Antibodies raised against rabbit seminal plasma bind to freshly ejaculated rabbit sperm, but fail to do so after exposure to capacitating conditions (Johnson and Hunter, 1972; Oliphant and Brackett, 1973), indicating that seminal plasma components on the sperm surface are removed or altered as a function of capacitation. Oliphant (1976) has shown that removal of seminal plasma components is essential for induction of the acrosome reaction in rabbit sperm. While it is true that seminal plasma components derive from both the epididymis and accesory sex glands, it has been shown using surface iodination techniques (Oliphant and Singhas, 1979) and antibodies directed against fibronectin (Koehler et al., 1980) that some surface components removed during capacitation are unique to the ejaculated cell.

Surface alterations associated with capacitation are not restricted to the extrinsic portion of the cell surface, but also involve modification of intrinsic membrane components. Freeze-fracture studies of guinea pig (Friend et al., 1977) and hamster (Kinsey and Koehler, 1978) sperm have shown that rearrangement of intramembranous proteins occurs during capacitation, resulting in formation of clear patches devoid of protein. Alterations in the membrane lipids also takes place during capacitation. Friend (1980) has shown a similar clearing of sterol components and Bearer and Friend (1982) have demonstrated an alteration in distribution of anionic phospholipids during capacitation of guinea pig sperm.

While a number of alterations in both extrinsic and intrinsic sperm surface properties can be documented, the functional significance of these changes during capacitation remains unclear. Clegg (1983) has reviewed extensively the possible mechansims by which modifications in membrane structure may impact on capacitation. In terms of functional alterations, perhaps the only firm evidence linking a specific extrinsic factor to capacitation involves seminal plasma. Chang (1957) was the first to demonstrate that seminal plasma could directly influence capacitation. Rabbit sperm when first capacitated by intrauterine incubation were "decapacitated" when reincubated in seminal plasma, i.e., they reversibly lost their ability to fertilize. When "decapacitated" sperm were re-introduced into the female reproductive tract, they were "recapacitated". It is now well-recognized that seminal plasma contains a decapacitation factor or factors (DF), although the biochemical nature and mode of action remains under debate (see review by Oliphant and Eng, 1981).

Human seminal plasma contains a DF-like substance that influences human sperm capacitation. Capacitation of both rabbit (Pinsker and Williams, 1968; McRorie and Williams, 1974) and mouse (Reddy et al., 1979, 1982) sperm is adversly affected by components of human seminal plasma. Kanwar et al. (1979) reported that human sperm penetration of zona-free hamster eggs was blocked by homologous seminal plasma. This effect was observed only when seminal plasma was present during both preincubation (capacitation) and insemination. No adverse effect was detected when seminal plasma was present during insemination alone, suggesting that seminal plasma blocks a preliminary step to sperm-egg fusion, i.e., capacitation or the acrosome reaction. Van der ven et al. (1982) obtained similar inhibitory effects with a high molecular weight factor obtained by ultracentrifugation of seminal plasma ($\sim$100,000g). This preparative method is similar to that employed by Reddy et al. (1982) for the isolation of a human seminal plasma fraction that inhibits mouse sperm capacitation, and is analogous to previously described procedures for the preparation of rabbit seminal plasma DF (Bedford and Chang, 1962).

How might the removal or alteration of seminal plasma components, such as DF, impact on capacitation? A plausible mechanism involves the regulation of Ca^{2+} flux activity at the sperm surface. Ca^{2+} is intimately associated with a variety of physiological events at fertilization. Increased intracellular Ca^{2+} levels are absolutely essential for induction of the acrosome reaction in both invertebrate and vertebrate species (Garbers and Kopf, 1980; Yanagimachi, 1981) and roles for Ca^{2+} in sperm attachment to the zona pellucida (Saling et al., 1978), sperm-egg fusion (Yanagimachi, 1978), and regulation of motility (Babcock and Lardy, 1982; Tash and Means, 1983) have been elucidated.

The role of Ca^{2+} in capacitation per se in lower mammals is unclear. Yanagimachi and Usui (1974), noting that synchronous acrosome reactions could be induced in guinea pig epididymal sperm by adding Ca^{2+} to sperm pre-incubated in the absence of extracellular Ca^{2+}, concluded that calcium was required for the acrosome reaction but not for capacitation. Fraser (1982) challenged this view, however, claiming a Ca^{2+} requirement for mouse sperm capacitation distinct from that of the acrosome reaction. In her study, sperm were incubated in Ca^{2+}-free media and introduced into media containing Ca^{2+} at half-hour intervals. Sperm had to be exposed to Ca^{2+} for at least 30 min. to complete capacitation as fertilization rates, acrosome reactions, and hyperactivated motility (all markers of capacitation in this species) were suppressed in sperm exposed to Ca^{2+} for less than this time period.

Perhaps of more relevance to the role of calcium in human sperm capacitation are recent findings in the bovine, involving both epididymal and ejaculated sperm (Babcock et al., 1979). Bovine epididymal sperm, low in endogenous Ca^{2+} content, are capable of Ca^{2+} uptake when washed into Ca^{2+} containing buffer. In contrast, ejaculated sperm, also low in Ca^{2+} content, do not accumulate calcium. Moreover, exposure of epididymal sperm to seminal plasma markedly reduces the ability of these cells to take up Ca^{2+}. Evidence has been presented for the existence of a specific calcium transport inhibitor protein in seminal plasma that is responsible for this effect (Rufo et al., 1982).

Comparative studies of Ca^{2+} flux regulation by human sperm are difficult since a direct comparison of epididymal and ejaculated cells is impractical. However, there is a suggestion that Ca^{2+} regulation in ejaculated human sperm is altered during capacitation (Byrd et al., 1983). When incubated under capacitating conditions, washed sperm (free of seminal plasma) show cyclic fluxes in Ca^{2+} uptake (Figure 5) and the time of removal from seminal plasma affects this behavior. Sperm allowed to liquify (i.e., remain in seminal plasma) for 30 minutes display four times greater Ca^{2+} uptake activity than sperm removed five minutes after ejaculation (Figure 6). This difference in Ca^{2+} flux activity may be related directly to sperm function since sperm exposed only briefly to seminal plasma display decreased penetration levels in the zona-free hamster egg bioassay relative to 30 minute exposed sperm (Figure 7). A hypothesis based on these findings is that: 1) the ability of sperm to regulate Ca^{2+} flux is altered as a critical step during capacitation, 2) human seminal plasma contains a Ca^{2+} transport regulatory protein, similar to the bovine, that associates with the sperm surface and limits Ca^{2+} uptake, 3) during liquifaction, this regulatory protein is removed directly or is modified such that the sperm gains the ability to regulate Ca^{2+} flux and, (4) the acquisition of a critical intracellular calcium level sets in motion the events culminating in an acrosome reaction. Available results are sparse and more information is clearly required. We need determinations of intracellular Ca^{2+} pools, particularly locally within the sperm head where the molecular events of capacitation and the acrosome reaction take place.

What would be the consequences of an increase in intracellular free Ca^{2+} during capacitation? At present, it is impossible to clearly distinguish between Ca^{2+} effects on capacitation from those required for initiation of the acrosome reaction. Yanagimachi (1981) and Clegg (1983) have reviewed several hypotheses concerning the role of Ca^{2+} in induction of the acrosome reaction. An overview of their discussions, integrated with our views concerning Ca^{2+} flux regulation is presented below.

The initial step in the capacitation-acrosome reaction sequence involves surface modifications that, in turn, permits Ca^{2+} to enter the cell. During capacitation, removal or modification of a seminal plasma DF-like component (a Ca^{2+} transport inhibitor protein?) occurs. Removal of this factor activates or exposes specific membrane transport mechanisms for Ca^{2+}, an ATPase (Gordon et al., 1978; Meizel, 1978) or specific Ca^{2+} transport proteins (Green, 1978; Yanagimachi, 1981). Clegg (1983) suggests that rather than activation of a Ca^{2+} ATPase, a

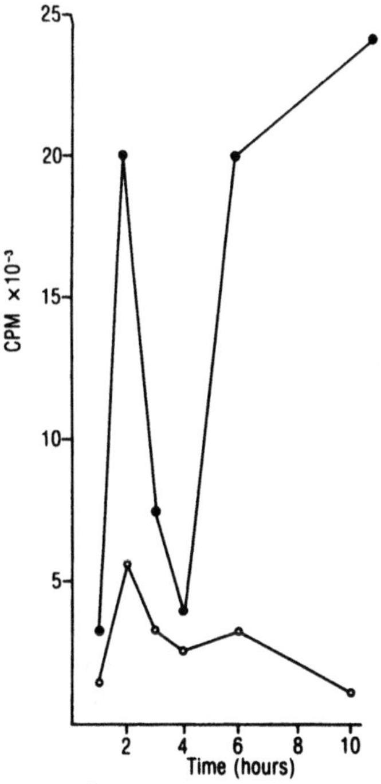

Figure 5

Calcium flux activity during incubation of human sperm. Sperm washed free of seminal plasma were incubated in BWW contining 3.5% (-o-) or 0.3% (-●-) HSA. At the indicated times aliquots were removed, incubated with $^{45}CaCl_2$ for 30 min., washed and the ^{45}Ca uptake was determined.

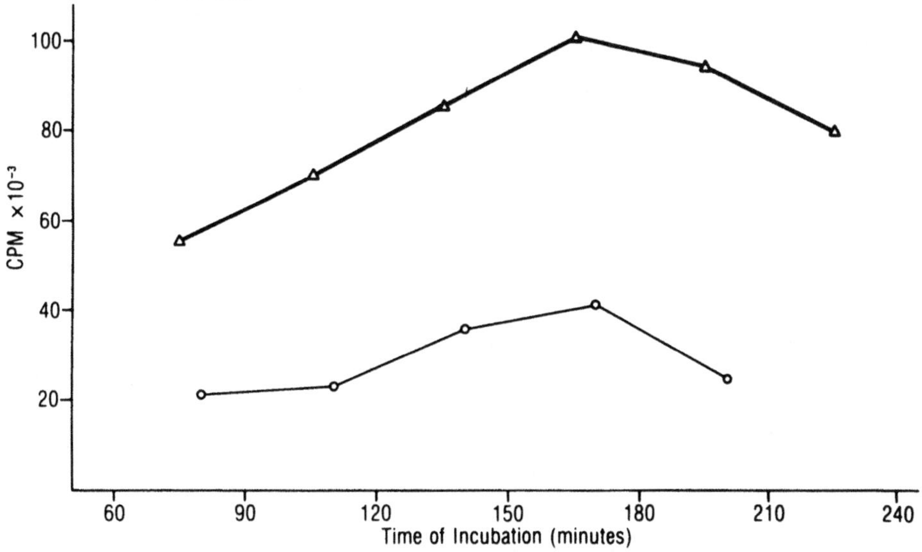

Figure 6

Seminal plasma effect on calcium uptake by human sperm. Sperm were washed free of seminal plasma 5 min. (-o-) or 30 min. (-Δ-) post-ejaculation and incubated in BWW contining 3.5% HSA. At the indicated times aliquots were removed, incubated with $^{45}CaCl_2$ for 30 min., washed and the ^{45}Ca uptake was determined.

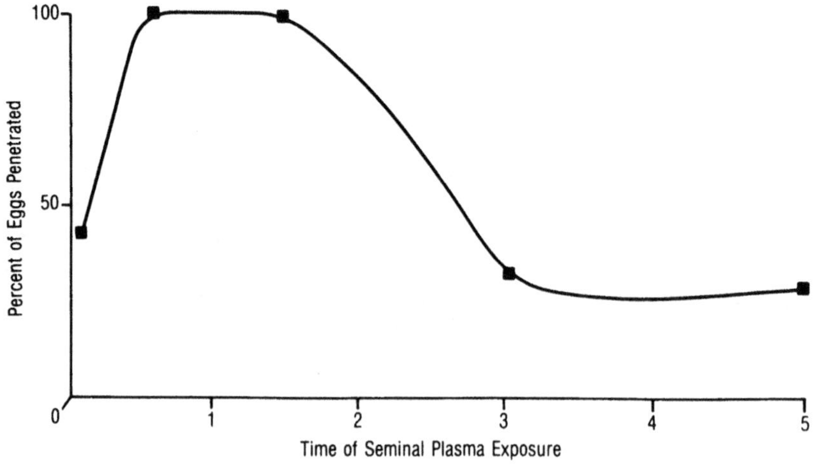

Figure 7

The influence of seminal plasma on human sperm penetration of zona-free hamster eggs. Sperm from a single ejaculate were washed free of seminal plasma at the indicated times following ejaculation, then pre-incubated (capacitated) for 3 hours in BWW containing 3.5% HSA. Freshly prepared zona-free hamster ova were inseminated with equivalent concentrations of sperm and finally scored for penetration after 3 hours.

"barrier" to Ca^{2+} influx is removed. The exposure of ion channels for Ca^{2+} may be reflected on a molecular level by structural modifications involving movement of membrane proteins or lipids (Friend et al., 1977; Bearer and Friend, 1982). The net result of this stage is the accumulation of free Ca^{2+} within the cell, particularly in the region between the plasma and outer acrosomal membranes.

Once a critical intracellular Ca^{2+} level is reached, Ca^{2+} participates in events that ultimately lead to fusion of the plasma and outer acrosomal membranes. In this regard, Ca^{2+} may play several roles. Yanagimachi (1981) has theorized that Ca^{2+} neutralizes opposing negative charges between the plasma and outer acrosomal membranes, allowing their close approximation as a pre-requisite to fusion. Gordon et al. (1978) and Meizel (1978) have suggested that an ATPase on the outer acrosomal membrane pumps Ca^{2+} into the acrosome proper. Once inside the acrosome, Ca^{2+}, possibly by affecting an increase in intra-acrosomal pH, activates the conversion of proacrosin to acrosin. Acrosin is a proteolytic enzyme that may have several functions during fertilization, including penetration of the zona pellucida (Stambaugh, 1978; See Chapter 12) and/or initiation of the acrosome reaction. Acrosin may enzymatically degrade membrane components leading to fusion, or activate other enzymes (phospholipase) that would promote membrane fusion (Meizel, 1978; Clegg, 1983). Alternatively, acrosin may solubilize the acrosomal matrix, resulting in increased internal osmotic pressure (Green, 1978). Yanagimachi (1981) proposed that Ca^{2+} inactivates a Mg^{2+}-ATPase on the plasma and/or outer acrosomal membrane, resulting in an influx of water into the acrosome.

Ca^{2+} may also mediate alterations in membrane lipid components. Yanagimachi (1981) suggests that Ca^{2+} binds to membrane phospholipids and causes a "phase transition" from a fluid to crystalline state, contributing to membrane destabilization as a prelude to fusion. This is in accord with the observations of O'Rand (1977), who demonstrated decreased mobility of a specific rabbit sperm surface antigen during capacitation. Another possibility is that Ca^{2+} would bind directly to membrane phospholipids, thereby inducing fusion. Since, as demonstrated by Friend (1980) and Bearer and Friend (1982), membrane phospholipids accumulate in focal regions of the plasma membrane during capacitation, this scheme accounts for the focal points of membrane fusion commonly observed (Clegg, 1983). Activation of phospholipase by Ca^{2+} (or acrosin) provides an additional role for Ca^{2+}. Phospholipase, by acting on membrane phospholipids, liberates substances such as lysophospholipid that act as fusogenic agents. Three observations are relevant here: 1) phospholipase inhibitors prevent hamster sperm acrosome reactions (Lui and Meizel, 1979); 2) phospholipase is released from acrosome-reacted hamster sperm (Llanos et al., 1982); and 3) exogenous lysophospholipids induce acrosome reactions in the guinea pig (Fleming and Yanagimachi, 1981). Finally, membrane lipid alterations may involve modification of cholesterol and sterol sulfate moieties that contribute to membrane destabilization (Davis et al., 1980; Langlais et al., 1981).

An increase in intracellular Ca^{2+} levels may influence cyclic nucleotide metabolism during capacitation and/or induction of the acrosome reaction. Garbers and Kopf (1980) and Clegg (1983) have reviewed the evidence supporting a role for cyclic AMP and related enzymes, such as adenylate cyclase, in capacitation and the acrosome reaction. Addition of cyclic AMP analogues or phosphodiesterase inhibitors to sperm preparations stimulates the induction of an acrosome reaction and/or fertilization *in vitro* (Reyes et al., 1978; Hyne and Garbers, 1979; Fraser, 1981; Bavister et al., 1983). In the human, there is some evidence that exogenous cAMP or phosphodiesterase inhibitors enhance capacitation rates as measured with the zona-free hamster egg bioassay (Perreault and Rogers, 1982b; Chan et al., 1983). However, whether or not cAMP mediates specific responses at the membrane level, or acts in a more general fashion by stimulating motility or metabolic activity, for example, remains open to question.

In summary, surface alterations take place during capacitation that allow the sperm to regulate Ca^{2+} uptake. When a critical intracellular level is reached, Ca^{2+}, through a number of potential pathways, promotes membrane fusion necessary for induction of the acrosome reaction.

CONCLUSIONS

The growing interest in IVF-ET for treatment of human infertility should be supported by a more thorough understanding of all aspects of the process. As detailed in this chapter, sperm must undergo capacitation to effect fertilization; however, the methodology for and molecular mechanisms of capacitation remain poorly defined. Recent advances in experimental techniques (monoclonal antibodies and other specific probes of cell function), together with methods adapted to study human sperm function directly (such as the zona-free hamster egg bioassay) provide the tools to support the investigation of human sperm capacitation on a molecular level. As our pool of information concerning the physiology of human fertilization increases, it is reasonable to expect that success in human IVF-ET will increase, and that the types of infertility treated will expand. It is when this expansion reaches male infertility directly attributable to sperm dysfunction that insights into the basic physiology of sperm function should prove invaluable.

REFERENCES

Aitken, R. J., Best, F.S.M., Richardson, D.W., Djahanbakhch, O., and Lees, M.M., 1982, The correlates of fertilizing capacity in normal fertile men, Fertil. Steril., 38:68.

Austin, C.R., 1951, Observations on the penetration of the sperm into the mammalian egg, Aust. J. Res. Sci. Ser.B., 4:581.

Austin, C.R., 1952, The "capacitation" of the mammalian sperm, Nature (London), 170:326.

Babcock, D.F., and Lardy, H.A., 1982, Alterations in membrane permeability to Ca^{2+} and their consequences during maturation of mammalian spermatozoa, in: " Membranes and Transport," Vol. 1, A.N. Martonosi, ed., Plenum Press, New York.

Babcock, D.F., Singh, J.P., and Lardy, H.A., 1979, Alteration of membrane permeability to calcium ions during maturation of bovine spermatozoa, Dev. Biol., 69:85.

Barros, C., Bedford, J.M., Franklin, L.E., and Austin, C.R., 1967, Membrane vesiculation as a feature of the mammalian acrosome reaction, J. Cell Biol., 34:C1.

Barros, C., Berrios, M., and Herrera, E., 1973, Capacitation in vitro of guinea pig spermatozoa in a saline solution, J. Reprod. Fert., 34:547.

Bavister, B.D., 1969, Environmental factors important for in vitro fertilization in the hamster, J. Reprod. Fert., 18:544.

Bavister, B.D., 1981a, Analysis of culture media for in vitro fertilization and criteria for success, in: "Fertilization and Embryonic Development In Vitro," L. Mastroianni, Jr. and J.D. Biggers, eds., Plenum Press, New York.

Bavister, B.D., 1981b, Substitution of a synthetic polymer for protein in a mammalian gamete culture system, J. Exp. Zool., 217:45.

Bavister, B.D., and Yanagimachi, R., 1977, The effects of sperm extracts and energy sources on the motility and acrosome reaction of hamster spermatozoa in vitro, Biol. Reprod., 16:228.

Bavister, B.D., Boatman, D.E., Leibfried, L., Loose, M., and Vernon, M.W., 1983, Fertilization and cleavage of rhesus monkey oocytes in vitro, Biol. Reprod., 28:983.

Bearer, E.L., and Friend, D.S., 1982, Modifications of anionic lipid domains preceeding membrane fusion in guinea pig sperm, J. Cell Biol., 92:604.

Bedford, J.M., 1970, Sperm capacitation and fertilization in mammals, Biol. Reprod., Suppl. 2:128.

Bedford, J.M., 1977, Sperm/egg interaction: The specificity of human spermatozoa, Anat. Rec., 188:477.

Bedford, J.M., 1983, Significance of the need for sperm capacitation before fertilization in eutherian mammals, Biol. Reprod., 28:108.

Bedford, J.M., and Chang, M.C., 1962, Removal of decapacitation factor from seminal plasma by high speed centrifugation, Am. J. Physiol., 202:179.

Bedford, J.M., and Cooper, G.W., 1978, Membrane fusion events in the fertilization of vertebrate eggs, in: "Cell Surface Reviews," Vol. 5, G. Poste and G.L. Nicolson, eds, North-Holland, Amsterdam.

Berger, T., Marrs, R.P., Saito, H., and Kletzky, O.A., 1983, Factors affecting human sperm penetration of zona-free hamster ova. Am. J. Obstet. Gynecol., 145:397.
Biggers, J.D., Whitten, W.K., and Whittingham, D.G., 1971, The culture of mouse embryos in vitro, in: "Methods of Mammalian Embryology," J.C. Daniel, Jr. ed., Freeman and Co. San Francisco.
Binor, Z., Sokoloski, J.E., and Wolf, D.P., 1980, Penetration of the zona-free hamster egg by human sperm, Fertil. Steril., 33:321.
Brackett, B.G., and Oliphant, G., 1975, Capacitation of rabbit spermatozoa in vitro, Biol. Reprod., 12:260.
Brackett, B.G., Bousquet, D., Boice, M.L., Donawick, W.J., Evans, J.F., and Dressel, M.A., 1982, Normal development following in vitro fertilization in the cow, Biol. Reprod., 27:147.
Bronson, R., Cooper, G., and Rosenfeld, D., 1981, Ability of antibody-bound human sperm to penetrate zona-free hamster ova in vitro, Fertil. Steril., 36:778.
Byrd, W., Sokoloski, J.E., and Wolf, D.P., 1983, Analysis of calcium uptake during incubation of human spermatozoa, Biol. Reprod. 28, Suppl. 1:103.
Chan, S.Y.W., Tang, L.C.H., and Ma, H.K., 1983, Stimulation of the human spermatozoal fertilizing ability by dibutyryl 3', 5'-cAMP and theophylline in vitro, Arch. Androl., 11:19.
Chang, M.C., 1951, Fertilizing capacity of spermatozoa deposited into the fallopian tubes, Nature, (London) 168:697.
Chang, M.C., 1957, A detrimental effect of seminal plasma on the fertilizing capacity of sperm, Nature, (London) 179:258.
Chang, M.C., and Hunter, R.H.F., 1975, Capacitation of mammalian sperm: biological and experimental aspects, in: "Handbook of Physiology," Section 7, R.O. Greep, and E.B. Astwood, eds., American Physiological Society, Washington, D.C.
Clegg, E.D., 1983, Mechanisms of mammalian sperm capacitation, in: "Mechanism and Control of Animal Fertilization," J.F. Hartmann, ed., Academic Press, New York.
Craft, I., McLeod, F., Bernard, A., Green, S., and Twigg, H., 1981, Sperm numbers and in vitro fertilization, Lancet, 2:1165.
Davis, B.K., 1976, Influence of serum albumin on the fertilizing ability in vitro of rat spermatozoa, Proc. Soc. Exp. Biol. Med., 151:240.
Davis, B.K., Byrne, R., and Bedigian, K., 1980, Studies on the mechanism of capacitation: Albumin-mediated changes in the plasma membrane lipids during in vitro incubation of rat sperm cells, Proc. Nat. Acad. Sci. USA, 77:1546.
Dor, J., Rudak, E., and Aitken, R.J., 1981, Antisperm antibodies: their effect on the process of fertilization studied in vitro. Fertil. Steril., 35:535.

Dravland, E., and Meizel, S., 1981, Stimulation of hamster sperm capacitation and acrosome reaction in vitro by glucose and lactate and inhibition by the glycolytic inhibitor α-chlorohydrin, Gamete Res., 4:515.

Edwards, R.G., Purdy, J.M., Steptoe, P.C., and Walters, D.E., 1981, The growth of human preimplantation embryos in vitro, Am. J. Obstet. Gynecol., 141:408.

Feichtinger, W., Kemeter, P., and Szalay, S., 1983, The Vienna program of in vitro fertilization and embryo transfer - a successful clinical treatment, Europ. J. Obstet. Gynec. Repro. Biol., 15:63.

Fleming, A.D., and Yanagimachi, R., 1981, Effects of various lipids on the acrosome reaction and fertilizing capacity of guinea pig spermatozoa with special reference to the possible involvement of lysophospholipids in the acrosome reaction, Gamete Res., 4:253.

Fraser, L.R., 1981, Dibutyryl cyclic AMP decreases capacitation time in vitro in mouse spermatozoa, J. Reprod. Fert., 62:63.

Fraser, L., 1982, Ca^{2+} is required for mouse sperm capacitation and fertilization in vitro, J. Androl., 3:412.

Fraser, L.R., and Quinn, P.J., 1981, A glycolytic product is obligatory for initiation of the sperm acrosome reaction and whiplash motility required for fertilization in the mouse, J. Reprod. Fert., 61:25.

Friend, D.S., Orci, L., Perrelet, A., and Yanagimachi, R., 1977, Membrane particle changes attending the acrosome reaction in guinea pig spermatozoa, J. Cell Biol., 74:561.

Friend, D.S., 1980, Freeze-fracture alterations in guinea pig sperm membranes preceeding gamete fusion, in: "Membrane-Membrane Interactions," N.B. Gilula, ed., Raven Press, New York.

Garbers, D.L., and Kopf, G.S., 1980, The regulation of spermatozoa by calcium and cyclic nucleotides, in: "Advances in Cyclic Nucleotide Research," Vol. 13, P. Greengard and G.A. Robison, eds., Raven Press, New York.

Go, K.J., and Wolf, D.P., 1983, The role of steroids in sperm capacitation, Adv. Lipid. Res., 20:317.

Gordon, M., Dandekar, P.V., and Eager, P.R., 1978, Identification of phosphatases on the membranes of guinea pig sperm, Anat. Rec., 191:123.

Gould, J.E., Overstreet, J.W., Yanagimachi, H., Yanagimachi, R., Katz, D.F., and Hanson, F.W., 1983, What functions of the sperm cell are measured by in vitro fertilization of zona-free hamster eggs?, Fertil. Steril., 40:344.

Green, D.P.L., 1978, The mechanism of the acrosome reaction, in: "Development in Mammals," Vol. 3, M. H. Johnson, ed., North-Holland, Amsterdam..

Hall, J.L., 1981, Relationship between semen quality and human sperm penetration of zona-free hamster ova, Fertil. Steril., 35:457.

Hanada, A., and Chang, M.C., 1972, Penetration of zona-free eggs by spermatozoa of different species, Biol. Reprod., 6:300.

Hoppe, P.C., 1976, Glucose requirement for mouse sperm capacitation in vitro, Biol. Reprod., 15:39.

Hoppe, P.C., and Whitten, W.K., 1974, An albumin requirement for fertilization of mouse eggs in vitro, J. Reprod. Fert., 39:433.

Hyne, R.V., and Garbers, D.L., 1979, Calcium-dependent increase in adenosine 3',5'-monophosphate and induction of the acrosome reaction in guinea pig spermatozoa, Proc. Natl. Acad. Sci. U.S.A., 76:5699.

Hyne, R.V., and Garbers, D.L., 1981, Requirement of serum factors for capacitation and the acrosome reaction of guinea pig spermatozoa in buffered medium below pH 7.8, Biol. Reprod., 24:257.

Jamil, K., and White, I.G., 1981, Induction of acrosomal reaction in sperm with ionophore A23187 and calcium, Arch. Androl., 7:283.

Johnson, M.H., 1975, The macromolecular organization of membranes and its bearing on events leading up to fertilization. J. Reprod. Fert., 44:167.

Johnson, W.L., and Hunter, A.C., 1972, Immunofluorescent evaluation of the male rabbit reproductive tract for sites of secretion and absorption of seminal antigens, Biol. Reprod., 6:13.

Kanwar, K. C., Yanagimachi, R., and Lopata, A., 1979, Effects of human seminal plasma on fertilizing capacity of human spermatozoa, Fertil. Steril., 31:321.

Karp, L.E., Williamson, R.A., Moore, D.E., Shy, K.K., Plymate, S.R., and Smith, W.D., 1981, Sperm penetration assay: Useful test in evaluation of male fertility, Obstet. Gynecol., 57:620.

Katz, D.F., and Yanagimachi, R., 1980, Movement characteristics of hamster spermatozoa within the oviduct, Biol. Reprod., 22:759.

Kinsey, W.H., and Koehler, J.K., 1978, Cell surface changes associated with in vitro capacitation of hamster sperm, J. Ultrastruc. Res., 64:1.

Koehler, J.K., 1978, The mammalian sperm surface: Studies with specific labelling techniques, Int. Rev. Cytol., 54:73.

Koehler, J.K., 1981, Lectins as probes of the spermatozoon surface, Arch. Androl., 6:197.

Koehler, J.K., DeCurtis, I., Stenchever, M.A., and Smith, D., 1982, Interaction of human sperm with zona-free hamster eggs: A freeze-fracture study, Gamete Res., 6:371.

Koehler, J.K., Nudelman, E.D., and Hakomori, S., 1980, A collagen-binding protein on the surface of ejaculated rabbit spermatozoa, J. Cell Biol., 86:529.

Langlais, J., Zollinger, M., Plante, L., Chapdelaine, A., Bleau, G., and Roberts, K.D., 1981, Localization of cholesteryl sulfate in human spermatozoa in support of a hypothesis for the mechanism of capacitation, Proc. Natl. Acad. Sci. U.S.A., 78:7266.

Lenz, R.W., Ball, G.D., Leibfried, M.L., Ax, R.L., and First, N.L., 1983, In vitro maturation and fertilization of bovine oocytes are temperature-dependant processes, Biol. Reprod., 29:173.

Llanos, M.N., Lui, C.W., and Meizel, S., 1982, Studies of phospholipase A_2 related to the hamster sperm acrosome reaction, J. Exp. Zool., 221:107.

Lopata, A., McMaster, R., McBain, J.C., and Johnston, W.I.H., 1978, In vitro fertilization of preovulatory human eggs, J. Reprod. Fert., 52:339.

Lopata, A., Johnston, I.W.H., Hoult, I.J., and Speirs, A.I., 1980, Pregnancy following intrauterine implantation of an embryo obtained by in vitro fertilization of a preovulatory egg, Fertil. Steril., 33:117.

Lui, C.W., and Meizel, S., 1977, Biochemical studies of the in vitro acrosome reaction inducing activity of bovine serum albumin, Differentiation, 9:59.

Lui, C.W., and Meizel, S., 1979, Further evidence in support of a role for hamster sperm hydrolytic enzymes in the acrosome reaction, J. Exp. Zool., 207:173.

Lui, C.W., Cornett, L.E., and Meizel, S., 1977, Identification of the bovine follicular fluid protein involved in the in vitro induction of the hamster sperm acrosome reaction, Biol. Reprod., 17:34.

Mahi, C.A., and Yanagimachi, R., 1973, The effects of temperature, osmolality, and hydrogen ion concentration on the activation and acrosome reaction of golden hamster spermatozoa, J. Repro. Fert., 35:55.

Mahi, C.A., and Yanagimachi, R., 1978, Capacitation, acrosome reaction, and egg penetration by canine spermatozoa in a simple defined media, Gamete Res., 1:101.

McMaster, R., Yanagimachi, R., and Lopata, A., 1978, Penetration of human eggs by human spermatozoa in vitro, Biol. Reprod., 19:212.

McRorie, R.A., and Williams, W.L., 1974, Biochemistry of mammalian fertilization, Ann. Rev. Biochem., 43:777.

Meizel, S., 1978, The mammalian sperm acrosome reaction, a biochemical approach, in: "Development in Mammals," Vol. 3, M. H. Johnson, ed., North-Holland, Amsterdam.

Mettler, L., Baukloh, V., and Seki, M., 1982, Human in vitro fertilization and sperm immunological animal experiments, in: "Follicular Maturation and Ovulation," Exerpta Medica, Amsterdam.

Miyamoto, H., and Chang, M.C., 1973a, The importance of serum albumin and metabolic intermediates for capacitation of spermatozoa and fertilization of mouse eggs in vitro, J. Reprod. Fert., 32:193.

Miyamoto, H., and Chang, M.C., 1973b, Effect of osmolarity on fertilization of mouse and golden hamster eggs in vitro, J. Reprod. Fert., 33:481.

Miyamoto, H., Toyoda, Y., and Chang, M.C., 1974, Effect of hydrogen ion concentration on in vitro fertilization of mouse, golden hamster, and rat eggs, Biol. Reprod., 10:487.

Munemasa, K.H., Cash, M.K.M., and Rogers, B.J., 1983, Inhibition of human sperm penetration into zona-free hamster eggs by glucose and fructose, Biol. Reprod., 28, Suppl. 1:39a.

Myles, D.G., and Primakoff, P., 1983, A guinea pig sperm surface antigen that migrates during capacitation, Biol. Reprod., 28, Suppl. 1:70a.

Oliphant, G., 1976, Removal of sperm-bound seminal plasma components as a prerequisite to induction of the acrosome reaction, Fertil. Steril., 27:28.

Oliphant, G., and Brackett, B.G., 1973, Immunological assessment of surface changes of rabbit sperm undergoing capacitation, Biol. Reprod., 9:404.

Oliphant, G., and Eng, L.A., 1981, Collection of gametes in laboratory animals and preparation of sperm for in vitro fertilization, in: "Fertilization and Embryonic Development In Vitro," L. Mastroianni, Jr and J. D. Biggers, eds. Plenum Press, New York.

Oliphant, G., and Singhas, C.A., 1979, Iodination of rabbit sperm plasma membranes: Relationship of specific surface proteins to epididymal function and sperm capacitation, Biol. Reprod., 21:937.

O'Rand, M.G., 1977, Restriction of a sperm surface antigen's mobility during capacitation, Dev. Biol., 55:260.

Overstreet, J.W., Yanagimachi, R., Katz, D.F., Hayashi, K., and Hanson, F.W., 1980a, Penetration of human spermatozoa into the human zona pellucida and the zona-free hamster egg: a study of fertile donors and infertile patients, Fertil. Steril., 33:534.

Overstreet, J.W., and Hembree, W.D., 1976, Penetration of the zona pellucida of non-living human oocytes by human spermatozoa in vitro, Fertil. Steril., 27:815.

Overstreet, J.W., Gould, J.E., Katz, D.F., and Hanson, F.W., 1980b, In vitro capacitation of human spermatozoa after passage through a column of cervical mucus, Fertil. Steril., 34:604.

Perreault, S.D., and Rogers, B.J., 1981, Effects of various sugars on the time course of human spermatozoal capacitation in vitro, J. Androl., 2:22.

Perreault, S.D., and Rogers, B.J., 1982a, Capacitation pattern of human spermatozoa, Fertil. Steril., 38:258.

Perreault, S.D., and Rogers, B.J., 1982b, Relationship between fertilizing ability and cAMP in human spermatozoa, J. Androl., 3:396.

Pinsker, M.C., and Williams, W.L., 1968, Spermatozoan decapacitation factor in human seminal plasma, Proc. Soc. Exp. Biol. Med., 129:446.

Plachot, M., Mandelbaum, J., Cohen, J., and Salat-Baroux, J., 1982, In vitro fertilization and embryo transfer in human during spontaneous cycles, in: "Follicular Maturation and Ovulation," Excerpta Medica, Amsterdam.

Purdy, J.M., 1982, Methods for fertilization and embryo culture in vitro, in: "Human Conception In Vitro," R.G. Edwards and J.M. Purdy, eds., Academic Press, New York.

Quinn, P., Stanger, J.D., and Whittingham, D.G., 1982, Effect of albumin on fertilization of mouse ova in vitro, Gamete Res., 6:305.

Reddy, J.M., Stark, R.A., and Zaneveld, L.J.D., 1979, A high molecular weight anti-fertility factor from human seminal plasma, J. Reprod. Fert., 57:437.

Reddy, J.M., Audhya, T.K., Goodpasture, J.C., and Zaneveld, L.J.D., 1982, Properties of a highly purified antifertility factor from human seminal plasma, Biol. Reprod., 27:1076.

Reyes, A., Goicoechea, B., and Rosado, A., 1978, Calcium ion requirement for rabbit spermatozoal capacitation and enhancement of fertilizing ability by ionophore A23187 and cyclic adenosine 3': 5'-monophosphate, Fertil. Steril., 29:451.

Rogers, B.J., 1978, Mammalian sperm capacitation and fertilization in vitro: a critique of methodology, Gamete Res., 1:165.

Rogers, B.J., and Yanagimachi, R., 1975, Retardation of guinea pig sperm acrosome reaction by glucose: the possible importance of pyruvate and lactate metabolism in capacitation and the acrosome reaction, Biol. Reprod., 13:568.

Rogers, B.J., Chang, L., and Yanagimachi, R., 1979a, Glucose effect on respiration: possible mechanism for capacitation in guinea pig spermatozoa, J. Exp. Zool., 207:107.

Rogers, B.J., Perreault, S.D., Bentwood, B.J., McCarville, C., Hale, R.W., and Soderdahl, D.W., 1983, Variability in the human-hamster in vitro assay for fertility evaluation, Fertil. Steril., 39:204.

Rogers, B.J., Van Campen, H., Ueno, M., Lambert, H., Bronson, R., and Hale, R., 1979b, Analysis of human spermatozoal fertilizing ability using zona-free ova, Fertil. Steril., 32:664.

Rufo, Jr., G.A., Singh, J.P., Babcock, D.F., and Lardy, H.A., 1983, Purification and characterization of a calcium transport inhibitor protein from bovine seminal plasma, J. Biol. Chem., 257:4627.

Russell, L., Peterson, R.N., and Freund, M., 1979, Morphological characteristics of the chemically induced acrosome reaction in human spermatozoa, Fertil. Steril., 32:87.

Saling, P.M., Storey, B.T., and Wolf, D.P., 1978, Calcium-dependant binding of mouse epididymal spermatozoa to the zona pellucida, Dev. Biol., 65:515.

Soupart, P., and Strong, P.A., 1974, Ultrastructural observations on human oocytes fertilized in vitro, Fertil. Steril., 25:11.

Stambaugh, R., 1978, Enzymatic and morphological events in mammalian fertilization, Gamete Res., 1:65.

Talbot, P., and Chacon, R.S., 1980, A new procedure for rapidly scoring acrosome reactions of human sperm, Gamete Res., 3:211.

Talbot, P., and Chacon, R.S., 1981, A triple stain technique for evaluating normal acrosome reactions of human sperm, J. Exp. Zool., 215:201.

Talbot, P., and Chacon, R.S., 1982, Ultrastructural observations on binding and membrane fusion between human sperm and zona pellucida-free hamster oocytes, Fertil. Steril., 37:240.

Tash, J.S., and Means, A.R., 1983, Cyclic adenosine 3', 5' monophosphate, calcium, and protein phosphorylation in flagellar motility, Biol. Reprod., 28:75.

Testart, J., Lassalle, B., and Frydman, R., 1982, Success of human in vitro fertilization in spontaneous or stimulated cycles and technical procedures used, in: "Follicular Maturation and Ovulation," Excerpta Medica, Amsterdam.

Testart, J., Lassalle, B., Frydman, R., and Belaisch, J.C., 1983, A study of factors affecting the success of human fertilization in vitro. II. Influence of semen quality and oocyte maturity on fertilization and cleavage, Biol. Reprod., 28:425.

Toyoda, Y., and Chang, M.C., 1974, Fertilization of rat eggs in vitro by epididymal sperm and the development of eggs following transfer, J. Reprod. Fert., 36:9.

Triana, L.R., Babcock, D.F., Lorton, S.P., First, N.L., and Lardy, H.A., 1980, Release of acrosomal hyaluronidase follows increased membrane permeability to calcium in the presumptive capacitation sequence for spermatozoa of the bovine and other mammalian species, Biol. Reprod., 23:47.

Trounson, A.O., Leeton, J.F., Wood, C., Webb, J., and Kovacs, G., 1980, The investigation of idiopathic infertility by in vitro fertilization, Fertil. Steril., 34:431.

Trounson, A.O., Mohr, L.R., Wood, C., and Leeton, J.F., 1982, Effect of delayed insemination on in vitro fertilization, culture and transfer of human embryos, J. Reprod. Fert., 64:285.

Tyler, J.P.P., Pryor, J.P., and Collins, W.P., 1981, Heterologous ovum penetration by human spermatozoa, J. Reprod. Fert., 63:499.

Van der Ven, H., Bhattacharyya, A.K., Binor, Z., Leto, S., and Zaneveld, L.J.D., 1982, Inhibition of human sperm capacitation by a high molecular weight factor from human seminal plasma, Fertil. Steril., 38:753.
Wolf, D.P., and Sokoloski, J.E., 1982, Characterization of the sperm penetration bioassay, J. Androl., 3:445.
Wolf, D.P., Sokoloski, J.E., Dandekar, P., and Bechtol, K.B., 1983, Characterization of human sperm surface antigens with monoclonal antibodies, Biol. Reprod., 29:713.
Wortham, Jr., J.W.E., Veeck, L.L., Witmyer, J., and Jones, Jr., H.W., 1983a, Vital initiation of pregnancy (VIP) using human menopausal gonadotropin and human chorionic gonadotropin ovulation induction: Phase I - 1981, Fertil. Steril., 39:785.
Wortham, Jr., J.W.E., Veeck, L.L., Witmyer, J., Sandow, B.A., and Jones, Jr, H.W., 1983b, Vital initiation of pregnancy (VIP) using human menopausal gonadotropin and human chorionic gonadotropin ovulation induction: Phase II-1981, Fertil. Steril., 40:170.
Yanagimachi, R., 1969, In vitro acrosome reaction and capacitation of golden hamster spermatozoa by bovine follicular fluid and its fractions, J. Exp. Zool., 170:269.
Yanagimachi, R., 1970, In vitro capacitation of golden hamster spermatozoa by homologous and heterologous blood sera, Biol. Reprod., 3:147.
Yanagimachi, R., 1972a, Penetration of guinea pig spermatozoa into hamster eggs in vitro, J. Reprod. Fert., 28:477.
Yanagimachi, R., 1972b, Fertilization of guinea pig eggs in vitro, Anat. Rec. 174:9.
Yanagimachi, R., 1977, Specificity of sperm-egg interaction, in: "Immunobiology of Gametes" M.H. Johnson and M. Edidin, eds., Cambridge University Press, London.
Yanagimachi, R., 1978, Calcium requirement for sperm-egg fusion in mammals, Biol. Reprod. 19:949.
Yanagimachi, R, 1981, Mechanisms of fertilization im mammals, in: "Fertilization and Embryonic Development In Vitro," L. Mastroianni, Jr. and J. D. Biggers, eds., Plenum Press, New York.
Yanagimachi, R., and Usui, N., 1974, Calcium dependance of the acrosome reaction and activation of guinea pig spermatozoa, Exp. Cell Res., 89:161.
Yanagimachi, R., Lopata, A., Odom, C.B., Bronson, R.A., Mahi, C.A., and Nicolson, G.L., 1979, Retention of biological characteristics of zona pellucida in highly concentrated salt solution: The use of salt-stored eggs for assessing the fertilizing capacity of spermatozoa, Fertil. Steril., 31:562.
Yanagimachi, R., Yanagimachi, H., and Rogers, B.J., 1976, The use of zona-free animal ova as a test-system for the assessment of the fertilizing capacity of human spermatozoa, Biol. Reprod., 15:471.

12

OOGENESIS, FERTILIZATION AND EARLY DEVELOPMENT

William Byrd and Don P. Wolf

The study of mammalian reproduction to date has led to an appreciation of some of the diverse fundamental processes and events associated with gamete maturation, fertilization and embryonic development. In this chapter, we will discuss both theoretical and practical aspects of these subjects limiting our attention to the human as much as possible.

OOGENESIS AND FOLLICULAR GROWTH - AN OVERVIEW

Before the discharge of a mature fertilizable oocyte at ovulation, a prolonged developmental sequence in both the oocyte and the follicle must occur. Oocytes enter into the prophase stage of the first meiotic division during development of the fetal ovary between the fourth and seventh month of gestation. Unless the follicle undergoes atresia, the oocytes are suspended in diplotene of the first meiotic division for years until recruited during the reproductive cycle. A model depicting the developmental sequence described below is presented in Figure 1. Several million oocytes are formed in the fetal ovary, but this number is reduced by atresia to 100,000 to 400,000 at puberty of which only approximately 400 are ever ovulated (Baker, 1972; Edwards, 1977, 1980; Chapter 5). The human immature oocyte at the primordial follicle stage is approximately 50-70 um in diameter (Baca and Zamboni, 1967). It develops a large prominant nucleus or germinal vesicle containing the chromosomes in the diplotene stage (also referred to as the dictyate or diffuse diplotene stage). Throughout the reproductive life of the female,

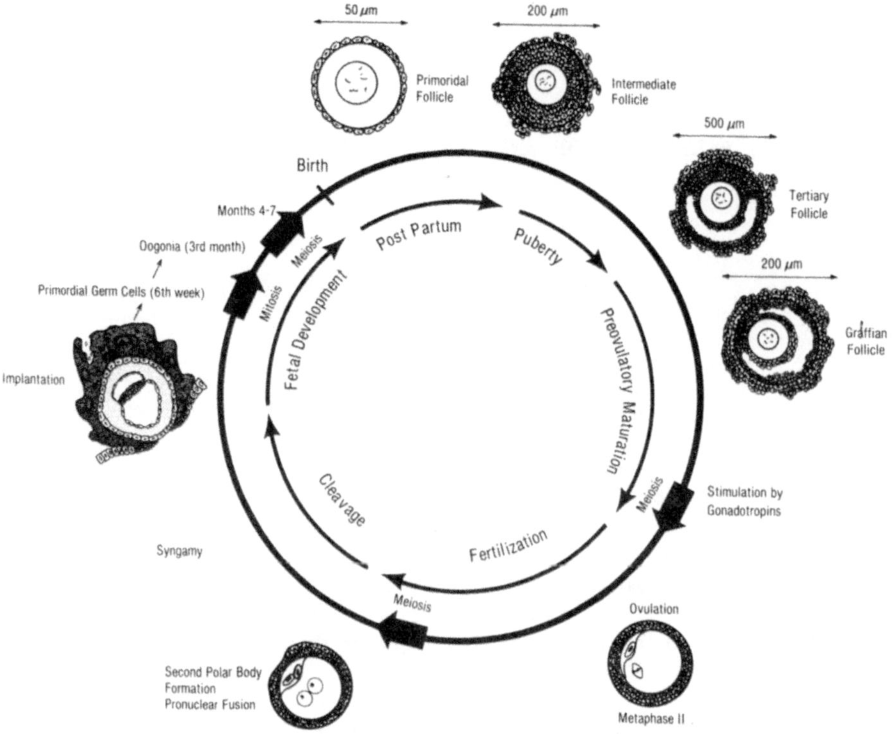

Figure 1

Oocyte maturation cycle

recruitment into actively growing follicles occurs from the pool of primordial follicles, independent of gonadotropin influence (Fritz and Speroff, 1982). During follicular growth, mitotic activity of the single layer of follicular cells surrounding the oocyte results in an increase to 3-5 cell layers. The outermost layers of follicular cells, apposed to the basement membrane which underlies the theca interna, comprise most of the granulosa cells in the maturing intermediate follicle (Figure 1). Granulosa cells surrounding the oocyte will form the cumulus oophorus. A deposition of material between the oocyte and the innermost follicular cells occurs forming the zona pellucida. This acellular layer of glycoproteins is initially discontinuous when laid down, but eventually forms a layered-porus structure (Stegner and Wartenberg, 1961; Dunbar, 1983). Processes from the surrounding granulosa or cumulus cells project or pass through the zona to form junctional complexes with the oocyte plasma membrane (Baca and Zamboni, 1967; Zamboni, 1971; Anderson, 1974; Anderson and Albertini, 1976; Szollosi and Gerard, 1983). Gap junctions between the cumulus cells and the plasma membrane of the oocyte provide a mechanism for regulating oocyte maturation by mediating passage of small molecules (Gilula et al., 1972). Since the membrana granulosa (cumulus oophorus) has no blood supply, the transport of hormones and nutrients and cell-cell communication between the cumulus and oocyte presumably occur through the gap junctions (Meck et al., 1973; Albertini et al., 1975; Amsterdam et al., 1976; Brower and Schultz, 1982). There is a highly significant contribution of nutrients to the oocyte from the granulosa cells suggesting metabolic cooperativity between these two cell types which supports oocyte growth (Heller et al., 1981).

The development of the mature graffian follicle containing the preovulatory oocyte is under strict gonadotrophic hormone control (Fritz and Speroff, 1982; Chapter 5). In each cycle approximately 20 to 50 follicles are recruited and enter into the secondary FSH dependent stage of development, but only three or fewer reach a size of 8 mm by midcycle at the time of ovulation. With each cycle of follicular recruitment, there are successive peaks of estrogen signaling the emergence of the dominant follicle. High levels of circulating estrogen in turn feedback to the pituitary and induce an LH surge.

Concomitant with the LH surge, meiosis is resumed and the oocyte enters diakinesis forming the first metaphase spindle (Edwards, 1965a,b; Mastroianni and Noriega, 1970; Steptoe and Edwards, 1970; Suzuki and Izuka, 1970). Due to the eccentric position of the metaphase spindle, one daughter cell will receive a disproportionate amount of the cytoplasm and become the first polar body upon completion of the first meiotic division. The oocyte rapidly begins the second meiotic division and arrests again at second metaphase prior to ovulation in most mammalian species. In addition to the morphological changes accompanying meiotic maturation, a decrease in metabolic activity occurs reflecting the termination of gap junctions (Schultz et al., 1978; Heller and Schultz, 1980). Resumption of meiotic maturation with the formation of the second polar body is dependent upon fertilization. If fertilization does not occur within a few hours following ovulation, the oocyte will degenerate (Edwards, 1980).

In response to the LH surge, cumulus cells transform into columnar shaped cells while their cellular processes retract from the perivitelline space and the zona pellucida (Eppig, 1979; Edwards, 1980). Disruption of gap junctions between these cells and the oocyte signals not only the resumption of meiosis but also a migration of cortical granules from the subcortical cytoplasm to the extreme periphery of the oocyte cortex. This process, referred to as cortical maturation, is important for subsequent events of fertilization (Szollosi and Gerard, 1983). The LH surge also triggers luteinization of granulosa cells, vacuolation and vascularization of the theca with an increase in antral fluid (liquor folliculi), the synthesis of prostaglandins and the initiation of other processes essential to follicular rupture (Fritz and Speroff, 1982).

With the resumption of meiosis, expansion and/or mucification of the cumulus is induced with a continuous accumulation of fluid in the antral chamber due to the secretory activity of the granulosa cells. This process causes a separation of the oocyte-cumulus mass from the follicular wall such that the complex is free-floating in the antrum of the follicle prior to ovulation (Peters and McNatty, 1980). The cumulus cells are embedded in a matrix of glycosaminoglycans and expansion is due to secretion of hyaluronic acid into this matrix. Before the LH surge in humans, the density of cumulus cells in this matrix is approximately 1.3 x 10^6 cells/mm^3. Following the LH peak, when the oocyte has arrested in the second meiotic metaphase awaiting ovulation, the cell density is less than 1 x 10^5 cells/mm^3, a tenfold decrease in density (Testart et al., 1982). In the mouse, this process *in vitro* is FSH, not LH, dependent (Eppig, 1979). Further work by Eppig (1981) suggests that prostaglandin PGE_2 may play an indirect role in the stimulation of cumulus expansion *in vivo*. Following ovulation, two to three layers of cumulus cells remain tightly adherent to the zona pellucida surrounding the oocyte and are referred to as the corona radiata.

PREOVULATORY OOCYTE MATURATION IN VIVO AND *IN VITRO*

In primates, oocytes are normally ovulated and fertilized at the second metaphase of meiosis (Longo, 1973). When oocytes in diplotene, liberated from the follicular environment, are maintained under appropriate culturing conditions, most will resume meiosis and a varied number of them will spontaneously mature. Maturation of these oocytes to the second metaphase occurs irrespective of the stage of follicular development from which they are released thus effectively separating meiotic maturation from folliculogenesis and ovulation. In the rabbit, oocytes mature *in vitro* at a rate similar to that *in vivo*, i.e., in a graafian follicle stimulated with gonadotropins (Chang, 1955). Pioneering work on maturation of human oocytes *in vitro* was begun in 1939 by Pincus and Sanders, while in recent times Edwards (1965a,b) is credited with extensive efforts to mature and fertilize ovarian oocytes. Based on studies of Edwards and several other investigators (Table 1), it is apparent that the culturing of human oocytes leads to a highly variable number of oocytes (8-73%) that spontaneously mature in vitro. In immature oocytes the stimulus to resume meiosis occurs with the liberation of the oocyte from the follicle; thus, if oocytes are cultured in vitro within intact follicles, meiotic maturation does not occur (Edwards, 1962).

While it is thought that preovulatory maturation, which is restricted to the dominant follicle, is induced by the preovulatory surge of LH, the mechanism is poorly understood. As indicated above, it has been suggested that termination of intercellular communication with the cumulus cells causes resumption of meiosis (Gilula et al., 1977). An equally plausible mechanism is that the reinitiation of meiosis reflects changes in follicular inhibitory factors (Tsafriri et al., 1976; Channing et al., 1983). A correlation between changes in oocyte maturation inhibitor in human preovulatory follicles and oocyte maturation and fertilizability was recently reported by Channing et al. (1983). They measured porcine oocyte maturation in follicular fluid recovered from patients undergoing IVF-ET and demonstrated that oocyte maturation in the IVF patient was associated with a decline in oocyte maturation inhibitor and an increase in estrogen in follicular fluid. These data suggest that decreasing oocyte maturation inhibitor and increasing estrogen may be responsible for oocyte maturation and rule out estrogen as a possible oocyte inhibitory factor as suggested by McGaughey (1977). In support of a role for estrogen in maturation, Jones et al. (1983) have presented evidence that the absolute level plus the pattern of the circulating E_2 response during follicular maturation has a critical influence on subsequent pregnancy rates. This could be due to variation in oocyte maturity or it could be mediated through an influence on the luteal phase. Lopata (1983) also suggests that the magnitude of the E_2 response influences fertilization but not the pregnancy rate.

In vitro, the composition of culturing media may influence maturation as well, as the addition of LH, estradiol or PGE increases the proportion of oocytes maturing while other components are inhibitory (Jagiello et al., 1975). Because of the limited success of in vitro meiotic maturation of immature oocytes recovered at different undefined stages of maturation, in vitro fertilization protocols rely on preovulatory oocytes that are aspirated after intrafollicular maturation.

Table 1. Timing of human oocyte maturation *in vitro*

	Number of Oocytes[c]	Percent of Oocytes Reaching Metaphase II		
		Hours in Culture		
		0-24	24-35.9	36
Edwards, (1965)				
a unspecified medium	41	-	-	17.0
b Medium 199	91	3.1	3.0	73.0
Kennedy and Donahue (1969)				
Medium 199	49	-	-	40.8
Ham's F-10	38	-	-	50.0
Mastroianni and Noriega (1970)	63	-	-	36.5
Ham's F-10				(40-50 hrs)
Zamboni et al. (1972)	159		15.2	39.2
Ham's F-10			(<37 hrs)	
Chang (1971)				
Medium 199 + BSA	109	-	-	8.2
Medium 199 + Follicular Fluid	140	-	-	31.4
Suzuki et al. (1981)				
Ham's F-10	117	-	-	54.7
Nishimoto et al. (1982)				
Krebs-Ringer-bicarbonate	16	-	-	37.5
				(40 hrs)

c. Oocytes were obtained from ovaries irrespective of the phase of the menstrual cycle.

Timing of Ovulation in Natural and hCG Treated Cycles

Successful recovery of fertilizable oocytes requires precise timing of both oocyte and follicular maturation since variation exists from cycle to cycle, even in the same patient. However, the introduction of follicular recruitment and ovulatory agents such as hMG, clomiphene citrate and hCG combined with timed laparoscopies has made the collection of mature preovulatory oocytes routine. In most in vitro fertilization programs where hCG is used to induce pre-ovulatory maturation, oocytes are recovered 35-36 hours after injection (Lopata et al., 1980; Trounson et al., 1981a). This timing is based on the observation that less than 5% of patients ovulate within 35-37 hours of hCG administration; this value increases to 35-42% by 37-39 hours (Edwards 1977; Testart et al., 1982b).

In natural or spontaneous cycles, ovulation normally occurs approximately 28-32 hours after the onset of the LH surge (Garcia et al., 1981) and follicular aspiration is performed anywhere from 18 to 28 hours later (Edwards, 1975; Steptoe et al., 1980; Garcia et al., 1981; Trounson et al., 1981a). As can be seen in Table 1 in vitro meiotic maturation of oocytes requires at least 36 hours between recovery and metaphase II (Edwards et al., 1970; Seibel et al., 1982). This is several hours longer than the interval between LH surge and follicular rupture, suggesting that oocyte maturation is initiated before the peak in circulating levels of LH is reached, probably at the time of the initial serum LH increase (Seibel et al., 1982; Zeilmaker and Alberda, 1982).

Maturation of the Immature Oocyte

Oocytes are usually mature when aspirated 18-28 hours after the LH surge in spontaneous cycles. When exogenous hormonal stimulation of the follicular cycle is used, oocytes of varied maturity are recovered (Testart et al., 1983a). Recovery of immature oocytes (i.e., those oocytes which have not undergone germinal vesicle breakdown) during laparoscopy necessitates a prolonged maturation in vitro. Insemination of immature oocytes which have not completed preovulatory meiotic maturation is characterized by a reduced fertilizability perhaps reflecting a spontaneous or premature release of cortical granules (Rosseau et al., 1977). In immature oocytes that undergo sperm-egg fusion, at least two undesirable events may occur. First, the sperm nucleus may fail to decondense and/or transform into a pronucleus (Edwards et al., 1969; Iwamatsu and Chang, 1971; Barros and Munoz, 1973; Overstreet and Hembree, 1976; Usui and Yanagimachi, 1976). Second, the oocyte may become polyspermic due to an incomplete maturation of cortical granules (Sathananthan and Trounson,

1982b). Immature oocytes have been matured in culture and fertilized with some success (Edwards et al., 1969; Thibault, 1972, 1977; Soupart and Morgenstern, 1973; Veeck and Garcia, 1983; Veeck et al., 1983) and upon transfer have resulted in pregnancy (Veeck et al., 1983).

OOCYTE RECOVERY AND CLASSIFICATION

Evaluation of oocyte maturity is based on the morphology of the cumulus mass, the surrounding corona cells and the presence of a germinal vesicle or polar body (when the ooplasm can be visualized). Classification is crucial since immature oocytes will require prolonged maturation *in vitro* before insemination. Mature oocytes are surrounded by large, macroscopic masses containing dispersed cumulus cells embedded in a matrix of glycosaminoglycans. The oocyte and its zona pellucida are enclosed by the corona radiata (Figure 2A,B). It is not possible to determine accurately the state of oocyte maturity based on cumulus dispersion. However, the degree of cumulus expansion is related to the follicular recruitment program used (Testart et al., 1983a). Greater than 90% of oocytes aspirated from spontaneous cycles display a fully expanded cumulus (grade ++; Testart et al., 1983a) compared to only 50% in oocytes aspirated following clomiphene citrate or hMG stimulation.

Aspiration of small follicles with an external diameter of 8-15 mm may result in the recovery of immature oocytes. These immature cells are characterized by the absence of a cumulus mass and the presence of several layers of tightly adhering granulosa cells (Figure 2C; grade "0", Testart et al., 1983a). Immature oocytes, usually present with a "tight" zona pellucida, i.e., with no apparent perivitelline space compared to mature eggs. The germinal vesicle in these oocytes is intact, but may be difficult to observe due to adhering granulosa cells. After culturing for 24 to 30 hours, the adherent cells dislodge and spread out over the surrounding surface and it is possible to confirm the presence or absence of a germinal vesicle. Germinal vesicle breakdown should occur during this time interval with, in some cases, the formation of the first polar body (Figure 2D).

Oocyte recovery rates for IVF-ET are dependent upon several factors including, but not restricted to, ovarian access, follicular size and operator skill. Success rates as a function of the follicular recruitment protocol employed in our IVF-ET program from 7-81 to 7-83 are presented in Table 2. The rationale for attempting different recruitment protocols was to maximize the number of recoverable, fertilizable oocytes and to evaluate the advantages and disadvantages of each protocol (Chapters 6 and 7). Depending upon the follicular recruitment regimen used, recovery rates ranged from 54.1% to 95.2%. In clomiphene citrate stimulated cycles (150 or 50 mg/day, days 5-9; Table 2), our rates were somewhat lower than those reported by other laboratories using similar protocols which may reflect our tendency to attempt aspiration of smaller follicles (Table 3). In contrast, our recoveries in hMG treated cycles were higher than those reported by other laboratories using hMG (Table 3). Our hMG treatment consisted of 4 ampules per day (1 amp contains 75 I.U. FSH and 75 I.U. LH), from day 3 until the day before hCG administration with hCG given on the day that at least 2 follicles, 16 mm or greater were present as determined by ultrasound. In hMG treated cycles, 7 out of 19 patients had "polyovular" follicles. Following aspiration two oocytes were recovered from each of seven follicles, three from each of three follicles and five from each of two follicles. The recovery of supernumerary oocytes accounts for the higher recovery rate in the hMG group. These "polyovular" follicles may well have resulted from simultaneous aspiration of several closely apposed smaller follicles. On a few occasions, as many as three oocytes have been found in the same cumulus mass suggesting that either the cumulus masses from three small follicles became interspersed during aspiration or that they originated from a true polyovular follicle. Similar observations of "polyovular" follicles were reported by Steptoe and Edwards (1970) who noted occasional aspiration of two or more oocytes from one follicle after hMG stimulation. Evidence has been cited by Jones (1968) that exogenous gonadotrophin stimulation may induce the inclusion of more than one oocyte in a follicle resulting in a "polyovular" follicle. Based on the results summarized in Table 3, oocyte recovery rates in clomiphene citrate stimulated patients are high, comparable with the spontaneous cycle while in hMG treatment cycles rates drop slightly. This may simply reflect differences in follicular size in the two cases.

The treatment regimen used in follicular stimulation also will influence the degree of maturity of the recovered oocytes. We have recovered populations of oocytes in which as many as 14% of the oocytes were immature (clomiphene citrate, 50 mg; Table 2). Similiarly, Testart et al. (1983a) classified 19-22% as immature following follicular recruitment with clomiphene citrate or hMG, but only 5% of the oocytes recovered from spontaneous cycles were immature. In an early study using clomiphene citrate, Lopata et al. (1978a) reported 41% of the oocytes recovered were non-ovulatory or immature, and with hMG stimulation, 16% of the oocytes aspirated were classified as immature (Wortham et al., 1983).

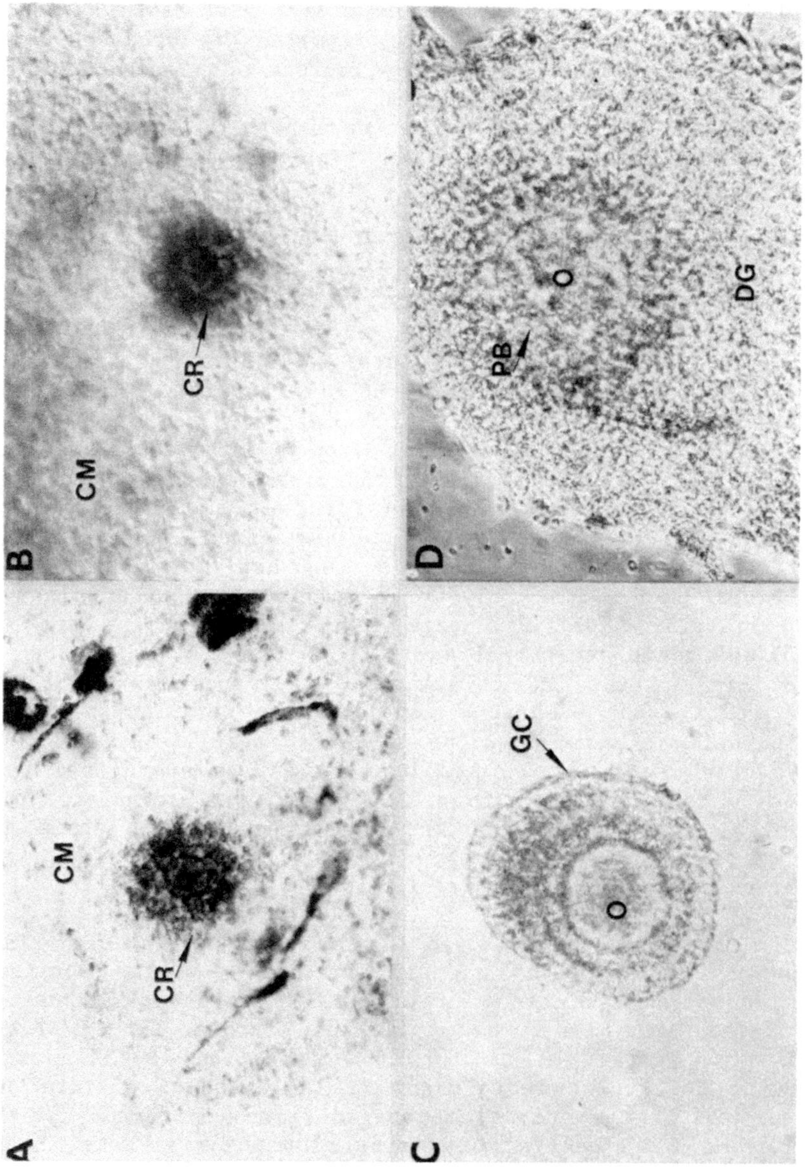
A
CM
CR
B
CM
CR
C
GC
O
D
PB
O
DG

Figure 2

Light microscopy of human ovarian oocytes; A) a preovulatory oocyte aspirated from a 20mm follicle following follicular recruitment with hMG; B) a preovulatory oocyte recovered from a 21mm follicle after clomiphene citrate stimulation (50mg/day); C) an Immature oocyte aspirated from a 12mm follicle and D) the immature oocyte from Figure 2C after culturing for 24 hours. Legends: CR = corona radiata; CM = cumulus mass; O = oocyte; GC = granulosa cells; PB = polar body; DG = dispersed granulosa. Magnification: 2A,B = 19X, 2C,D = 47X.

Table 2. Summary of oocyte recovery and classification results for the U.T. Houston IVF-ET Program

Follicular Recruitment Protocol	Number Patients Undergoing Laparoscopy	Number Follicles Aspirated	Number Eggs Recovered	Percent Egg Recovery	Number Eggs (Total) Mature	Number Eggs (Total) Immature	Percent Mature
Clomiphene Citrate (150mg)[b]	39	120 (3.07±1.34)[a]	65 (1.76±1.15)	54.1%	65	0	100.0%
Clomiphene Citrate (50mg)[b]	89	252 (2.79±1.05	149 (1.71±1.05)	59.1%	128	21	85.9%
Clomiphene Citrate + hMG[c]	18	103 (4.77±2.04)	64 (3.0 ±1.71)	62.1%	56	8	87.5%
hMG[d]	19	85 (4.47±2.22)	81 (4.36±2.85)	95.2%	74	7	91.3%

a = mean ± S.D.
b = clomiphene citrate; cycle days 5–9
c = clomiphene citrate; cycle days 5–9, hMG 2 amps/day, days 6,8,10; 1 amp hMG = 75 I.U. FSH and 75 I.U. LH
d = hMG; 4 amps day, cycle day 3 until day before hCG

Table 3. Summary of oocyte recovery rates for various IVF-ET programs

Type of Cycle	Reference	Number Follicles Aspirated	Number Eggs Recovered	Egg Recovery %
Spontaneous	Edwards, 1981	109	95	87
	Mettler et al., 1981	18	11	61
	Johnston et al., 1981	62	36	58
	Testart et al., 1983a	27	21	78
Clomiphene Citrate				
(50-100mg)	Renou et al., 1981	54	35	65
(50-100mg)	Trounson et al., 1981	31	25	81
(100-150mg)	Lopata, 1983			
	Data from 1980	211	157	74
	1981	684	512	75
	1982	590	369	63
(150mg)	Testart et al., 1983a	188	130	69
Clomiphene Citrate/hMG (50-100mg C+hMG)	Lopata, 1983	1336	1009	76
hMG	Edwards et al., 1980	-	45	66(per patient)
	Mettler et al., 1982	217	88	41
	Testart et al., 1983	58	31	53
	Jones et al., 1983	771	526	68

FERTILIZATION: AN OVERVIEW

The fundamentals of fertilization of mammalian oocytes *in vitro* have been studied extensively; however, detailed mechanisms *in humans* remain unknown. Fertilization is a multi-step process with many interrelated steps (Figures 3 and 4). Information will be included from both *in vivo* and *in vitro* studies where instructive i.e., to help clarify the sequence of events. A review of sperm capacitation is presented in Chapter 11.

The first reported fertilization of human oocytes *in vitro* was published in 1944 by Rock and Menkin (also Menkin and Rock, 1948). Several other early claims of human *in vitro* fertilization resulting in cleavage should also be cited (Shettles, 1955; Hyashi, 1963). Because unfertilized ova can fragment or activate and cleave parthenogenetically these early reports are considered inaccurate by many (Mastroianni and Noriega, 1970; Blandau, 1980). The first unequivocal IVF-ET success was the birth of baby Louise Brown reported by Steptoe and Edwards (1978), soon followed by successes in Australia by Lopata et al., (1980), and Trounson et al. (1981 a,b). The cumulative effect of these successes resulted in the acceptance of IVF-ET as a treatment for infertility in humans.

Sperm Transport

Sperm can reach the oviduct within five minutes of coitus, a rate that far exceeds their swimming speed (Settledge et al., 1973). Sperm transport in women above the endocervix is largely passive, dependent upon the muscular activity of the reproductive tract (Alhgren, 1981). Overstreet and Tom (1982) have demonstrated that non-motile sperm are transported to the oviducts within 15 minutes following insemination in rabbits. They suggest that seminal plasma contributes indirectly to the initial transport by stimulating vaginal contractions and that in the uterus sympathetic control may facilitate transport. However, not all sperm are transported to the oviducts. The cervix and the uterotubal junction constitute sperm reserviors from which slow release can occur over prolonged time periods (Hafez, 1975). Sperm may retain their fertilizing capability for as long as 120 hours (Ferin et al., 1973), thus extending the possible time between coitus and fertilization.

Penetration of the Cumulus Mass

The ovulated oocyte is surrounded by a mass of cumulus cells embedded in a matrix of hyaluronic acid (Piko, 1969; Figure 2). One function of the cumulus mass and associated hyaluronic acid is

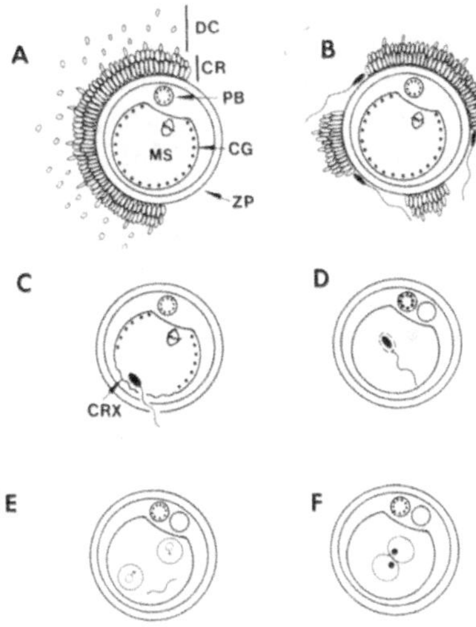

Figure 3

Schematic representation of the successive steps in fertilization of the human oocyte; A) Preovulatory oocyte with associated cumulus (DC) and corona radiata cells (CR), the oocyte is in the second meiotic metaphase with one polar body (PB); B) following insemination and dispersion of the cumulus cells, sperm bind to the zona pellucida (ZP); C) the sperm undergoes the acrosome reaction, penetrates the zona, fuses with the egg plasma membrane and enters the ooplasm. Fusion initiates the cortical reaction (CRX) at the site of sperm penetration which then spreads around the oocyte surface. Extruded contents of the egg cortical granules induced a zona reaction which helps prevent additional sperm penetration; D) extrusion of the 2nd polar body and sperm head decondensation; E) formation of pronuclei and F) central migration of pronuclei. Fertilization is completed at syngamy when the pronuclear membranes breakdown and the maternal and paternal chromosomes intermingle in preparation for the first mitotic division.

to aid in transport of the egg to the ampulla (Blandau, 1969, 1971). The fimbria of the oviduct is closely apposed to the surface of the ovary and, at midcycle, fimbrial cilia sweep the ovarian surface. If an ovulated oocyte is present, it is carried from the ovary into the ampulla.

The precise role of the cumulus in fertilization is unknown. The presence of the cumulus mass is neither necessary to nor a prerequisite for fertilization as cumulus-free oocytes have been fertilized in vivo (Moore and Bedford, 1978) or in vitro in several mammals (Yanagimachi, 1977, 1981). The fertility of these eggs compared to controls is somewhat lower; thus, the cumulus may play a minor role perhaps by enhancing sperm capacitation or the acrosome reaction. In the human it has been suggested, but not documented, that the cumulus assists in in vitro fertilization (Soupart and Morgenstern, 1973).

Sperm penetration of the cumulus and dissolution of the matrix is aided by hyaluronidase and possibly other sperm acrosomal enzymes (Bradford et al., 1976; Zaneveld, 1976;). Hyaluronidase acts by depolymerizing the hyaluronic acid matrix. Indirect evidence that hyaluronidase is required for cumulus penetration includes the finding that antibodies raised against hyaluronidase, when added to insemination mixtures containing rabbit sperm and cumulus masses, block dispersion of the cumulus and sperm penetration (Dunbar et al., 1976). Moreover, a synthetic inhibitor of hyaluronidase (myocrisin) will block the in vitro fertilization of mouse oocytes with intact cumulus or follicle cells (Reddy et al., 1979). If the cumulus cells are removed, myocrisin treated sperm will penetrate suggesting that the specific action of this enzyme is on sperm penetration of the cumulus. At the same myocrisin concentration, there is apparently no effect on motility or the acrosome reaction in guinea pig sperm (Reddy et al., 1979). Myocrisin has no effect on human acrosin in vitro suggesting it is specific for hyaluronidase (Reddy et al., 1979).

In view of the apparent dispersal of the cumulus by sperm acrosomal hyaluronidase, the question arises as to when and where the acrosome reaction occurs that results in the release of this activity. It has been proposed that the initial step in sperm-egg interaction in mammals is a loose attachment between the zona pellucida and the sperm head which precedes a much tighter binding to the zona (Hartmann et al., 1972; Hartmann, 1983). A number of studies indicate that an intact acrosome is essential for binding; however, the state of the sperm acrosome at the time of binding is somewhat controversial and is species specific (Gwatkin, 1977; Green, 1978; Meizel, 1978; Dale and Monroy, 1981). In the mouse

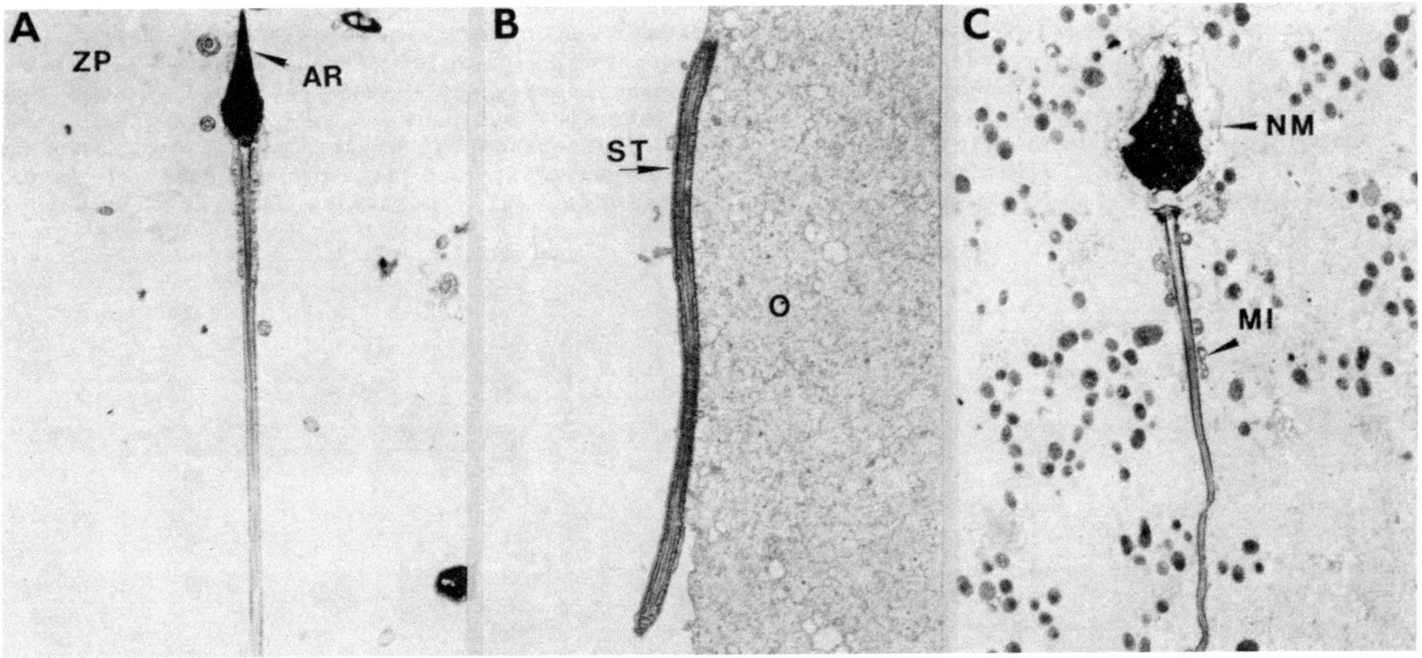

Figure 4 A, B & C

Ultrastructure of the fertilization process in human ova inseminated *in vitro*; A) A spermatozoan which has undergone the acrosome reaction (AR) in the zona pellucida (ZP) Mag = 3900X; B) Incorporation of the sperm tail (ST) into the oocyte (O) of a Zona-free oocyte. Mag = 1200X (reprinted with permission, Soupart and Strong, 1975); C) Decondensation of the sperm pronucleus in the ooplasm with the breakdown of the nuclear membrane (NM). Mitochondria are being discarded from the midpiece of the flagella. Mag = 7800X;

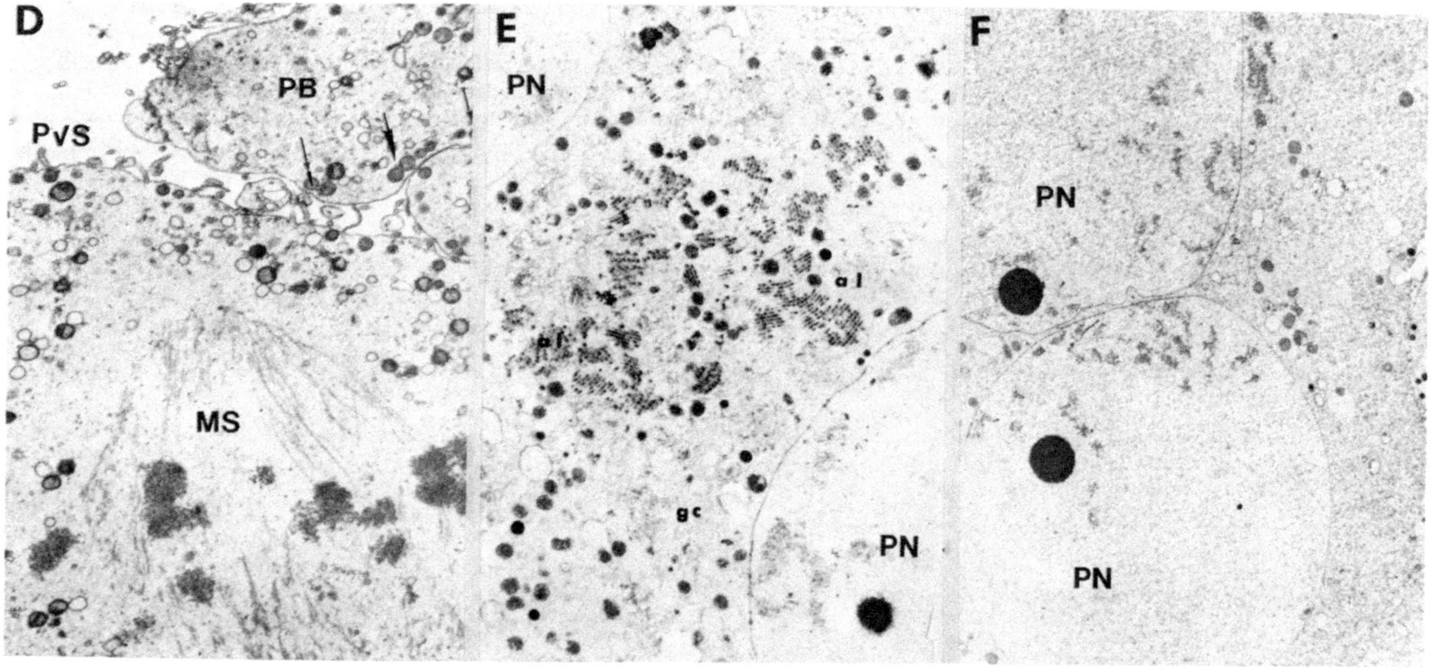

D) Second polar body formation. The first polar body (PB) with its cortical granules (see arrows) is apparent in the perivitelline space. The mitotic spindle (MS) of the second metaphase is perpendicular to the oocyte surface. Mag = 3900X; E) Migration of male and female sperm pronuclei. Stacks of annulate lamellae (AL) and Golgi complexes (GC) are seen between the advancing pronuclei. Mag = 6500X (reprinted with permission, Soupart and Strong, 1974) and F) Male and female pronuclei prior to syngamy and first cleavage. Mag = 4500X.

NOTE: These figures are from the Pierre Soupart Memorial Archives generously donated to the University of Texas Medical School by Mrs. P. Soupart.

(Saling and Storey, 1979; Saling et al., 1979; Florman and Storey, 1982; Bleil and Wassarman, 1983) and in the hamster, (Phillips and Shalgi, 1980) acrosome reacted sperm do not bind to the zona. In contrast to these findings, Huang et al. (1981) found that in the guinea pig, only acrosome reacted sperm bound to the zona. Yanagimachi (1981) has reported that both intact and reacted sperm bind to the zona pellucida in the hamster. In a later report, Cummins and Yanagimachi (1982) suggest that in the hamster in vivo acrosome reactions begin shortly before contact with the cumulus and are completed shortly before or after contact with the zona. This appears to be the case in the rabbit where sperm undergo the acrosome reaction while passing through the cumulus (Bedford, 1971, 1972). In humans (McMaster et al., 1978), intact spermatozoa may also be found attached to the zona.

One must ask what is the source of hyaluronidase if only intact sperm are present on the zona? Are there sperm which contact the cumulus, undergo the acrosome reaction and release hyaluronidase without reaching the surface of the oocyte? One possiblity is that sperm undergo an "intermediate" stage in the acrosome reaction where the plasma membrane is intact, but the outer acrosomal membrane vesiculates (Chapter 11, Figure 2B) permitting release of soluble acrosomal enzymes through pores in the plasma membrane. Early work by Talbot and Franklin (1974) demonstrated that hyaluronidase was liberated from hamster spermatozoa before acrosomal or plasma membrane vesiculation occurred. Evidence cited by Blandau (1980) suggests that uncapacitated rodent sperm can also cause dissolution of the cumulus mass. Thus, when epididymal sperm are added to freshly ovulated eggs, the cumulus masses are dispersed within a few minutes.

Binding to the Zona Pellucida

Following penetration of the cumulus, sperm bind to the surface of the zona pellucida, a glycoprotein coat surrounding the egg (Figures 3 and 4). The zona pellucida is an acellular envelope (approximately 5-15 um thick) secreted by the oocyte which provides a variety of functions during fertilization and preimplantation development before being shed prior to implantation. (Bleil and Wassarman, 1980a,b,c; Bousquet et al., 1981; Dunbar, 1983; Wassarman, 1983). The zona surface is characterized by a number of "holes" or fenestrations which appear rather irregular in size and shape when viewed by scanning electron microscopy (Gwatkin et al., 1976; Jackowski and Dumont, 1979; Phillips and Shalgi, 1980a). Biochemical analysis of zonae of pig, rabbit, human and mouse has shown that these layers are comprised predominantly of protein and carbohydrate with at least three major macromolecular components (Bleil and Wassarman, 1980b; Dunbar et al., 1980; Dunbar 1983; Sacco et al., 1983,).

Several lines of evidence suggest that sperm binding to the zona surface may be mediated by specific sperm receptors on or in the zona. Binding to the surface of the zona is relatively species specific (Hanada and Chang, 1972; Hartmann et al., 1972; Yanagimachi, 1977; Gwatkin and Williams, 1977; Schmell and Gulyas, 1980a) except in the rabbit (Bedford, 1977; Swenson and Dunbar, 1982) and is altered dramatically following fertilization (Gwatkin et al., 1973) without any corresponding dramatic ultrastructural change (Meyerhofer et al., 1977). Binding of sperm to the zona can be interferred with or blocked by treatment of the zona with proteases (Hartmann and Gwatkin, 1971) or lectins (Oikawa et al., 1973) which presumably alter or mask surface receptors. Again, there are species differences as sperm binding to the mouse zona is impervious to trypsin exposure (Inoue and Wolf, 1975). Binding to the zona in vivo and in vitro is also inhibited by pretreatment of the zona with antisera against whole eggs or ovaries (Shivers and Dudkiewicz, 1974; Mahi and Yanagimachi, 1979; Trounson et al., 1980b). Zona preparations from unfertilized eggs block sperm binding to hamster eggs whereas zona from fertilized oocytes are completely inactive (Gwatkin and Williams, 1977). The inner and outer surfaces of the zona also display different sperm binding characteristics. The inner layer of the mouse zona does not bind sperm in vitro (Phillips and Shalgi, 1980b) while binding occurs to both the inner and the outer surface of the hamster zona (Gwatkin and Williams, 1977).

The isolation of specific sperm receptors has been reported from hamster (Gwatkin, 1982) and mouse zonae (Bleil and Wassarman, 1980a,b, 1983). One of the three glycoproteins of the mouse zona ZP3, has been associated with sperm receptor activity and acrosome reaction induction. Fertilization modifies ZP3 so that it can no longer serve as a receptor (Bleil and Wassarman, 1983). The other two zona proteins, ZP1 and ZP2, have little effect on sperm binding or induction of the acrosome reaction but may play some role in the hardening reaction discussed below.

The Acrosome Reaction and Penetration of the Zona Pellucida

For sperm, a crucial step in fertilization is capacitation and induction of the acrosome reaction (Chapter 11) since both of these events are obligatory to penetration of oocyte investments and sperm-egg fusion. The apparent site of the acrosome reaction in humans is on or near the zona (Figure 3a). Ultrastructural studies have demonstrated that in human oocytes fertilized in vitro, 100% of the sperm located within the zona are acrosome reacted (McMaster et al., 1978). Moreover, there is an increase in the proportion of acrosome-reacted sperm that bind to the zona surface as compared to unbound sperm, and that proportion increases with the length of incubation. Following one hour of incubation approximately 10% of bound sperm showed a reaction which increased to 85% at three hours (McMaster et al., 1978). In the mouse, the binding and induction of the acrosome reaction has been characterized extensively. Earlier we discussed evidence that acrosome intact sperm bind to the surface of the mouse zona. Additional support for this conclusion comes from a study in which the acrosome reaction is inhibited by the cholinergic antagonist 3-quinuclidinyl benzilate (Florman and Storey, 1981). Inhibited sperm bind to the zona pellucida but they do not penetrate, thereby effectively separating zona binding from the acrosome reaction and zona penetration. Wassarman and coworkers clarified the molecular mechanisms of binding and induction of the acrosome reaction when they discovered that the zona glycoprotein ZP3, the sperm receptor, mediated both of these events (Bleil and Wassarman, 1983). Isolated ZP3 from unfertilized but not from fertilized zona can induce the acrosome reaction *in vitro*.

In human sperm the acrosome reaction *in vitro* is characterized by membrane vesiculation and loss of the plasma and outer acrosomal membranes (Jamil and White, 1981; Wolf et al., 1983; Chapter 11). In other mammals, this reaction releases the acrosomal contents including the zona lysin, acrosin, and permits dissolution and penetration of the zona and sperm entry into the perivitelline space (McRorie and Williams, 1974; Hartree, 1977; Stambaugh, 1978).

Acrosin, a trypsin-like enzyme, is stored in the acrosomal vesicle as an inactive zymogen, proacrosin, which is converted to acrosin during or after capacitation (Brown and Hartree, 1974; Meizel and Murkejee, 1976; Meizel, 1978; Mack et al., 1983). Some of the active enzyme is tightly bound to the inner acrosomal membrane and is retained after the acrosome reaction (Bhattacharyya et al., 1979). A large body of indirect evidence suggests that acrosin is required for zona penetration and that the proteolytic activity of acrosin is responsible for the formation of penetration slits in the zona (Rogers and Bentwood, 1982). Trypsin inhibitors suppress sperm penetration and fertilization both *in vivo* and *in vitro* (Stambaugh et al., 1969; Zaneveld, 1976; Wolf, 1977; Beyler and Zaneveld, 1982) and the zonalytic action of acrosin *in vitro* has been established by dissolving isolated zona with acrosin fractions (Stambaugh et al., 1965; Stambaugh and Buckley, 1969; Zaneveld, 1976). Some investigators still consider that the role of acrosin is open to debate (Bedford and Cross, 1978; Yanagimachi, 1981; Moore and

Bedford, 1983). Zona penetration *per se* is, however, likely to involve a combination of biochemical (proteolysis) and physical (motility) activities.

Sperm-Egg Plasma Membrane Fusion

After penetration of the zona pellucida, sperm enter the perivitelline space and contact the oocyte plasma membrane. This membrane is characterized by a number of short microvilli (0.3 to 1.0 um long) overlying a cortical granule-containing cortex except for the surface adjacent to the second metaphase spindle (Schmell et al., 1983). The point of fusion is probably the segment of the sperm plasma membrane remaining over the restricted equatorial region and a microvillar rich region of the oocyte surface (Bedford et al., 1979; Shalgi and Phillips, 1980). Sperm cease motility soon after contacting the plasma membrane, perhaps due to egg membrane depolarization or ion flux activity as occurs in invertebrate species (Epel, 1978). The sperm are engulfed, but not phagocytized, by the microvilli of the egg surface which may play an active role in drawing the sperm into the ooplasm (Yanagimachi, 1977). The post-acrosomal membrane fuses with the oolemma to form a mosaic plasma membrane. These interaction events in fertilization are thought to be rapid, as sperm are seldom observed in the matrix of the zona pellucida, in the perivitelline space or in the process of fusion when examined at fixed time points by transmission electron microscopy. The actual time requirement for induction of the acrosome reaction, penetration of the zona and fusion with the plasma membrane in the human has not been established. The length of time reported for capacitation and penetration of the zona of mature human oocytes ranges from 2.5 hours (McMaster et al., 1978) to 7 hours (Edwards et al., 1969). Fusion of sperm and egg membranes triggers three key reactions necessary for development: the cortical reaction blocking further sperm penetration, nuclear activation allowing completion of meiosis in the egg, and metabolic derepression of the egg.

Cortical Reaction and the Block to Polyspermy

Polyspermy *in vivo* is considered a rare but lethal event in mammals (Austin and Bishop, 1957). The cumulative effect of several factors serve to limit multiple sperm penetration: 1) the restricted number of sperm reaching the site of fertilization as the female reproductive tract serves a sieving function; 2) the protective effect of the egg's associated cumulus and corona cells; and 3) the egg's block to polyspermy responses *per se* - the zona reaction, the egg plasma membrane block to polyspermy and the elimination of supernumerary sperm by abstriction in ooplasmic blebs (Yu and Wolf, 1981). The egg's responses are initiated by sperm-egg fusion and mediated, at least in part, through a cortical reaction. Ultrastructurally this reaction can be viewed as a fusion of cortical granules (300-600nm diameter) underlying the egg surface with the egg plasma membrane and the exocytotic release of granule contents into the perivitelline space (Figure 5). Cortical granule membrane is then incorporated into the egg plasma membrane resulting in the formation of a mosaic membrane (Figure 5; Barros and Yanagimachi, 1971; Schuel, 1978; Wolf, 1978, 1981; Gulyas, 1980; Yanagimachi, 1981). The cortical granules in unfertilized mammalian eggs are polarized in an irregular layer underlying the plasma membrane with the greatest concentration found in the cortex away from the meiotic spindle (Zamboni, 1971; Nicosia et al., 1977; Gulyas, 1980). It is unclear at this time which event initiated by sperm-egg fusion triggers the cortical reaction. By analogy to invertebrates, release of internally sequested calcium may be involved (Epel, 1980). This release could be regulated by ion fluxes at the plasma membrane or the release of calcium from the sperm at the point of sperm fusion. A localized increase in calcium ions, then, could serve to effect additional calcium release in a reaction propagated around the entire surface of the egg (Epel, 1978, 1980).

Formation and exocytosis of cortical granules have been examined ultrastructurally in human oocytes fertilized _in vitro_; granules release either at the surface individually or after coalescence of 2-6 granules (Sathananthan and Trounson, 1982). The contents of the cortical granules blend with the inner zona pellucida to form deposits or striae of dense material on the inner surface.

A molecular basis for the zona reaction, i.e., the block to sperm penetration at the level of the zona, involves cortical granule induced loss of sperm receptor activity in the zona pellucida so that binding and penetration of supplemental sperm is blocked (Braden and Austin, 1954; Barros and Yanagimachi, 1971; Soupart and Strong, 1975; Gwatkin, 1977; Wolf and Hamada, 1977). If unfertilized eggs are exposed to cortical granule contents collected from fertilized eggs, they are rendered impermeable to capacitated sperm (Barros and Yanagimachi, 1971; Gwatkin et al., 1973; Wolf and Hamada, 1977). Since the cortical granule activity can be blocked by both trypsin inhibitors as well as by heat, a trypsin-like protease is implicated in the reaction (Gwatkin and Williams, 1974; Wolf and Hamada, 1977). Following cortical granule exocytosis there is also an increased resistance of the zona pellucida to enzymatic and chemical digestion, referred to as zona hardening (Wolf, 1981). There is histochemical evidence suggesting that hardening of the zona of mouse eggs occurs via an

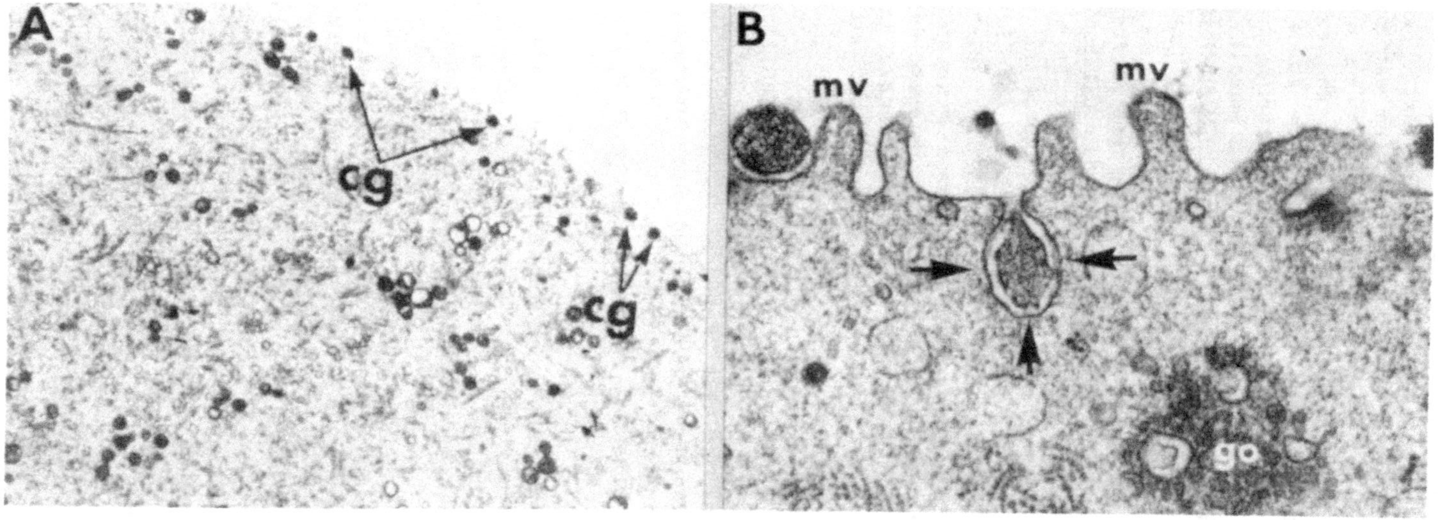

Figure 5

A) Zona-free mouse egg prior to insemination. Cortical granules are present beneath the plasma membrane. Mag = 7100X (reprinted with permission from Wolf et al., 1979); B) Tubal mouse egg after incubation with sperm for 30 minutes. There is a pit (labeled by arrows) suggestive of cortical granule discharge; microvilli (mv) and Golgi complexes (go) are present. Mag = 40,000X (reprinted with permission from Nicosia et al., 1977).

ovoperoxidase catalyzed cross-linking of tyrosine residues in zona glycoproteins. This activity has been associated with cortical granules (Schmell and Gulyas, 1980b). A role for zona hardening in polyspermy prevention has not been demonstrated. Indeed, in rabbit eggs, zona hardening occurs in the absence of a block to polyspermy at the level of the zona (Schmell et al., 1983). Since rabbit eggs remain monospermic in the presence of several sperm in the perivitelline space, a block must occur in this species at the level of the plasma membrane (Braden et al., 1954; Austin and Bishop, 1957; Overstreet and Bedford, 1974).

Direct experimental evidence for an egg plasma membrane block to polyspermy in mammals is limited to the rabbit, gopher and mole, where it is the exclusive response, and to rodents and cats where a zona reaction is also important (Austin and Bishop, 1957; Austin, 1975). In vitro studies of zona-free mouse oocytes suggest that a polyspermy block at the level of the plasma membrane is established 60 minutes or less following sperm-egg fusion (Wolf, 1978; Sato, 1979). As in the zona reaction, this block is species specific since zona-free hamster eggs do not show it (Usui and Yanagimachi, 1976; Binor et al., 1982). Evidence against the involvement of cortical granule exocytosis in the plasma membrane block is available in the mouse (Wolf et al., 1979). When cortical granule exocytosis in zona-free mouse eggs was triggered by mechanical stimulation or by exposure to the calcium ionophore A23187, there was a 50-100% loss of cortical granules as documented by ultrastructural analysis, yet the fertilizability of these cortically activated eggs was identical to that of controls.

In invertebrates and some vertebrates, there is evidence that electrical depolarization of the egg membrane controls sperm entry (Jaffe, 1976; Gould-Somero et al., 1979; Hagiwara and Jaffe, 1979; Cross and Elinson, 1980). Physical correlates to depolarization could involve alterations in membrane fluidity or the migration or diffusion of membrane components such as sperm receptors, enzymes, ion gates or channels. In the mammalian egg, studies on electrical depolarization indicate that the plasma membrane polyspermy block is not electrically mediated (Miyazaki and Igusa, 1981; Jaffe et al., 1983; McCulloh et al., 1983).

The human oocyte relies primarily on the zona reaction to control polyspermy; it is not clear whether a plasma membrane block might also be involved (Soupart and Strong, 1975; Edwards et al., 1981). However, polyspermy does occur at a relatively high frequency in vitro under the high sperm concentrations employed (Evans et al., 1980; Trounson et al., 1980a). The presence of swollen sperm heads in the perivitelline space is consistent with the conclusion that polyspermy results from the lack of a zona reaction perhaps reflecting delayed cortical granule release (Sathananthan and Trounson, 1982a,b).

HUMAN IN VITRO FERTILIZATION

We have used four different follicular recruitment protocols during 1981-1983 in an effort to study follicular recruitment and oocyte recovery. Laboratory protocols for fertilization and embryo transfer have remained essentially the same with the exception of the sperm concentration and the transfer media. Clomiphene citrate (50 mg/day, days 5-9) and clomiphene citrate-hMG (50mg/day, days 5-9; 2 amps hMG, days 6,8,10) were the most successful treatments as measured by fertilization (84-87%) rates (Table 4). The first follicular recruitment trial used at U.T. Houston was clomiphene citrate (150 mg/day, days 5-9) patterned after Lopata et al. (1977, 1978a). Two notable results of this trial (N=39) were the absence of clinical pregnancies and a relatively low egg recovery rate. The former may reflect possible antagonistic effects of clomiphene citrate on pregnancy establishment (Chapter 6); however, this effect of high clomiphene citrate apparently has not been experienced by other laboratories. The low recovery rate may, in part, reflect our inexperience in IVF-ET during this early phase. Following this trial, we lowered the clomiphene citrate dose to 50 mg/day; with this treatment we have 10 pregnancies (17.2% of transfers) including 8 live births and two continuing pregnancies. In a more recent series, we used paired randomized, double blind trials to compare clomiphene citrate (50 mg/day) to clomiphene citrate-hMG (50 mg/day days 5-9; 2 amps hMG, days 6, 8, 10) or to hMG alone (4 amps/day days 3 to hCG). We have not had a pregnancy in the hMG ovarian stimulation trial (N=19; Table 4). Possible explanations for this outcome are discussed in Chapter 7. However, in the clomiphene citrate-hMG series we have two pregnancies; (12.5% of transfers) two live births (twins) and one continuing pregnancy. While preclinical or "biochemical" pregnancies were experienced with these protocols, the most useful parameter clearly is the number of continuing pregnancies, therefore, we have recorded here only pregnancies that have progressed beyond 12 weeks of gestation. To date we have not had any spontaneous abortions.

By way of comparison and summary, the pregnancy rates (5-24% of patients undergoing transfers) reported by other IVF laboratories are presented in Table 5. These percentages include all pregnancies irregardless of embryo wastage. A breakdown into preclinical and clinical pregnancies can be made for some (Table 6). Of the 176 pregnancies listed in Table 6, only 56% can be classified as term or ongoing pregnancies. Greater than 50% of the reported wastage represents preclinical or biochemical pregnancies. Analysis of results in the future would be benefited if biochemical pregnancies were reported separately. Another parameter that should be reported is the etiology of infertility, since only pregnancies established in women with complete tubal occulsion can be attributed unequivocally to IVF-ET.

Motile Sperm Number and In Vitro Fertilization

In mammals, sperm deposited in the female reproductive tract undergo extensive dilution as they penetrate the cervical mucus, uterine lumen, and uterotubal junction before reaching the ampulla, the site of fertilization. The normal human ejaculate contains on the average 200 x 10^6 sperm. However, fewer than 200 sperm reach the site of fertilization as evidenced by the number found in flushings of the ampulla between 2 and 34 hours post-coitus (Ahlgren, 1971, 1975, 1981). Sperm remain motile and fertile in the oviduct for at least 48 hours although they may persist as motile sperm for much longer time periods in the lower reproductive tract (Austin, 1975; Ferin et al., 1973).

We have used sperm concentrations ranging from 1 x 10^4 to 5 x 10^5 motile sperm/ml to achieve successful fertilization. Initially we conducted a systematic evaluation of the effects of concentration on fertilization by inseminating eggs from the same patient at different concentrations (Wolf et al., manuscript in preparation). A summary of these results are presented in Table 7 and Figures 6 and 7. A comparison between the fertility of oligospermic and normal males in IVF-ET is presented in Table 7 without regard to the follicular recruitment program used. A breakdown of fertilization success at different sperm concentrations and follicular recruitment programs is seen in Figure 6. We are now using 5 x 10^4 motile sperm/ml as our standard inseminating concentration since it supports the highest fertility rates with the lowest degree of polyspermy. Lowering the motile sperm concentration to 25,000 in a limited trial was associated with a decrease in the fertilization rate to 50% (N=6) and at 10,000 motile sperm the fertilization rate in a very limited number of eggs was 33% (N=3). Craft et al. (1981) also reported successful fertilization at 10,000 motile sperm. Obviously, the ideal number for fertilization of preovulatory oocytes, has yet to be determined but for the normal husband it is not as high as the 100-500 x 10^5 levels used in the initial IVF-ET protocols.

The difference in sperm-egg ratios _in vivo_ (10^2:1) and _in vitro_ (10^4 to 10^6:1) raises the possibility of a high

Table 4. The fertilization and cleavage *in vitro* of eggs recovered at U.T. Houston

Follicular Recruitment Protocol	Number Patients Undergoing Laparoscopy	Number Eggs Fertilized: Mature Number/Percent	Number Eggs Fertilized: Immature Number/Percent	Percent Of Mature Fertilized Eggs That Cleaved	Percent of Fertilized Eggs Transferred
Clomiphene Citrate (150mg)	39	42/64.6	0/0	100	95.2
Clomiphene Citrate (50mg)	89	108/84.3	6/28.5	91.6	92.1
Clomiphene Citrate (50mg)+hMG	18	49/87.5	3/37.5	77.5	88.4
hMG	19	52/70.3	2/28.6	88.0	90.7

Follicular Recruitment Protocol	Embryos Transferred per Follicles Aspirated %	Pregnancies per Embryos Transferred %	Pregnancies per Patients Receiving Transfers %	Pregnancies per Laparoscopies %
Clomiphene Citrate (150mg)	61.5	0	0	0
Clomiphene Citrate (50mg)	64.4	9.5	17.2	11.2
Clomiphene Citrate (50mg)+hMG	56.2	5.4	12.5	11.1
hMG	55.5	0	0	0

Note: Data includes all eggs and follicles, regardless of size and differs slightly from those presented in Chapter 6, Table 3.

Table 5. Summary of reported IVF-ET results for the period 1980-1983

Follicular Recruitment Protocol	Reference %	Embryos Transferred Per Follicles Aspirated %	Pregnancies Per Embryos Transferred %	Pregnancies Per Patients Receiving Transfers %	Pregnancies Per Laparoscopies %
Clomiphene Citrate					
100mg	Johnston et al., 1981	30	7	9	3
100mg	Feichtinger and Kemeter, 1983	72	8	16	9
150mg	Kerin et al., 1983	-	-	24	-
150mg + hMG	Kerin et al., 1983	63	11	20	18
100-150mg	Lopata, 1983				
	data for 1980	29	7	9	3
	1981	41	8	11	7
	1982	59	8	15	15
150mg	Trounson and Wood, 1981	-	-	-	14
150mg	Trounson et al., 1981b	81	12	12	10
	Fishel et al., 1983	-	17	23	-
	Edwards et al., 1983	-	-	21	15

hMG					
5 amps	Edwards et al., 1980a	-	-	5	-
2 amps	Jones et al., 1983	46	14	24	19
Clomiphene Citrate + hMG					
150mg + hMG	Kerin et al., 1983	-	-	23	-
50-100mg + hMG	Lopata 1983	43	9	24	18
Spontaneous					
	Testart et al., 1983a	-	-	29	8
	Trounson et al., 1981b	85	0	0	0
	Trotnow et al., 1983	56	-	-	-
	Edwards et al., 1983	-	-	16	10

Notes: Some literature citations were excluded if the data was summarized in more recent papers. Pregnancies may include biochemical or preclinical cases. In several cases the reported results did not allow calculation of Table entries.

Table 6. Embryonic wastage in IVF-ET

Reference	Total Pregnancies	Wastage Preclinical:Clinical	Term Pregnancies or Ongoing Pregnancies	Wastage Percent
Trounson and Wood (1981)	16	4:3	9	44
Feichtinger et al., (1983)	18	6	12	33
Houston 1982-1983	15	3:0	12	20
Jones et al. (1983)	33	8:4	21	36
Kerin et al. (1983)	20	3	17	15
Lopata, (1983)				
1980	3	2	1	67
1981	17	14	3	82
1982	55	14:11	30	45
Testart et al. (1983)	8	6	2	75
Trotnow et al. (1983)	6	3	3	50

frequency of polyspermy in vitro. Following natural conceptions there is a high incidence of triploidy in aborted fetuses. In a study of 1499 abortuses by Boué et al. (1975), 38.5% of the karyotypes were abnormal and 25% of abnormal karyotypes were either triploids or polyploids. Another major factor contributing to polyspermy frequency is oocyte maturation (Trounson et al., 1982). Several eggs in our IVF-ET program were classified as polyspermic based on the presence of 3 pronuclei 16 to 18 hours after insemination. In eggs inseminated at 100,000 (N=117) and 50,000 (N=153) motile sperm/ml the polyspermy rates were 5.98 and 1.26%, respectively ($p < 0.001$). In these cases, sperm had been preincubated more than 5 hours before insemination. In our initial protocol, sperm were preincubated for only 2 hours and employed at 500,000 motile cells/ml. In this case only 1.12% of the eggs (N=89) were clearly polyspermic; however, a significant fragmentation rate was also seen at this concentration. Additionally, high sperm concentrations may expose oocytes to metabolic and degenerative by-products from the sperm which may have a negative effect on fertilization and development.

Most IVF-ET programs, our own included, select for motile sperm by taking only sperm that remain in suspension as they undergo capacitation. The percentage of motile sperm in these selected fractions increases markedly over the original ejaculate and is usually well above 60% (Figure 7). So long as the progression is good and the percentage of motile cells in the selected population is greater than 40%, there is no influence of motility on fertilization (Figure 7). However, when the percentage of motile sperm is in the 20-40% range a significant decrease in fertilization is observed. Since we inseminate with equivalent concentrations of motile cells, this drop off at the lower end of the motility curve may reflect the effect of lower progressive motility or an unrecognized sperm-related dysfunction.

We have also used IVF-ET as a treatment modality for oligospermic males; oligospermia being defined as a sperm count of less than 20×10^6 sperm/ml in the original ejaculate. Based on the results of a limited series there was a definite and dramatic drop in fertilizability when sperm concentrations below 5×10^5 motile sperm/ml were employed (Table 7). Since oligospermic males have a lower initial sperm concentration ($10.4 \times 10^6 \pm 4.3$ sperm/ml) a relatively large volume of the sperm suspension, up to 1:10 (v:v) must be added to achieve concentrations of 500,000 motile sperm/ml. The percent motility of washed-incubated sperm in these males (59.8% $\pm$ 16.7 S.D.) was comparable to normal ranges (Figure 6) although the motility dropped to as low as 22% in one case. Males with normal semen parameters but low sperm concentrations in the washed, preincubated fraction ($9.0 \times 10^6 \pm$ 1.9 S.D.) still show high fertilizability (85% of oocytes

Table 7. Fertilization success at different sperm concentrations at U.T. Houston IVF-ET

	Sperm Concentration Motile Sperm/ml	Number of eggs Inseminated	Sperm Concentration In Whole Semen	Percent Fertilized[a]
Oligospermic Males	500,000	26	$< 20x10^6$ sperm/ml	61.5
	100,000	9	"	22.0
	50,000	2	"	0
Normal Males	500,000	89	$> 20x10^6$ sperm/ml	66.2
	100,000	117	"	69.2
	50,000	153	"	71.2

a). Student T Test: all values differ from each other ($P < .01$)

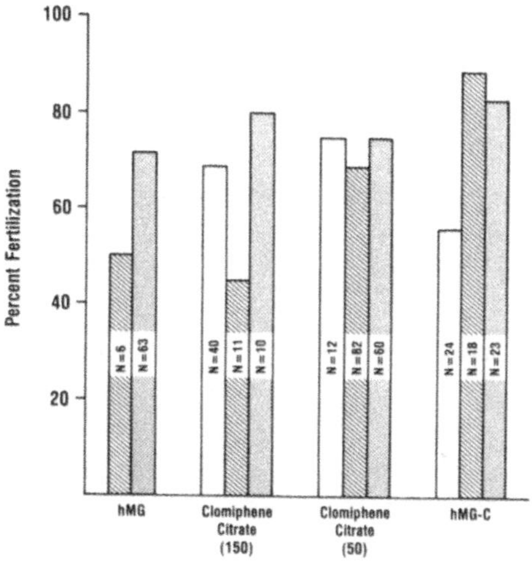

Figure 6

Sperm concentration dependency in the fertilization of human oocytes recovered by follicular aspiration following four different recruitment trials. Legends: Open bar = 500,000 motile sperm/ml of insemination medium (one ml of insemination medium per egg); hatched bar = 100,000 motile sperm/ml; dotted bar = 50,000 motile sperm/ml.

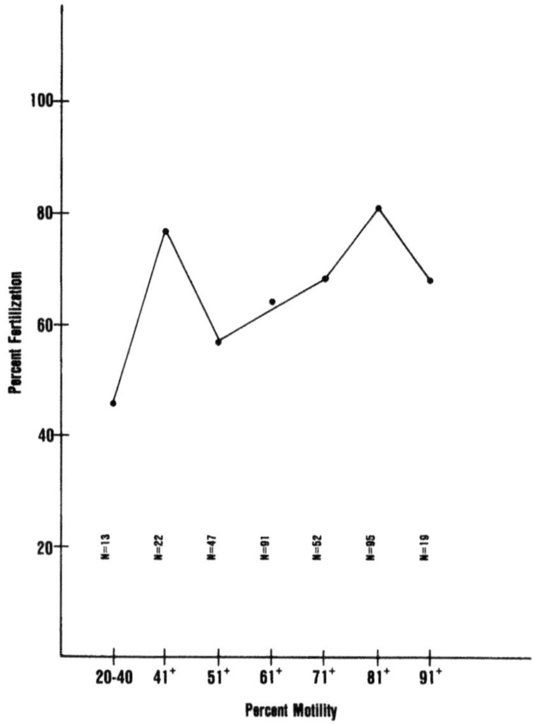

Figure 7

Fertilization of recovered oocytes as a function of different sperm motilities. Sperm motility was measured in washed sperm preparations prior to insemination.

recovered fertilized, N=22). Fishel and Edwards (1982) have reported fertilization rates (65%) in oligospermic males at a concentration of 8 x 10^5 sperm/ml. They report at least two patients with oligospermic husbands who have delivered normal infants. Testart et al. (1983b) have reported a significant difference in in vitro development ($p < .001$) using sperm from males with abnormal as opposed to normal semen analysis. They report a pregnancy rate per number of transfers when semen parameters are normal of 23.1% (26 transfers, 61 eggs inseminated). However, in a series of males with abnormal semen analysis 40 eggs were inseminated but none developed normally. When male fertility potential is tested using the zona-free hamster egg bioassay (Chapter 14) the oligospermic patient often scores poorly, again indicating that sperm parameters other than number, motility and progression must be important to penetration or fertilization.

Fertilization of Immature Oocytes Matured In Vitro

Using sperm concentrations ranging from 50,000 to 500,000 motile cells per ml, we have attempted fertilization of a number of immature eggs (graded by the absence of a cumulus mass, the presence of an intact germinal vesicle or both, N=33; see Figure 2C). We routinely culture immature eggs for 24-30 hours before examining eggs for the presence of a germinal vesicle or polar body. Eggs are inseminated at this time regardless of their state of maturity. Sperm penetration and pronuclear development is dependent upon sperm concentration, but not in the expected fashion. No immature eggs were fertilized when inseminated with 500,000 motile sperm/ml (N=6) while 28.5% of the eggs inseminated with 100,000 sperm/ml (N=14) and 46.1% of those inseminated at 50,000 motile sperm/ml (N=13) showed pronuclear development. Based on this small sample, high sperm concentrations may adversely affect the final stages of oocyte maturation or fertilization per se. Veeck et al. (1983) reported fertilization rates of 59.4% for immature eggs matured in vitro prior to insemination. Fertilization was based on either pronuclear development or cleavage prior to transfer. The lowered fertilizability of immature as opposed to preovulatory eggs probably reflects the presence of immature oocytes that do not mature (Veeck et al., 1983b). Recall from Table 1 that only about 50% of oocytes cultured in vitro mature spontaneously.

The question concerning immature oocytes is their ability to support clinical pregnancies. Veeck et al. (1983a,b) report that immature oocytes fertilized in vitro contribute to successful pregnancies. Eight pregnancies were established as a result of transfer of both immature and mature oocytes and in two cases pregnancies resulted from the transfer of only in vitro matured oocytes. We have not yet established a pregnancy with the transfer of only immature oocytes.

DEVELOPMENT IN VITRO

Sperm Decondensation, Pronuclear Formation and Fusion

After fusion with the plasma membrane, the sperm nucleus is incorporated into the ooplasm carrying with it the basal body, centriole, mitochondria and tail components (Szollosi, 1965; Longo, 1973). The pronucleus of the sperm differentiates within a few hours concomitant with the resumption of meiotic maturation in the egg resulting in the formation of the second polar body and haploid female pronucleus. The steps of differentiation of the male pronucleus consist of breakdown of the nuclear membrane, decondensation of chromatin, turnover of nuclear protamines, deposition of histones and formation of the pronuclear membrane. Except for decondensation, these events are sequential (see Figures 3 and 4 for depiction of some of these events).

Morphologically dramatic transformations of the incorporated sperm head within the egg begin with a breakdown or dispersion of the sperm nuclear membrane along the periphery of the midregion which then progresses in an anterior and posterior fashion (Bedford, 1970; Yanagimachi and Noda, 1970a,b). Breakdown of the sperm nuclear membranes exposes the condensed chromatin to the cytoplasm with resultant chromatin dispersion and DNA synthesis (Szollosi, 1966; Longo, 1973). Little is known about the mechanism of these events in vivo, but in vitro release of DNA template restriction and nuclear swelling are dependent upon both endogenous proteolytic activity as well as disulfide-bond reduction (Zirkin and Chang, 1977). Disulfide bond reduction is required for decondensation of mature sperm (Mahi and Yanagimachi, 1976; Zirkin and Chang, 1977), while an acrosin-like protease associated with the sperm nucleus may be involved in both protamine degradation and nuclear decondensation (Zirkin et al., 1982). The dispersed chromatin is then enclosed within a pronuclear envelope formed from the aggregation of vesicles into elongate cisternae which eventually make the double membrane structure of the nuclear membrane (Longo, 1973; Soupart and Strong, 1975). The nucleus increases in size and forms approximately eight nucleoli (Soupart and Strong, 1974). The flagellum is rapidly dispersed; however, axial filaments remain intact for at least 24 hours and provide one criteria for fertilization, at least in fixed-stained whole mounts or thin sections. The female pronucleus develops near the site of second polar body extrusion in a fashion similar to that occurring with the male pronucleus. There is a dispersal of chromatin, coalescence of vesicles and formation of the nuclear membrane. Both nuclei become active metabolically as evidenced by the large number of nucleoli that appear shortly after pronuclear formation.

Pronuclear fusion occurs following migration of the pronuclei into the interior of the egg (Longo, 1973). Fusion takes place in three steps: 1) association, but not actual fusion, of the pronuclei; 2) interdigitation of pronuclear membranes; and 3) vesiculation of the nuclear envelopes allowing formation of the mitotic spindle and subsequent cleavage. Fertilization is considered complete at syngamy when the maternal and paternal chromosomes become associated with each other.

Metabolic Activation

Metabolically, the ovulated mammalian oocyte is relatively inactive awaiting the stimulus of fertilization or parthenogenetic activation. Following sperm-egg fusion there is activation of a variety of metabolic pathways concomitant with increased protein and nucleic acid synthesis (Wolf, 1982). Metabolic requirements of the zygote and early cleavage stage embryos are satisfied in large measure by preformed materials, such as proteins and ribonucleic acids, stored during oogenesis. The fertilized ovum is capable of sustaining protein synthesis in the absence of early RNA synthesis presumably reflecting the presence of maternal messenger RNA. Considerable effort has been spent defining the nature and quantity of preformed materials and evaluating their function.

The molecular mechanisms of metabolic activation at fertilization have been studied extensively in the invertebrate egg and similar molecular correlates are believed to operate in mammals. Two potential effectors of oocyte activation have been identified. First, permeability changes occur in the plasma membrane resulting in an influx of calcium or a release of calcium from internal stores. Evidence for the role of calcium in egg activation comes from work on invertebrate, hamster and mouse ova. Eggs from these species can be activated with calcium ionophore A23187 which causes cortical granule release, metabolic activation and DNA synthesis (Steinhardt et al., 1974; Epel, 1980; Cuthbertson et al., 1981; Winkler, 1982). Second, ion flux (inward sodium influx coupled with a hydrogen efflux) causes an alkalinization of the egg cytoplasm. This increase in internal pH plays a major role in protein and DNA synthesis (Winkler, 1982) and although it follows calcium release, it is thought to be the controlling step in metabolic activation. If eggs are activated with calcium ionophore in zero-sodium sea water, no activation takes place since internal alkalinization of the egg cannot occur (Epel, 1980; Winkler, 1982). However, if sodium is added back to the medium activation results. The calcium involvement in activation can be bypassed by treating eggs with ammonia or other weak penetrating bases which raise cytoplasmic pH by combining directly with hydrogen as the uncharged species come to equilibrium (Winkler, 1982). Eggs treated in this manner will activate metabolically and undergo DNA synthesis. However, despite these insights, it is likely that several coupled events including calcium release and cytoplasmic alkalinization, regulate activation of eggs, since no parthenogenetic agent by itself will induce both activation and cleavage.

Evaluation of Fertilization and Development In Vitro

The human embryo can be cultured from the pronuclear stage to the hatching blastocyst in vitro (Steptoe et al., 1971). The initial culturing of human embryos was carried out using media developed for mouse embryos (Edwards et al., 1970). Later, more complex media were introduced such as Ham's F-10 supplemented with human or fetal calf serum (Edwards et al., 1970; Steptoe et al., 1971). Pregnancies have been obtained in a variety of different media (Chapter 13) including modified Tyrodes, Ham's F-10 with serum (Edwards et al., 1980; Lopata, 1982; Lopata et al., 1980a; Trounson et al., 1981b), Earle's solution (Purdy, 1982), modified Whitten's medium (Trounson et al., 1980a, 1982), Whittingham's T6 medium (Trounson et al., 1982) and Menezo's B_2 medium (Feichtinger et al., 1983; Testart et al., 1983a,b). At present, a data base is not yet available that allows evaluation of whether or not the culture medium used contributes significantally to fertilization, development or implantation rates. In a controlled trial of four different media, Trounson (1983) concluded that none of the media tested (Ham's F-10; Whitten's, Whittingham's T-6; Earle's) showed any distinct advantage as expressed by implantation rates.

Evaluation of fertilization requires visualization of the oocyte at approximately 18 hours post-insemination after the remaining adherent granulosa cells are mechanically removed from the oocyte (Chapter 13, Figure 2). The presence of two pronuclei are taken as presumptive evidence of fertilization. We do not use the presence of two polar bodies as a criterion for fertilization since spontaneous division of the first polar body has been observed in human oocytes (Ortiz et al., 1983). Spontaneous activation of the oocyte may occur; in these rare cases 2-cell embryos can be observed as early as 16 hours. The presence or absence of a sperm tail in the cytoplasm cannot be used as a reliable criterion of fertilization as visualization is not possible in the living cell.

The ultimate indication of embryonic viability is the establishment of a clinical pregnancy after transfer. Short of this indicator, the rate of cleavage and the morphological quality of the embryo must be used. Little information is available on the cleavage of human embryos in vivo (Hertig et al., 1954). However, in spite of differing culture conditions, there is a fairly consistent pattern to human embryonic development in vitro (Figure 8) with a window observed at the first (Avg. 37.8 hrs; range 31-43 hrs) and second (Avg. 44.8 hrs; range 38-53 hrs) cleavage stages. Retarded cleavage rates may reflect reduced embryo viability in the human (Trounson, 1982; Trounson et al., 1982b; Mohr et al., 1983) and in some animals while faster cleavage rates are more frequently associated with the establishment of pregnancies (Trounson et al., 1982a). As evidence of the latter observation, Mohr et al. (1983) reported that 50% of the embryos which resulted in pregnancies were at the

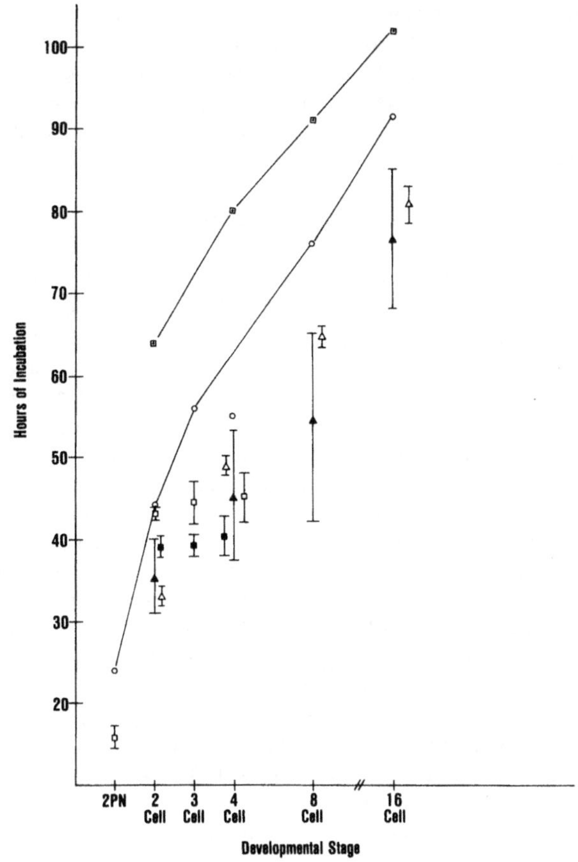

Figure 8

Preimplantation development rates for embryos produced by IVF. Legends: (⊡) = Lauritsen, 1982; (○) = Sundstrom et al., 1981; (Δ) = Edwards et al., 1981; (▲) = Trounson et al., 1982; (■) = U.T. Houston 1982-1983; (□) = Wortham et al., 1983.

4-cell stage by 32-40 hours post-insemination. Another parameter which may influence cleavage rates is the time of insemination. Lopata (1982) reported that oocytes inseminated four to six hours after recovery cleaved much more rapidly than those inseminated immediately. In addition, there is evidence that eggs recovered from clomiphene/hCG treatment cleave somewhat faster than their counterparts from natural or clomiphene alone cycles. Fishel et al. (1983) reported that 89% of fertilized eggs recovered after clomiphene-hCG treatment were at the 8-cell stage by 65 hours, whereas this percentage was 63% in clomiphene and 61% in the unstimulated cycle.

Detailed information on oocyte integrity can be obtained by transmission electron microscopy (Sundstrom et al., 1981; Mohr and Trounson, 1982, Sathananthan and Trounson, 1982); however, application of this technique is of limited value in IVF-ET where we rely on light microscopy and non-destructive techniques. Micrographs of normal cleavage stages of human embryos have been published by Trounson et al. (1982) and Edwards (1977, 1980). While the relationship between embryo quality and the establishment of pregnancy has not been documented, it is assumed that higher pregnancy rates are associated with higher quality embryos, a tenant established in bovine embryo transfer (Shea, 1981). Spiers et al. (1983) transfer embryos only if they appear healthy on the basis of dividing blastomeres of equal size which occupy most of the space within the zona. Moreover, cell division must be progressive and within established limits (Figure 8). On the other hand, the totipotency of 2-8 cell blastomeres should be considered (Zeilmaker and Alberda, 1982). Mohr et al. (1983) found that the transfer of embryos containing a few anucleate fragments and otherwise normal blastomeres or even blastomeres which appear multinucleated is compatible with subsequent normal development and implantation. In our own experience, we have achieved pregnancies with the transfer of embryos of relatively low quality containing uneven blastomeres and anucleate fragments and therefore of a relatively low quality. We are currently grading embryos (on a scale of 1-5) as suggested by Mohr et al. (1983), considering cell size and shape, the presence of fragments or other debris in the perivitelline space and the gross quality of the cytoplasm. Another possible approach to embryo assessment that has not been exploited in the human involves the use of fluorescein diacetate (Mohr et al., 1983).

EMBRYO TRANSFER

Pregnancies have resulted following transfer of pronuclear (Veeck et al., 1983), 2 to 4 cell (Edwards et al., 1980; Trounson et al., 1981; Trounson and Wood, 1981) 8-cell (Edwards et al., 1980; Lopata et al., 1980a; Wood et al., 1981) and 16-cell embryos (Edwards et al., 1980) into the uterine cavity (Chapter 16). At this time, there is no clear information on the optimal stage of embryo development for transfer, but the transfer of morula embryos has not resulted in pregnancy (Edwards et al., 1980). The normal transport of ova in women requires a time period of 96-120 hours post-LH surge before eggs reach the uterus. Based on this, embryos in synchrony with the receptive uterus would be approximately at the 16-32 cell stage.

With the optimization of ovarian stimulation protocols in IVF-ET, the transfer of multiple embryos has become routine (Table 8). The success rate for IVF-ET when only one embryo is transferred is 12%, well below the estimated 25-30% natural fecundity rate (Leridon, 1977). At this time, we do not understand the reasons for the lower rate, but certainly embryo quality (Trounson, 1983) and the effects of ovarian stimulation upon the reproductive tract must be considered as primary candidates. It is clear at this time that there is a marked improvement in the pregnancy rate (2x) when two embryos are transferred, and this improvement does not carry a significant risk of twinning (Table 8). With the transfer of 3 embryos the mean pregnancy rate shows a further increase from 24 to 33%. The transfer of 4 embryos also carries a 33% chance of pregnancy but now the incidence of multiple gestation is unacceptably high.

PARTHENOGENESIS

Fertilization has two primary functions: establishment of the diploid genome and metabolic activation of the egg. Pincus and Enzmann (1936) were the first to show that the activation of rabbit oocytes can be accomplished without fertilization. Since then, oocytes from a variety of mammalian species have been induced experimentally to undergo parthenogenesis by a wide variety of treatments: chilling, electrical shock, aging, hyaluronidase or calcium ionophore A23187 exposure (Beatty, 1970; Tarkowski et al., 1970; Graham, 1971, 1974; Steinhardt et al., 1974, Kaufman and Sachs, 1976). Parthenogenetic mammalian embryos may survive to blastocysts or even to limbbud stages post-implantation (Chang, 1955; Tarkowski, 1971).

We have recovered four preovulatory oocytes which have presumably undergone parthenogenetic activation. All were recovered from patients stimulated with hMG and were evaluated as parthenogenic based on morphology. Three oocytes, each from a different patient, showed one pronucleus and one apparent polar body when examined by Nomarski optics (example Figure 9A). Two of these oocytes cleaved, one reaching the 4-cell stage and the other reaching 8 cells before fragmenting. The fourth displayed two irregular blastomeres at 16.5 hours with a nucleus in each (Figure 9A). This oocyte did not continue development. Non-human primate oocytes have been stimulated <u>in vitro</u> to undergo parthenogenesis

Table 8. The relationship between the number of embryos transferred and pregnancy rates in various IVF-ET programs

	Pregnancy Success[a]				
	Number of Embryos Transferred				
Reference	1	2	3	4	5
Fishel et al., 1983	19% N=120	33% N=36	-	-	-
Feichtinger and Kemeter, 1983	12% N=34	30% (b) N=30	36% (c,e) N=11	-	-
Houston IVF-ET[f] 5/82 - 6/83	10% N=31	19% N=27	10% N=10	33% (b) N=6	50% N=2
Johnston et al., 1983	7% N=135	16% N=82	31% N=13	50% N=6	-
Jones et al., 1983	17% N=107	26% N=102	41% N=29	36% N=11	-
Kerin et al., 1983	0 N=29	31% (d) N=32	39% (b) N=18	50% (c,e) N=6	- -
Speirs et al., 1983	10% N=60	22% N=49	19% N=37	35% (c) N=23	0 N=1
Trounson, 1983	7% N=43	25% N=44	23% N=44	0 N=9	-
Mean Pregnancy Success	12% N=559	24% N=402	33% N=162	33% N=61	33% N=3
Percent of Transfers Resulting in Multiple Pregnancies	0	1%	3%	10%	0

a) total pregnancies reported, b) 1 set of twins, c) 2 sets of twins, d) 3 sets of twins, e) 1 set of triplets, f) clinical pregnancies progressing beyond first trimester and live births only (clomiphene 50 $\pm$ hMG trials)

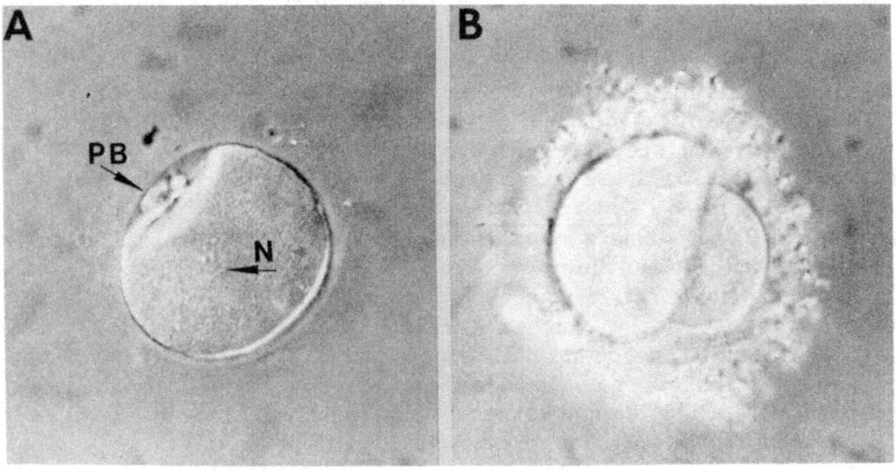

Figure 9

Parthenogenetically activated eggs; A) Oocyte with two possible polar bodies and one pronucleus; B) Oocyte undergoing premature cleavage within 16 hours of recovery. Mag = 96X

(Abramczuk et al., 1977). The majority (29%) underwent extrusion of a single polar body and formation of a single pronucleus similar to Figure 9A. Of these oocytes, 48% underwent cleavage. While there is no evidence that human parthenogenetic embryos develop normally, the results from our study suggest that human oocytes can activate parthenogentically, undergo at least the first meiotic division with pronuclear formation and cleavage _in vitro_.

REFERENCES

Abramczuk, J., Stark, R.A., Konwinski, M., Solter, D., Mastrioanni, L. and Koprowski, H., 1977, Parthenogenetic activation of rhesus monkey follicular oocytes _in vitro_, _J. Embryol. Exp. Morph._, 42:115.

Albertini, D.F., and Anderson, E., 1974, The appearance and structure of intercellular connections during the ontogeny of the rabbit ovarian follicle with particular reference to gap junctions, _J. Cell Biol._, 63:234.

Albertini, D.F., Fawcett, D.W., and Olds, P.T., 1975, Morphological variation in gap junctions of ovarian granulosa cells, Tissue Cell, 7:389.

Alhgren, M., 1971, "Number of Spermatozoa in the Ampulla of the Human Fallopian Tube," Abstract 7th World Congress on Fertility and Sterility, Tokyo.

Alhgren, M., 1975, Sperm transport to and survival in the human fallopian tube, Gynecol. Invest., 6:206.

Alhgren, M., 1981, Sperm migration throughout the female genital tract, in: "Human Reproduction," K. Semm and L. Mettler, eds., Excerpta Medica, Princeton.

Amsterdam, A., Josephs, R., Liberman, M.E., and Linder, H.R., 1976, Organization of intramembranous particles in freeze-cleaved gap junctions of rat graffian follicles., J. Cell Sci. 21:93.

Anderson, E., 1974, Comparative aspects of the ultrastructure of the female gamete, Int. Rev. Cytol., Suppl., 4:1.

Anderson, E., and Albertini, D.F., 1976, Gap junctions between the oocyte and companion follicle cells in the mammalian ovary, J. Cell Biol., 71:680.

Austin, C. R., 1975, Membrane fusion events in fertilization, J. Reprod. Fert., 44:155.

Austin, C. R., and Bishop, M. W. H., 1957, Fertilization in mammals, Biol.Rev., 32:296.

Baca, M., and Zamboni, L., 1967, The fine structure of human follicular oocytes, J. Ultrastruct. Res., 19:354.

Baker, T.G., 1972, Gametogenesis, in: "The Use of Non-Human Primates in Research on Human Reproduction," E. Diezfalusy and C.C. Standley, eds., Karolinska Institute, Stockholm.

Barros, C., and Yanagimachi, R., 1971, Induction of zona reaction in golden hamster eggs by cortical granule material Nature (London), 233,268.

Barros, C., and Munoz, G., 1973, Sperm-egg interaction in immature hamster oocytes, J. Exp. Zool., 186:73.

Beatty, R.A., 1970, The genetics of the mammalian gamete, Biol. Rev., 45:73.

Bedford, J. M., 1970, Sperm capacitation and fertilization in mammals, Biol.Reprod., Suppl., 2:128.

Bedford, J. M., 1972, An electron microscopic study of sperm penetration into the rabbit egg after natural mating, Am. J. Anat., 133:213.

Bedford, J.M., 1977, Sperm-egg interaction: the specificity of human spermatozoa, Anat. Rec., 188:477.

Bedford, J.M., and Cross, N.L., 1978, Normal penetration of rabbit spermatozoa through a trypsin and acrosin-resistant zona pellucida, J. Reprod. Fert., 54:385.

Bedford, J. M., Moore, H.D.M., and Franklin, L.E., 1979, Significance of the equatorial segment of the acrosome of the spermatazoon in eutherian mammals, Exp. Cell Res., 119:119.

Beyler, S.A., and Zaneveld, L.J.D., 1982, Inhibition of in vitro fertilization of mouse gametes by proteinase inhibitors, J. Reprod. Fert., 66:425.

Bhattacharyya, A. G., Goodpasture, J. C., and Zaneveld, L. J. D., 1979, Acrosin of mouse spermatozoa, Am. J. Physiol., 237:40.

Blandau, R.J., 1969, Gamete transport, in: "The Mammalian Oviduct," E.S.E. Hafez, and R.J. Blandau, eds., Univ. of Chicago Press, Chicago.

Blandau, R.J., 1971, Normal egg transport through the oviducts of mammals, in: "Pathways to Conception," A.I. Sherman, ed., C. C. Thomas Co., Springfield,

Blandau, R. J., 1980, In vitro fertilization and embryo transfer, Fertil.Steril., 33:3.

Bleil, J. D., and Wasserman, P. M., 1980a, Mammalian sperm-egg interaction: Identification of a glycoprotein in mouse egg zonae pellucidae possessing receptor activity for sperm, Cell, 20:873.

Bleil, J. D., and Wasserman, P. M., 1980b, Structure and function of the zona pellucida: Identification and characterization of the proteins of the mouse oocyte's zona pellucida, Dev. Biol., 76:185.

Bleil, J.D., and Wassarman, P.M., 1980c, Synthesis of zona pellucida proteins by denuded and follicle-enclosed mouse oocytes during culture in vitro, Proc. Natl. Acad. Sci., U.S.A. 77:1029.

Bleil, J., and Wassarman, P.M., 1983, Sperm-egg interactions in the mouse. Sequence of events and induction of the acrosome reaction by a zona pellucida glycoprotein, Dev. Biol., 95:317.

Boue, J., Boue, A., and Lazar, P., 1975, Retrospective and prospective epidemiological studies of 1500 karyotyped spontaneous human abortions, Teratology, 12:11.

Bousquet, D., Leveille, M-C., Roberts, K.D., Chapdelaine, A., and Bleau, G., 1981, The cellular origin of the zona pellucida antigen in the human and hamster, J. Exp. Zool., 215:215.

Braden, A.W.H., and Austin, C.R., 1954, The number of sperm about the eggs in mammals and its significance for normal fertilization, Aust. J. Biol. Sci., 7:543.

Braden, A.W.H., Austin, C.R., and David, H.A., 1954, The reactions of zona pellucida to sperm penetration, Aust. J. Biol. Sci., 7:391.

Bradford, M.M., McRorie, R.A., and Williams, W.L., 1976, Involvement of esterases in sperm penetration of the corona radiata of the ovum, Biol. Reprod., 15:102.

Brower, P.T., and Schultz, R.M., 1982, Intercellular communication between granulosa cells and mouse oocytes: existence and possible nutritional role during oocyte growth, Dev. Biol., 90:144.

Brown, C. R., and Hartree, E. F., 1974, Distribution of trypsin-like proteinase in the ram spermatozoa, J. Reprod. Fertil., 36:195.

Chang, M.C., 1955, Maturation of rabbit oocytes in culture and their maturation activation fertilization and subsequent development in the fallopian tubes., J. Exp. Zool., 128:379.

Channing, C.P., Liu, C-Q., Jones, G.S., and Jones, H., 1983, Decline of follicular oocyte maturation inhibitor coincident with maturation and achievement of fertilizability of oocytes recovered at mid-cycle of gonadrotropin-treated women, Proc. Natl. Acad. Sci., U.S.A., In Press.

Craft, I., McLeod, F., Bernard, A., Green, S., and Twigg, H., 1981, Sperm numbers and in vitro fertilization, Lancet, 2:1165.

Cross, N.L., and Elinson, R.P., 1980, A fast block to polyspermy in frogs mediated by changes in membrane potential., Dev. Biol., 75:187.

Cummins, J.M., and Yanagimachi, R., 1982, Sperm-egg ratios and the site of the acrosome reaction during in vivo fertilization in the hamster, Gamete Res., 5:239.

Cuthbertson, K.S.R., Whittingham, D.G., and Cobbold, P.H., 1981. Free Ca^{2+} increases in exponential phases during mouse oocyte activation, Nature, (London) 275:217.

Dale, B., and Monroy, A., 1981, How is polyspermy prevented?, Gamete Res., 4:151.

Dunbar, B.S., 1983, Morphological, biochemical and immunochemical characterization of the mammalian zona pellucida, in: "Mechanism and Control of Animal Fertilization," J. F. Hartmann, ed., Academic Press, New York.

Dunbar, B.S., Liu, C., and Sammons, D.W., 1981, Identification of the three major proteins of porcine and rabbit zonae pellucida by high resolution 2-D gel electrophoresis, Biol. Reprod., 24:1111.

Dunbar, B. S., Munoz, C. G. Cordle, C. T., and Metz, C. B., 1976, Inhibition of fertilization in vitro by treatment of rabbit spermatozoa with univalent isoantibodies to rabbit sperm hyaluronidase, J. Reprod. Fertil., 47:381.

Dunbar, B. S., Wardrip, N. I., and Hedrick, J. I, 1980, Isolation, physiochemical properties, and macromolecular composition of zona pellucida from porcine oocytes, Biochemistry, 19:356.

Edwards, R.G., 1962, Meiosis in ovarian oocytes of adult mammals, Nature (London), 196:446.

Edwards, R. G., 1965a, Maturation in vitro of human ovarian oocytes, Lancet, 2:926.

Edwards, R. G., 1965b, Maturation in vitro of mouse, sheep, cow, pig, rhesus monkey and human ovarian oocytes, Nature (London), 208:349.

Edwards, R. G., 1977, Early human development: from the oocyte to implantation, in: "Scientific Foundations of Obstetrics and Gynecology, 2nd Edition," E. E. Phillip, J. Barnes, M. Newton, W. Heineman, eds., Medical Books Ltd., Chicago.

Edwards, R. G., 1980, "Conception in the Human Female," Academic Press, New York.

Edwards, R.G., 1981, Test tube babies, Nature (London); 293:253.

Edwards, R. G., and Steptoe, P. C., 1975, Induction of follicular growth, ovulation and luteinization in the human ovary, J. Reprod. Fert, Suppl. 22:121.

Edwards, R. G., Donahue, R. P., Baramki, T. A., and Jones, H. W., 1966, Preliminary attempts to fertilize human oocytes matured in vitro, Amer. J. Obstet Gynecol., 96:192.

Edwards, R. G., Bavister, B. D., and Steptoe, P. C., 1969, Early stages of fertilization in vitro of human oocytes mature in vitro," Nature (London), 221:632.

Edwards, R. G. Steptoe, P. C., and Purdy, J. M., 1970, Fertilization and cleavage in vitro of preovulatory human oocytes, Nature (London), 227:1307.

Edwards, R. G. Steptoe, P. C. Fowler, R. E., and Baillie, J., 1980, Observations on preovulatory human ovarian follicles and their aspirates, Brit. J. Obstet. Gynaecol., 87:769.

Edwards, R. G., Purdy, J. M., Steptoe, P. C., and Walters, D. E., 1981, The growth of human preimplantation embryos in vitro, Am. J. Obstet. Gynecol., 141:408.

Edwards, R.G., Fishel, S.B., and Purdy, J.M., 1983, In vitro fertilization of human eggs: analysis of follicular growth, ovulation and fertilization, in: "Fertilization of the human egg in vitro, H.M. Beier and H.R. Linder, eds., Springer-Verlag, Berlin,.

Epel, D., 1978, Mechanisms of activation of sperm and egg during fertilization of sea urchin gametes, Current Topics Dev. Biol., 12:185.

Epel, D., 1980, Ionic triggers in the fertilization of sea urchin eggs, New York Acad. Sci., 339:74.

Eppig, J. J., 1979, FSH stimulates hyaluronic acid synthesis by oocyte cumulus cell complexes from mouse preovulatory follicles, Nature (London), 261:483.

Eppig, J. J., 1981, Prostagland in E_2 stimulates cumulus expansion and hyaluronic acid synthesis by cumuli oophori isolated from mice, Biol. Reprod., 25:191.

Feichtinger, W., Kemeter, P., and Szalay, S., 1983, The Vienna program of in vitro fertilization and embryo transfer: a successful clinical treatment, Europ. J. Obstet. Gynec. Reprod. Biol., 15:63.

Ferin, J., Thomas, K., and Johansson, E.D.B., 1973, in: "Human Reproduction: Conception and Contraception," E.S.E. Hafez and T.N. Evans, eds., Harper and Row, New York.

Fishel, S.B., and Edwards, R.G., 1982, Essentials of fertilization, in: "Human Conception In Vitro," R.G. Edwards and J.M. Purdy, eds., Academic Press, New York.

Fishel, S. B., Edwards, R. G., and Purdy, J. M., 1983, In vitro fertilization of human oocytes: factors associated with embryonic development in vitro, replacement of embryos and pregnancy, in: "Fertilization of the Human Egg In Vitro," H. M. Beier and H. R. Linder, eds., Springer-Verlag, Berlin.

Florman, H.M., and Storey, B.T., 1981, Inhibition of in vitro fertilization of mouse eggs: 3-guinuclidinyl benzilate specifically blocks penetration of zonae pellucidae by mouse spermatozoa, J. Exp. Zool., 216:159.

Fowler, R. E., and Edwards, R. G., 1973, The genetics of early human development, J. Prog. Med. Genetics, 9:49.

Fritz, M.A., and Speroff, L., 1982, The endocrinology of the menstrual cycle: the interaction of folliculogenesis and neuroendocrine mechanisms, Fertil. Steril., 38:509.

Garcia, J.E., Jones, G.S., and Wright, G.L., Jr., 1981, Prediction of the time of ovulation, Fertil. Steril., 36:308.

Gilula, N.B., Reeves, O.R., and Steinbach, A., 1972, Metabolic coupling, and cell contacts, Nature (London), 235:262.

Gilula, N. B., Epstein, M. L., and Beers, W. H., 1977, Cell to cell communication and ovulation. A study of the cumulus-oocyte comples, J. Cell Biol., 78:58.

Gould-Somero, M., Jaffee, L.A., and Holland, L. Z., 1979, Electrically mediated fast polyspermy block in eggs of the marine worm, Urechis caupo, J. Cell Biol., 82:426.

Graham, C.F., 1971, Experimental early parthenogenesis in mammals, in: "Symposium on Intrinsic and Extrinsic Factors in Early Mammalian Development," G. Raspe, ed., Vol. 6, Perganon Press, New York.

Graham, C.F., 1974, The production of parthenogenetic mammalian embryos and their use in biological research, Biol. Rev., 49:399.

Green, D.P.L., 1978, The mechanism of the acrosome reaction, in: "Development in Mammals," vol. 3, M.H. Johnson, ed., North-Holland, Amsterdam, 3:65.

Gulyas, B.J., 1980, Cortical granules of mammalian eggs, Int. Rev. Cytol., 63:357.

Gulyas, B.J., and Schmell, E.D., 1980, Ovoperoxidase activity in ionophore treated mouse eggs. I. Electron microscopic localization, Gamete Res., 3:267

Gwatkin, R.B.L., 1977, Fertilization Mechanisms in Man and Mammals, Plenum Press, New York.

Gwatkin, R.B.L., 1982, Receptor for sperm on the mammalian ovum, in: "In Vitro Fertilization and Embryo transfer," E. S. E. Hafez and K. Semm, eds., A. R. Liss, Inc., New York.

Gwatkin, R.B.L. and Williams, D.T., 1977, Receptor activity of the hamster and mouse solubilized zona pellucida before and after the zona reactions, J. Reprod. Fert., 49:55.

Gwatkin, R.B.L., Carter, H.W., and Patterson, H., 1976, Association of mammalian sperm with cumulus cells and the zona pellucida studied by scanning, in: "Scanning Electron Microsc.," Vol. 2, H. Johari and R.P. Decker, eds., IIT Res. Inst. Chicago.

Gwatkin, R.B.L., Williams, D.T., Hartmann, J.F., and Kniazuk, M., 1973, The zona reaction of hamster and mouse eggs: Production in vitro by a trypsin-like protease from cortical granules, J. Reprod. Fertil., 32:259.

Hafez, E.S.E., 1975, Sperm transport, in: "Progress in Infertility," 2nd ed., S.J. Behrman and R.C.O. Kistuery, eds., Little, Brown and Co., Boston.

Hagiwara, S., and Jaffe, L.A., 1979, Electrical properties of egg cell membranes, Ann. Rev. Biophys. Bioeng., 8:385.

Hanada, A., and Chang, M.C., 1972, Penetration of zona-free eggs by spermatozoa of different species, Biol. Reprod., 6:300.

Hartmann, J. F. and Gwatkin, R. B. I., 1971, Alteration of sites on the mammalian sperm surface following capacitation, Nature, (London), 234:479.

Hartmann, J.F., Gwatkin, R.B.L., and Hutchinson, C.F., 1972, Early contact interactions between mammalian gametes in vitro: Evidence that the vitellus influences adherence between sperm and zona pellucida, Proc. Natl. Acad. Sci., U.S.A. 69:2767.

Hartmann, J.F., 1983, Mammalian fertilization: gamete surface interactions in vitro, in: "Mechanism and Control of Animal Fertilization," J. F. Hartmann, ed., Academic Press, New York.

Hartree, E. F., 1977, Spermatozoa, eggs and proteinases, J. Biochem. Soc. Trans., 5:375.

Hayashi, M., 1963, Fertilization in vitro using human ova, in: "Seventh Conference of the International Planned Parenthood Federation," Excerpta Medica, Amsterdam.

Heller, D.T., and Schultz, R.M., 1980, Ribonucleoside metabolism by mouse oocytes: metabolic cooperativity between the fully grown oocyte and cumulus cells, J. Exp. Zool., 214:355.

Heller, D.T., Cahill, D.M., and Schultz, R.M., 1981, Biochemical studies of mammalian oogenesis: metabolic cooperativity between granulosa cells and growing mouse oocytes, Dev. Biol., 84:455.

Hertwig, A. T., Rock, J., Adams, E. C., and Mulligan, W. J., 1954, On the preimplantation stages of the human ovum, J. Contri. Embryol., 240:201.

Huang, T.T.F., Fleming, A.D., and Yanagimachi, R., 1981, Only acrosome-reacted spermatozoa can bind to and penetrate zona pellucida: a study using the guinea pig, J. Exp. Zool., 217:287.

Inoue, M., and Wolf, D. P., 1975, Comparative solubility properties of rat and hamster zonae pellucidae, Biol. Reprod., 12:535.

Iwamatsu, T., and Chang, M. C., 1971, Factors involved in the fertilization of mouse eggs in vitro, J. Reprod. Fertil., 26:197.

Jackowski, S., and Dumont, J.N., 1979, Surface alterations of the mouse zona pellucida and ovum following in vivo fertilization: correlation with the cell cycle., Biol. Reprod. 20:150.

Jaffe, L.A., 1976, Fast block to polyspermy in sea urchin eggs is electrically mediated, Nature (London), 261:68.

Jaffe, L.A., Sharp, A.P., and Wolf, D.P., 1983, Absence of an electrical polyspermy block in the mouse, Dev. Biol., 96:317.

Jagiello, G., Ducayen, M., Miller, W., Graffeo, T., and Fang, J.S., 1975, Stimulation and inhibition with LH and other hormones of female mammalian meiosis in vitro., Reprod. Fert., 43:9.

Jamil, K., and White, I. G., 1981, Induction of acrosome reaction in sperm with ionophore A23187 and calcium, Arch. Androl., 7:283.

Johnston, I., Lopata, A., Speirs, A., Gronow, M., Martin, M., and Olivia, K., 1983, Current status of an in vitro fertilization programme and early pregnancy diagnosis, in: "Fertilization of the Human Egg In Vitro," H. M. Beier and H. R. Linder, eds., Springer-Verlag, Berlin.

Jones, G.S., 1968, Induction of ovulation, Ann. Rev. Medicine, 19:351.

Jones, H. W., Jr., 1983, Factors influencing implantation and maintenance of pregnancy following embryo transfer, in: "Fertilization of the Human Egg In Vitro," H. M. Beier and H. R. Linder, eds., Springer-Verlag, Berlin.

Kaufman, M.H. and Sachs, L., 1976, Complete preimplantation development in culture of parthenogenic mouse embryos, J. Embryol. Exp. Morph., 35:179.

Kennedy, J. F., and Donahue, R. P., 1969, Human oocytes: Maturation in chemically defined media, Science, 164:1292.

Kerin, J.F., Warnes, G.M., Quinn, P.J., Jeffrey, R., Kirby, C., Matthews, C.D., Seamark, R.F., and Cox, L.W., 1983, Incidence of multiple pregnancy following human in vitro fertilization and embryo transfer, Lancet, 2:531.

Lauritsen, J.G., 1982, Results of in vitro fertilization and culture of human ova, in: "Follicular Maturation and Ovulation," Excerpta Medica, Amsterdam.

Leridon, H., 1977, Human Fertility: The Basic Components, University of Chicago Press, Chicago.

Longo, F. J., 1973, Fertilization: A comparative ultrastructural review, Biol. Reprod. 9:149.

Lopata, A., 1982, Factors influencing the growth of human implantation embryos in vitro, in: "Human Conception In Vitro," R.G. Edwards and J.M. Purdy, eds., Academic Press, New York.

Lopata, A., 1983, Concepts in human in vitro fertilization and embryo transfer, Fertil. Steril., 40:289.

Lopata, A., Brown, J. B., Johnston, I. W., Leeton, J., McTalbot, J., and Wood, C., 1977, In vitro fertilization and embryo transfer in infertile patients treated with clomiphene and gonadotrophins, Theriogenology, 8:155.

Lopata, A., Brown, J. B., Leeton, J. F., McTalbot, J., and Wood, C., 1978a, In vitro fertilization of preovulatory oocytes and embryo transfer in infertile patients treated with clomiphene and human chorionic gonadotropin, Fertil. Steril., 30:27.

Lopata, A., McMaster, R., McBain, J. C., and Johnston, W. I. H., 1978b, In vitro fertilization of preovulatory human eggs, J. Reprod. Fert., 52:339.

Lopata, A., Johnston, I.W.H., Hoult, I.J., and Speirs, A.I., 1980a, Pregnancy following intrauterine implantation of an embryo obtained by in vitro fertilization of a preovulatory egg, Fertil. Steril., 33:117.

Lopata, A., Sathananthan, A. H., McBain, J. C., Johnston, W.I.H., and Speirs, A.L., 1980b, The ultrastructure of the preovulatory human egg fertilized in vitro, Fertil. Steril., 33:12.

Mack, S., Bhattacharyya, A.K., Joyce, C., Van Der Ven, H., and L.J.D. Zaneveld, 1983, Acrosomal enzymes of human spermatozoa before and after in vitro capacitation, Biol. Reprod., 28:1032.

Mahi, C.A., and Yanagimachi, R., 1975, Induction of nuclear decondensation of mammalian spermatozoa in vitro, J. Reprod. Fert., 44:293.

Mahi, C.A., and Yanagimachi, R., 1979, Prevention of in vitro fertilization of canine oocytes by anti-ovary antisera: a potential approach to fertility control in the bitch, J. Exp. Zool., 210:129.

Mastroianni, L., Jr., and Noriega, C., 1970, Observations on human ova and the fertilization process, Am. J. Obstet. Gynecol. 107:682.

McCulloh, D.H., Rexroad, C.E., and Levitan, H., 1983, Insemination of rabbit eggs is associated with slow depolarization and repetitive diphasic membrane potentials, Dev. Biol., 95:372.

McGaughey, R.W., 1977, The maturation of porcine oocytes in minimal defined media with varied macro-molecular supplements and varied osmolarity, Exp. Cell. Res., 109:25.

McMaster, R., Yanagimachi, R., and Lopata, A., 1978, Penetration of human eggs by human sperm in vitro, Biol. Reprod., 19:212.

McRorie, R. A., and Williams, W. L., 1974, Biochemistry of mammalian fertilization, Ann. Rev. Biochem., 43:777.

Meck, F.B., Albright, J.T., and Botticelli, C.R., 1973, The fine structure of granulosa cell nexus in rat ovarian follicles, Anat. Rec., 175:107.

Meizel, S., 1978, The mammalian sperm acrosome reaction: A biochemical approach, in: "Development in Mammals," Vol. 3, M. H. Johnson, ed., North-Holland, Amsterdam.

Meizel, S., and Mukerji, S. K., 1976, Biochemical studies of proacrosin and acrosin from hamster cauda epididymal spermatozoa, Biol. Reprod., 14:444.

Menkin, M. F., and Rock, J. 1948, In Vitro Fertilization and Cleavage of human ovarian eggs, Amer. J. Obstet. Gynecol., 55:440.

Mettler, L., Baukloh, V., and Kil, M.S., 1982, Human in vitro fertilization and sperm immunological animal experiments, in: "Follicular Maturation and Ovulation," Excerpta Medica, Amsterdam.

Miyazaki, S., and Igusa, Y., 1981, Fertilization potential in golden hamster eggs consists of recurring hyperpolarization, Nature (London), 290:702.

Mohr, L. R., Trounson, A. O., Leeton, J. F., and Wood, C., 1983, Evaluation of normal and abnormal embryo development during procedures in vitro, in: "Fertilization of the Human Egg In Vitro," H. M. Beier and H. R. Linder, eds., Springer-Verlag, Berlin.

Moore, H.D.M., and Bedford, J.M., 1978, An in vivo analysis of factors influencing the fertilization of hamster eggs, Biol. Reprod., 19:879.

Moore, H.D.M. and Bedford, J.M., 1983, The interaction of mammalian gametes in the female, in: "Mechanism and Control of Animal Fertilization," J.F. Hartmann, ed., Academic Press, New York.

Nicosia, S.V., Wolf, D.P., and Inoue, M., 1977, Cortical granule distribution and cell surface characteristics in mouse eggs., Dev. Biol., 57:56.

Nishimoto, T., Yamada, I., Niwa, K., Mori, T., Nishimura, T., and Iritani, A., 1982, Sperm penetration in vitro of human oocytes matured in a chemically defined medium, J. Reprod. Fert., 64:115.

Niwa, K., and Chang, M.C., 1975b, Fertilization of rat eggs in vitro at various times before and after ovulation with special reference to fertilization of ovarian oocytes matured in vitro, J. Reprod. Fertil., 43:435.

Oikawa, T., Yanagimachi, R., and Nicolson, G. L., 1973, Wheat germ agglutinin blocks mammalian fertilization, Nature (London), 241:256.

Overstreet, J.W., 1983, Transport of gametes in the reproductive tract of the female mammal, in: "Mechanism and Control of Animal Fertilization," J.F. Hartmann, ed., Academic Press, New York.

Overstreet, J.W., and Bedford, J.M., 1974, Comparison of the penetrability of the egg investments in follicular oocytes, unfertilized and fertilized ova of rabbit, Dev. Biol., 41:185.

Overstreet, J. W., and Hembree, W. C., 1976, Penetration of the zona pellucida of non-living human oocytes by human spermatozoa in vitro, Fertil. Steril., 27:815.

Overstreet, J.W., and Tony, R.A., 1982, Experimental studies of rapid sperm transport in rabbits, J. Reprod. Fert., 66:601.

Peters, H., and McNatty, K.P., 1980, "Ovulation in the Ovary", University California Press, Los Angeles.

Phillips, D.M., and Shalgi, R., 1980a, Surface architecture of mouse and hamster zona pellucida and oocyte, J. Ultrastruct. Res., 72:1.

Phillips, D.M., and Shalgi, R., 1980b, Surface properties of the zona pellucida, J. Exp. Zool., 213:1.

Piko, L., 1969, Gamete structure and sperm entry in mammals, in: "Fertilization," Vol. 2, C. B. Metz and A. Monroy, eds., Academic Press, New York.

Pincus, G., and Enzmann, E.V., 1936, The comparative behavior of mammalian eggs in vivo and in vitro. II. Activation of tubal eggs of the rabbit, J. Exp. Zool., 73:195.

Pincus, G., and Saunders, B., 1939, The comparative behavior of mammalian eggs in vivo and in vitro VI. The maturation of human ovarian ova., Anat. Rec., 75:537.

Purdy, J.M., 1982, Methods for fertilization and embryo culture in vitro, in: "Human Conception In Vitro," R.G. Edwards and J.M. Purdy, eds., Academic Press, New York.

Quigley, M.M., Maklad, N.F., and Wolf, D.P., 1983. Comparison of two clomiphene citrate dosage regimens for follicular recruitment in an in vitro fertilization program, Fertil. Steril., 40:178.

Reddy, J. M., Joyce, C., and Zaneveld, L.J.D., 1979, Role of hyaluronidase in fertilization; the antifertility activity of myocrisin, a nontoxic hyaluronidase inhibitor, J. Androl., 1:28.

Rock, J., and Menkin, M.F., 1944, In vitro fertilization and cleavage of human ovarian eggs, Science, 100:105.

Rogers, B.J., and Bentwood, B.J., 1982, Capacitation, acrosome reaction and fertilization, in: "Biochemistry of Mammalian Reproduction," L.J.D. Zaneveld and R.T. Chatterson, eds., John Wiley and Sons, New York.

Rosseau, P., Meda, P., Lecart, C., Hammont, S., and Ferin, J., 1977, Cortical granule release in human follicular oocytes, Biol. Repro., 16:104.

Sacco, A.G., Yurewicz, E.C., Subramanian, M.G., and Demayo, F.J., 1983, Zona pellucida composition: species cross reactivity and contraception potential of antiserum to a partially purified pig zona antigen, Biol. Reprod., In Press.

Saling, P. M., and Storey, B. T., 1979, Mouse gamete interaction during fertilization in vitro, J. Cell Biol., 83:544.

Saling, P. M., Sowinski, J., and Storey, B. T., 1979, An ultrastructural study of epididymal mouse spermatozoa binding to zonae pellucidae in vitro: Sequential relationship to the acrosome reaction, J. Exp. Zool., 209:229.

Sathananthan, A.H., and Trounson, A.O., 1982a., Ultrastructural observations on cortical granules in human follicular oocytes cultured in vitro, Gamete Res., 5:191.

Sathananthan, A. H., and Trounson, A. O., 1982b, Ultrastructure of cortical granule release and zona interaction in monospermic and polyspermic human ova fertilized in vitro, Gamete Res., 6:225.

Sathananthan, A. H., Trounson, A. O., Wood, C., and Leeton, J. F., 1982, Ultrastructural observations on the penetration of human sperm into the zona pellucida of the human egg in vitro, J. Androl., 3:356.

Sato, K., 1979, Polyspermy-preventing mechanisms in mouse eggs fertilized in vitro, J. Exp. Zool., 210:353.

Schmell, E.D., and Gulyas, B.J., 1980a, Mammalian sperm-egg recognition and binding in vitro., Biol. Reprod., 23:1075.

Schmell, E.D., and Gulyas, B.J., 1980b, Ovoperoxidase activity in ionophore treated mouse eggs. II. Evidence for the enzymes role in hardening the zona pellucida, Gamete Res., 3:279.

Schmell, E.D., Gulyas, B.J., and Hedrick, J.L., 1983, Egg surface changes during fertilization and molecular mechanisms of the block to polyspermy, in: "Mechanisms and Control of Animal Fertilization," J.F. Hartmann, ed., Academic Press, New York.

Schuel, H, 1978, Secretory functions of egg cortical granules in fertilization and development: a critical review, Gamete Res., 1:299.

Schultz, R.M., LaMarca, M.J., and Wassarman, P.M., 1978, Absolute ratio of protein synthesis during meiotic maturation of mammalian oocytes in vitro, Proc. Natl. Acad. Sci., U.S.A., 75:4160.

Seibel, M.M., Smith, D.M., Levesque, L., Borton, M., and Taymor, M.L., 1982. The temporal relationship between the luteinizing hormone surge and human oocyte maturation, Am. J. Obstet. Gynecol., 142:568.

Settledge, D.S.F., Motoshima, M., and Tredway, D.R., 1973, Sperm transport from the external cervical os to the fallopian tubes in women: a time and quantitative study, Fertil Steril., 24:655.

Shalgi, R., and Phillips, D. M., 1980, Mechanics of sperm entry in cyclic hamster, J. Ultrastruct. Res., 71:154.

Shea, B.F., 1981, Evaluating the bovine embryo, Theriogenology, 15:31.

Shettles, L. B., 1955, A morula stage of human ova develop in vitro, Fertil Steril., 6:287.

Shivers, C. A., and Dudkiewicz, A. B., 1974, Inhibition of fertilization with specific antibodies, in: "Physiology and Genetics of Reproduction, Part B," E. M. Coutinho and F. Fuchs, eds., Plenum Press, New York.

Soupart, P., and Morgenstern, L. L., 1973, Human sperm capacitation and in vitro fertilization, Fertil. Steril., 24:462.

Soupart, P., and Strong, P. A., 1974, Ultrastructural observation on human oocytes fertilized in vitro, Fertil. Steril., 25:11.

Soupart, P., and Strong, P. A., 1975, Ultrastructural observations on polyspermic penetration of zona pellucida-free human oocytes inseminated in vitro, Fertil. Steril., 36:523.

Stambaugh, R., and Buckley, J., 1968, Zona pellucida dissolution enzymes of the rabbit sperm head, Science, 161:585.

Stambaugh, R., Brackett, B.G., and Mastrioanni, L., 1969, Inhibition of in vitro fertilization of rabbit ova by trypsin inhibitors, Biol. Reprod., 1:223.

Stambaugh, R., 1978, Enzymatic and morphological events in mammalian fertilization, Gamete Res., 1:65.

Stegner, H.E., and Wartenberg, H., 1961, Elektronenmi Kroskopische mnd histochemische untersuchen uber struk fur und bildung der zona pellucida menshlicher Linzellen., Z. Zellforsch. Mikrosk. Anat., 53:702.

Steptoe, P. C., and Edwards, R. G., 1970, Laparascopic recovery of preovulatory human oocytes after priming of ovaries with gonadotrophins, Lancet, 1:683.

Steptoe, P. C., and Edwards, R. G., 1978, Birth after the reimplantation of a human embryo, Lancet, 2:366.

Steptoe, P. C., Edwards, R. G., and Purdy, J. M., 1971, Human blastocysts grown in culture, Nature (London), 229:132.

Steptoe, P.C., Edwards, R.G., and Purdy, J.M., 1980, Clinical aspects of pregnancies established with cleaving embryos grown in vitro., Brit. J. Obstet. Gynaecol., 87:757.

Steinhardt, R.A., Epel, D., Carroll, E.J., and Yanagimachi, R., 1974, Is calcium ionophore a universal activator for unfertilized eggs?, Nature (London), 252:41.

Sundstrom, P., Nilsson, O., and Liedholm, P., 1981, Cleavage rate and the morphology of early human embryos obtained after artificial fertilization and culture, Acta Obstet Gynecol. Scand., 60:109.

Suzuki, S., and Iizuka, R., 1970, Maturation of human ovarian follicular oocytes in vitro, Experientia., 26:640.

Suzuki, S., Kitai, H., Tojo, R., Seki, K., Oba, M., Fujiwara, T., and Iizuka, R., 1981, Ultrastructure and some biologic properties of human oocytes and granulosa cells cultured in vitro, Fertil. Steril., 35:142.

Swenson, C.E., and Dunbar, B.S., 1982, Specificity of sperm-zona interaction, J.Exp. Zool., 219:97.

Szollosi, D., 1965, The fate of sperm middle-piece mitochondria in the rat egg, J. Exp. Zool., 159:367.

Szollosi, D., and Gerard, M., 1983, Cytoplasmic changes in the mammalian oocytes during the preovulatory period, in: "Fertilization of the human egg in vitro," H. M. Beier and H. R. Linder, eds., Springer-Verlag, Berlin.

Talbot, P., and Franklin, L. E., 1974, Hamster sperm hyaluronidase, II. Its release from sperm in vitro in relation to the degenerative and normal acrosome reaction, J. Exp. Zool., 189:321.

Tarkowski, A.K., Witowska, A., and Nowicka, J., 1970, Experimental parthenogenesis in the mouse, Nature (London), 222:162.

Tarkowski, A.K., 1971, Recent studies on parthenogenesis in the mouse, J. Reprod. Fert. Suppl. 14:31.

Testart, J., Thebault, A., Frydman, R., and Papiernik, E., 1982a, Oocyte and cumulus oophorus changes inside the human follicle cultured with gonadotropins, in: "In Vitro Fertilization and Embryo Transfer," E.S.E. Hafez and K. Semm, A. R. Liss, Inc., New York.

Testart, J. Lassalle, B., and Frydman, R., 1982b, Success of human in vitro fertilization in spontaneous or stimulated cycles and technical procedures used, in: "Follicular Maturation and Ovulation," Elsevier North Holland Inc., New York.

Testart, J., Frydman, R., DeMouzon, J., Lassalle, and Belaisch, J. C., 1983a, A study of factors affecting the success of human fertilization in vitro. I. Influence of ovarian stimulation upon the number and condition of oocytes collected, Biol. Reprod., 28:415.

Testart, J., Lassalle, B., Frydman, R., and Belaisch, J.C., 1983b, A study of factors affecting the success of human fertilization in vitro. II. Influence of semen quality and oocyte maturity on fertilization and cleavage, Biol. Reprod., 28:425.

Thibault, C., 1969, In vitro fertilization of the mammalian egg, in: "Fertilization," Vol. 2, C. B. Metz and A. Monroy, eds., Academic Press, New York.

Thibault, C., 1972, Physiology and physiopathology of the fallopian tube, Int. J. Fertil., 17:1.

Thibault, C., 1977, Are follicular maturation and oocyte maturation independent processes?, J. Reprod. Fert., 51:1.

Tobias, P. S., and Schumacher, G.F.B., 1976, The extraction of acrosin from human spermatozoa, Biol. Reprod., 15:187.

Trotnow, S., Al-Hasani, S., Kinewald, T., Becker, H., and Hunlich, T., 1983, Transfer of human embryos at early cleavage stages, in: "Fertilization of the Human Egg In Vitro," H. M. Beier and H. R. Linder, eds., Springer-Verlag, Berlin.

Trounson, A.O., 1982, Factors influencing the success of fertilization and embryonic growth in vitro, in: "Human Conception In Vitro," R.G. Edwards and J.M. Purdy, eds., Academic Press, New York.

Trounson, A. O., Leeton, J. F., Wood, C., Webb, J., and Kovacs, G., 1980a, The investigation of idiopathic infertility by in vitro fertilization, Fertil. Steril., 34:431.

Trounson, A. O., Shivers, C. A., McMaster, R., and Lopata, A., 1980b, Inhibition of sperm binding and fertilization of human ova by antibody to porcine zona pellucida and human sera, Arch. Androl., 4:29.

Trounson, A., and Wood, C., 1981, Extracorporeal fertilization and embryo transfer, Clinics in Obstet. and Gynecol., 8:681.

Trounson, A.O., Leeton, J.F., Wood, C., Buttery, B., Webb, J., Wood, J., Jessup, D., McTalbot, J., and Kovaco, G., 1981a, A programme of successful in vitro fertilization and embryo transfer in the controlled ovulatory cycle, in: "Human Reproduction," K. Semm and L. Mettler, eds., Excerpta, Medica, Princeton.

Trounson, A. O., Leeton, J. F., Wood, C., Webb, J., and Wood, J., 1981b, Pregnancies in humans by fertilization in vitro and embryo transfer in the controlled ovulatory cycle, Science, 212:681.

Trounson, A. O., Leeton, J. F., and Wood, C., 1982 In vitro fertilization and embryo transfer in the human, in: "Follicular Maturation and Ovulation," Elsevier North Holland, Inc., New York.

Trounson, A. O., Mohr, L. R., Wood, C., and Leeton, J. R., 1982b, Effect of delayed insemination on in vitro fertilization and transfer of human embryos, J. Reprod. Fert., 64:285.

Trounson, A., 1983, Factors controlling normal embryo development and implantation of human oocytes fertilized in vitro, in: "Fertilization of the Human Egg In Vitro," H. M. Beier and H. R. Linder, eds., Springer-Verlag, Berlin.

Tsafriri, A., Pomerantz, S.H., and Channing, C., 1976, Inhibition of oocyte maturation by porcine follicular fluid: partial characterization of the inhibitor, Biol. Reprod., 14:511.

Usui, N., and Yanagimachi, R., 1976, Behavior of hamster sperm nuclei incorporated into eggs at various stages of maturation, fertilization and early development: The appearance and disappearance of factors involved in sperm chromatin decondensation in egg cytoplasm, J. Ultrastruct. Res., 57:276.

Veeck, L.L., and Garcia, J.E., 1983a, The contribution to pregnancy by pronuclei or post-nuclear concepti developed from morphologically immature human oocytes., Biol. Reprod., 28:73a.

Veeck, L.L., Wortham, J.W.E., Witmyer, J., Sandow, B.A., Acosta, A.A., Garcia, J.E., Jones, G.S., and Jones, H.W., Jr., 1983, Maturation and fertilization of morphologically immature human oocytes in a program of in vitro fertilization, Fertil. Steril., 39:594.

Wasserman, P., 1983, Oogenesis: synthetic events in the developing mammalian egg, in: "Mechanisms and Control of Animal Fertilization," J. F. Hartmann, ed., Academic Press, New York.

Winkler, M.M., 1982, Regulation of protein synthesis in sea urchin eggs by intracellular pH, in: "Intracellular pH: Its Measurement, Regulation and Utilization in Cellular Functions," R. Nuccitelli and D.W. Deamer, eds., Alan R. Liss, Inc., New York.

Wolf, D.P., 1977, Involvement of a trypsin-like activity in sperm penetration of zona-free mouse ova, J. Exp. Zool., 199:149.

Wolf, D. P., 1978, The block to sperm penetration in zona-free mouse eggs, Dev. Biol., 64:1.

Wolf, D.P., 1981, The mammalian egg's block to polyspermy, in: "Fertilization and Early Embryonic Development In Vitro," L. Mastroianni and J. D. Biggers, eds., Plenum Press, New York.
Wolf, D.P., 1982, The ovum before and after fertilization, in: "Biochemistry of Mammalian Development," L.J.D. Zaneveld and R.T. Chatterton, eds., Wiley and Sons, New York.
Wolf, D.P., and Hamada, M., 1977, Induction of zonal and egg plasma membrane blocks to sperm penetration in mouse eggs with cortical granule exudate, Biol. Reprod., 17:350.
Wolf, D.P., Nicosia, S.V., and Hamada, M., 1979, Premature cortical granule loss does not prevent sperm penetration of mouse eggs, Dev. Biol., 71:22.
Wolf, D.P., Byrd, W., and Boldt, J., 1983, Monoclonal antibodies against acrosomal cap antigens of human ejaculated sperm, J. Cell Biol., Abstract in Press.
Wood, C., Trounson, A., Leeton, J., McTalbot, J., Buttery, B., Webb, J., Wood, J., and Jessup, D., 1981, A clinical assessment of nine pregnancies obtained by in vitro fertilization and embryo transfer, Fertil. Steril., 35:502.
Wortham, J.W.E., Veeck, L.L., Witmyer, J., and Jones, H.W., 1983, Vital initiation of pregnancy using human menopausal gonadotropin and human chorionic gonadotropin ovulation induction: Phase 1-1981, Fertil. Steril., 39:785.
Yanagimachi, R., 1977, Specificity of sperm-egg interaction, in: "Immunobiology of Gametes," M. Edidin and M. H. Johnson, eds., Cambridge Univ. Press, New York.
Yanagimachi, R., 1981, Mechanisms of fertilization in mammals, in: "Fertilization and Embryonic Development In Vitro," L. Mastrioanni, Jr, Ed, and J. D. Biggers, eds., Plenum Press, New York.
Yanagimachi, R., and Noda, Y. D., 1970a, Ultrastructural changes in the hamster sperm head during fertilization, J. Ultrastruct. Res., 31:465.
Yanagimachi, R., and Noda, Y. D., 1970b, Physiological changes in the post-nuclear cap region of mammalian spermatozoa: A necessary preliminary to the membrane fusion between sperm and egg cells, J. Ultrastruct. Res., 31:486.
Yanagimachi, R., and Noda, Y. D., 1970c, Fine structure of the hamster sperm head, Am. J. Anat., 128:367.
Yanagimachi, R., and Noda, Y. D., 1970d, Electron microscopic studies of sperm incorporation into golden hamster egg, Am. J. Anat., 128:429.
Yu, S.F., and Wolf, D.P., 1981, Polyspermic mouse eggs can dispose of supernumerary sperm, Dev. Biol., 82:203.
Zamboni, L., 1971, "Fine Morphology of Mammalian Fertilization," Harper & Row, New York.
Zamboni, L., Thompson, R. S., and Smith, D. M., 1972, Fine morphology of human oocyte maturation in vitro, Biol. Reprod., 7:425.

Zaneveld, L.J.D., 1976, Sperm enzyme inhibitors as antifertility agents, *in*: "Human Semen and Fertility Regulation in Men," E.S.E. Hafez, ed., C.V. Mosby Co., St. Louis.

Zeilmaker, G.H., and Alberda, A. Th., 1982, Some observations on human oocyte maturation and fertilization and a consideration of the risks involved in employing the technique of *in vitro* fertilization, *in*: "Follicular Maturation and Ovulation," Excerpta Medica, Amsterdam.

Zirkin, B.R., and Chang, T.S.K., 1977, Involvement of endogenous proteolytic activity in thiol-induced release of DNA template restrictions in rabbit sperm nuclei, *Biol. Reprod.*, 17:131.

Zirkin, B.R., Chang, T.S.K., and Heaps, J., 1980, Involvement of an acrosin-like proteinase in the sulfhydryl-induced degradation of rabbit sperm nuclear protamine, *J. Cell Biol.*, 85:116.

Zirkin, B.R., Soucek, D.A., and Chang, T.S.K., 1982, Sperm nuclear packing and regulation during spermatogenesis and fertilization, *Johns Hopkins Med. J.*, 151:101.

13

LABORATORY DETAILS IN AN *IN VITRO* FERTILIZATION AND EMBRYO TRANSFER PROGRAM

Joseph E. Sokoloski and Don P. Wolf

In this chapter, the details of the IVF-ET program at UT-Houston are presented. This is done not only to introduce the complexities of IVF-ET but also with the objective of moving towards a standardization of protocols. Initially, standardization requires a complete description of the techniques, equipment, and supplies employed. Even with the most minute attention to detail, duplication of results by other laboratories will not necessarily be obtained. The protocols described here are certainly not unique to the UT program and credit as well as appreciation is expressed to Dr. Alex Lopata and co-workers (Lopata et al., 1980). Dr. Lopata visited Houston in the very early phases of our program and was kind enough to examine our protocols and modify them where appropriate. Additionally, references have been added throughout the chapter where modifications can be directly attributed to the contributions of others. IVF-ET is an exceedingly complex undertaking and the parameters which may contribute to success are virtually infinite. Although success rates in the most active groups have steadily improved over the past several years, the number of variables makes it appear unlikely that a major breakthrough will occur. Rather the most likely scenario is continued and gradual improvements in techniques and protocols resulting in higher egg recoveries, fertilization, development, implantation and clinical pregnancy rates. To our minds, one way to enhance the rate of improvement of IVF-ET protocols is to share details to the extent that many of the parameters can be standardized and unknowns can be varied one at a time in a controlled setting.

In contemplating the laboratory component of an IVF-ET program, experience with mammalian gametes and aseptic technique is mandatory. A basic introduction to these subjects can be found in: "Tissue Culture Methods and Applications", (P. F. Kruse and M. K. Patterson, Jr., eds) Academic Press, New York, 1973 and Mammalian Embryo Culture B. Minz, in: "Methods in Developmental Biology" (F. M. Wilt and N. K. Wessells, eds) Crowell, New York 1967. Human IVF-ET culture conditions are reviewed by Purdy (1982).

MAJOR EQUIPMENT ITEMS

Incubator

The water-jacketed incubator employed should have a stable temperature control mechanism with less than a 1.5°C fluctuation. Internal thermometers are recommended in any warm environment, and daily temperature checks should be done before the incubators are opened in the morning. Of course, when small volume culturing is done, the incubator chamber must have saturated humidity. The internal water reservoir should be cleaned regularly, and only recommended additives such as zephiran or copper sulfate should be used to prevent contamination. There are many models of incubators with a variety of air flow systems, only a few of which are designed to handle the mixing of three gasses. Moreover, a 3-gas incubator is not always designed so that all the gasses are under pressure and strictly regulated. We use an incubator which mixes filtered medical grade CO_2, nitrogen, and room air to give the desired mixture of 5% CO_2, 5% O_2, 90% N_2. Alternatively, 5% CO_2 in air can be employed (Jones et al., 1982; Feichtinger et al., 1983). Direct port measurements of CO_2 and O_2 should be conducted daily. This can be done conveniently with a Fyrite detector (Bacharach Co., Pittsburgh, PA). A double chambered incubator provides the additional option of separating a patient's eggs, when there are several, into completely independent incubators for protection in the event of incubator failure.

Microscopes

Dissecting microscopes with trinocular capabilities for simultaneous video recording are highly recommended. We are currently employing a Wild (M8) stereo zoom trinocular head and a Nikon base and light source (Figure 1). Twenty magnification eyepieces allow magnification over the range of 12 to 100 X. Coupled with this system we use color video micrographic equipment which allows simultaneous viewing and recording for permanent record. For photomicrographic recording at high resolution, an inverted microscope is also desirable.

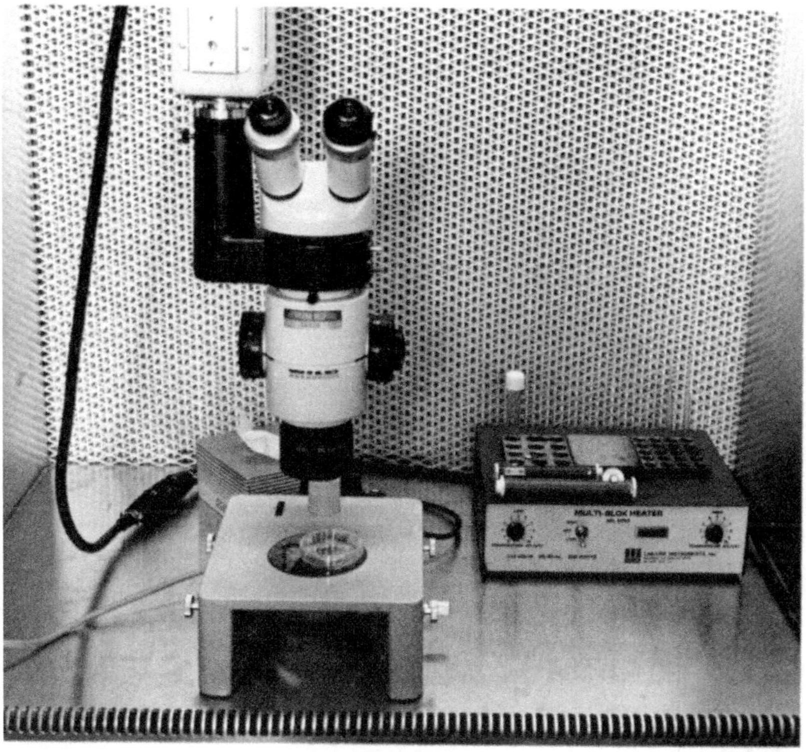

Figure 1

Dissecting microscope with video capability used for ovum recovery and handling.

Hoods

All procedures are conducted in horizontal laminar flow hoods containing germicidal lights. Surfaces are cleaned periodically with 70% ethanol and germicidal lights are left on when hoods are not in use.

CULTURE MEDIA

The IVF-ET program in Houston currently utilizes a modified Ham's F-10 medium. Several other culture media have been used successfully for human IVF-ET; Earles medium (Purdy, 1982), Menezo's B_2 (Testart et al., 1983), Whittinghams T-6 medium and a modified Whittens medium (Trounson, 1983). For comparative purposes, the composition of these media are listed in Table 1.

Table 1. Composition of culture media utilized for human *in vitro* fertilization

Constituent	Modified Earle's[1]	Modified Whittens[2]	Menezo's B_2[3]	Modified Ham's F-10[4]	Whittingham's T6[5]
	(mM)				
$CaCl_2$	1.80	-	-	0.29	1.78
KCl	5.36	4.77	3.82	3.82	1.42
$MgSO_4$	0.81	1.19	0.81	0.62	-
NaCl	116.34	87.94	89.92	126.6	97.84
NaH_2PO_4	1.01	-	-	-	
Na_2HPO_4	-	-	0.43	1.10	0.36
KH_2PO_4	-	1.19	0.44	0.61	-
$NaHCO_3$	25.0	22.62	29.76	25.0	25.0
Ca lactate	-	1.71	1.62	0.79	-
Na pyruvate	0.09	0.23	2.27	1.0	0.47
Glucose	5.55	5.55	6.66	6.11	5.55
Na lactate (60% syrup)	-	19.80	-	-	24.88
$MgCl_2$	-	-	-	-	0.47
Penicillin	Yes	Yes	Yes	Yes	Yes
Streptomycin	No	Yes	Yes	Yes	Yes
Albumin	Yes	Yes	Yes	Yes	Yes
Amino Acids, vitamins and other constituents	No	No	Yes	Yes	No

(1) Purdy (1982)
(2) Hoppe and Pitts (1973)
(3) Testart et al., (1983)
(4) Lopata et al., (1980)
(5) Quinn et al., (1982)

Stock Medium Preparation

Preparation of modified Ham's F-10 media - Standard tissue culture techniques are employed: No mouth pipetting; all procedures are confined to laminar flow hoods; aseptic technique throughout; all pipettes, catheters and filters are pre-rinsed with culture medium immediately prior to use.

Chemicals Required:

Ham's F-10 (1L/pkg)
Penicillin G (75 mg)
Streptomycin Sulfate (50 mg)
Calcium lactate 1.5 H_2O (245.2 mg)
Sodium bicarbonate (2.106g)
5X glass redistilled water (1 liter) (See Appendix A)

Equipment Required:

Osmometer
Analytical balance
Stirring mechanism
Sterile disposable syringes; 30-50cc capacity
Sterile filter; 0.22 μm

Glassware-Plasticware Required:

1 liter glass beaker; IVF washed (See Appendix A)
50 ml glass beaker; IVF washed
1 liter volumetric flask; IVF washed
10 ml pipettes; sterile, tissue culture grade plastic
250 ml flasks; sterile, tissue culture grade plastic
100 ml graduated cylinder; IVF washed

Procedure:

1. Dissolve 1 package of powdered Ham's F-10 in approximately 250 ml of 5X water
2. Add the penicillin-G and streptomycin. Mix well.
3. Dissolve the sodium bicarbonate in approximately 40 ml of 5X water.
4. Dissolve the calcium lactate in approximately 40 ml of 5X water.
5. Add the sodium bicarbonate solution to the Ham's F-10. Mix well.
6. SLOWLY add the calcium lactate solution to the Ham's F-10 with mixing.
7. Transfer the mixture to a volumetric flask and add 5X water to a final volume of 1 liter.

8. Determine the osmolarity and adjust to 275-280 mOsmol/kg: Usually the initial unadjusted value is 290-305 mOsmol/kg. To adjust osmolarity use the following formula: Initial reading (mOsmol/kg) - 280 (mOsmol/kg) / initial reading (mOsmol/kg) x 1 (V in liters) = volume in liters of medium to be removed and replaced with 5X water
9. Re-check osmolarity.
10. Filter medium through a sterile 0.22 µm filter into four 250 ml sterile tissue culture grade flasks (Falcon 3024).
11. Store at 4° C.
12. Use within 4 weeks of preparation.

Working Media

Chemicals Required:

Modified Ham's F-10 Stock (see above) (106 ml)
Maternal preovulatory serum - collected prior to receiving hCG and heat inactivated for 30 minutes at 56-60° C. (16 ml)
Sodium heparin (3000 IU)

Equipment Required:

Sterile disposable syringes; 30-50 ml capacity.
Sterile filters: 0.22 µm; 0.45 µm.

Glassware-Plasticware Required:

100 ml glass graduated cylinder; IVF washed
250 ml sterile flask; tissue culture grade plastic.
50 ml sterile flask; tissue culture grade plastic.
12 x 75 mm sterile tube with cap; tissue culture grade plastic.
16 x 125 mm sterile tube with cap; tissue culture grade plastic.
10 ml sterile pipette; tissue culture grade plastic.

Comment:

The media used for sperm washing and insemination are the same (i.e., Ham's F-10 with 7.5% patient serum). They are prepared simultaneously but are separated upon filtration into individual flasks for convenience and to assist in maintaining sterility throughout the procedure. The needle flushing medium is the same but also contains 100 IU/ml of heparin. All samples are identified by patient name and date on color coded tape.

Procedure:

Insemination, Sperm Washing and Flushing Media:

1. Add 92.5 ml of Ham's F-10 stock to a 100 ml graduated cylinder.
2. Add 7.5 ml of patient serum. Mix well.
3. Filter 45 ml of medium through a 0.22 μm filter into a sterile flask (Falcon 3013) labeled INSEMINATION I and cap tightly.
   Note: Occasionally, filtering the serum containing medium directly through the 0.22 μm filter may be difficult. If this occurs, prefilter the medium through a 0.45 um or larger filter. The 0.45 and 0.22 μm filters can even be attached together (piggy backed) for this purpose.
4. Filter 10 ml of medium into a sterile tube (Falcon 3013) labeled INSEMINATION II and cap tightly.
5. Filter 22 ml of medium into a sterile flask (Falcon 3013) labeled SPERM WASH I and cap tightly.
6. Filter 3 ml of medium into a sterile tube (Falcon 2003) labeled SPERM WASH II and cap tightly.
7. To the remaining 30 ml of medium, add 3000 IU of sodium heparin. Mix well.
8. Filter the heparin medium into a sterile flask (Falcon 3013) labeled FLUSHING and cap tightly.

Growth Medium:

1. Add 12.75 ml of Ham's F-10 stock to a flask.
2. To this add 2.25 ml of patient serum. Mix well.
3. Filter into a sterile flask (Falcon 3013) labeled GROWTH MEDIUM and cap tightly.

Transfer Medium: (Modified from Feichtinger et al., 1983).

1. Add 3.0 ml of Ham's F-10 stock to a test tube or flask.
2. Add 3.0 ml of patient serum and mix.
3. Filter into a sterile tube (Falcon 3033) labeled TRANSFER MEDIUM and cap tightly.

Transfer all of the filtered media from the laminar flow hood to the incubator and LOOSEN all caps. Incubate the media for approximately 16 hours at 37°C in a humidified atmosphere of 5% O_2: 5% CO_2: 90% N_2. Under these conditions the media should equilibrate to a pH of 7.4-7.6 (a change in color from pink to amber). If time does not permit or the color does not seem right, measure the pH and bubble the media with the above gas mixture until the proper pH is attained. Make sure you use filtered gases and STERILE pipettes and equipment if the bubbling procedure is used.

SPERM PROCESSING

The husband is instructed to abstain sexually for 48 hours prior to producing a sample for IVF. We do not use antibiotics prophylactically nor do we conduct routine microbiologic screens of semen. He is given a sterile specimen container and asked to bring the sample to the laboratory within one hour of collection on the day of the laparoscopy. Occasionally a husband has had difficulty in producing a sample, particularly if asked for the specimen after his wife has undergone surgery. We now routinely prepare the sperm before the scheduled laparoscopy. This alleviates some of the anxiety and also allows for a longer capacitation period. This longer capacitation time may contribute to our success with lower sperm concentrations (see Chapter 12). If the husband is anticipating a problem in producing a sample, a specimen can be obtained a few days before surgery and stored in liquid nitrogen, although we would still request a fresh sample on the day of egg retrieval. We have never had to use a frozen sample. Liquified ejaculates for freezing are diluted 1:1 (v/v) with a modified Krebs-Ringer bicarbonate medium containing 15% glycerol and incubated for 15 minutes at 37°C. Aliquots (0.5 ml) are transferred to plastic ampules, cooled to -20°C, suspended in nitrogen vapor for 2 to 7 minutes, and finally lowered into liquid nitrogen for storage until use. A sample is thawed by placing the ampule in a 37°C water bath for 20 minutes. Sperm are then processed for insemination following the procedure described for a fresh semen sample.

A prolonged preincubation (6-8 hrs) of sperm is not absolutely essential as pregnancies have resulted from samples preincubated for intervals under one hour.

Chemicals Required:

SPERM WASH I
SPERM WASH II

Equipment Required:

Microscope; for semen analysis.
Hemacytometer; for sperm count.
Clinical centrifuge; swinging bucket rotor capable of 500 x g.

Glassware-Plasticware Required:

Pasteur pipettes; sterile, IVF washed.
10 ml pipettes; sterile, disposable, tissue culture grade plastic.
Conical centrifuge tubes 15 ml; sterile, disposable, tissue culture grade plastic.

Comments:

We prepare 2 sperm suspensions (usually 1 ml each) from every ejaculate. Both are handled identically. One tube remains untouched in the incubator and is used as the sperm stock for insemination. The other is removed from the incubator just prior to the insemination and a sperm count and motility is made. The insemination volume required for the desired final motile sperm concentration is then calculated. This allows maintainance of a sterile environment for the inseminating sperm and provides an emergency backup of the sperm stock.

Procedure:

1. Upon receipt of the specimen in the laboratory, the container is immediately labeled, on color coded tape, with the patient's name and time of collection. If it has been less than 30 minutes since collection, the specimen is placed in a 37°C incubator for the remainder of the liquifaction period. Otherwise, it can be used immediately. Sperm are usually processed between 30 and 120 minutes of collection.
2. One ml aliquots of the liquified ejaculate are transferred to each of two sterile centrifuge tubes (Falcon 2095). In the case of the oligospermic patient, larger volumes, if available, should be processed.
3. To each tube add 3 ml of SPERM WASH I. Mix well with a sterile pasteur pipette.
4. Centrifuge the tubes at 500 X g for 10 minutes.
5. Either before processing the sample or while the sperm suspensions are spinning, record the total volume of the ejaculate and perform a standard semen analysis making particular note of the sperm motility, progression and concentration. Our observed ranges for all IVF patients processed to date (mean ± SEM) are: Volume; 1.6-5.6 cc (3.6± 0.2); Motility; 48-67% (57.6 ± 0.9); Progression, 2-4 (3.5) and Concentration 12-307 x 10^6 sperm/ml (86 ± 12 x 10^6).
6. As soon as the centrifuge stops, carefully remove the supernatant with a pasteur pipette.
7. Add 3 ml of SPERM WASH I to each pellet and resuspend the sperm by fairly vigorous agitation in a pasteur pipette.
8. Recentrifuge the sperm suspension at 500 X g for 10 minutes.
9. Remove the supernatant as before and resuspend the pellets in 1 ml SPERM WASH II using fresh pipettes. In the case of the oligospermic patient, sperm concentrations can be increased at this point by reconstituting the pellet in smaller volumes of SPERM WASH II.
10. Transfer sperm suspensions to the IVF incubator, loosen caps and place at a 30-45° angle. The sperm will remain in this state until insemination or approximately 5-7 hours. NOTE: When more than 1 specimen is processed EXTREME CAUTION must be taken to avoid cross contamination.

OOCYTE RECOVERY AND PREINCUBATION

Chemicals required:

FLUSHING MEDIUM
INSEMINATION MEDIUM I; INSEMINATION MEDIUM II

Equipment Required:

Pipettor; 5 ml capacity
Dissecting microscope
Pipettor; 10 ml capacity
Warming block; 37°C, with individual tube supports

Glassware-Plasticware required:

Pasteur pipette; 5 3/4 inch, sterile, IVF washed
5 ml pipette; sterile, disposable, tissue culture grade plastic
35 x 10 mm petri dish; sterile, disposable, tissue culture grade plastic.
60 x 15 mm petri dish; sterile, disposable, tissue culture grade plastic.
60 x 15 mm organ culture dish; sterile, disposable, tissue culture grade plastic.

Comment:

The follicular aspirate is handled exclusively in a laminar flow hood and every attempt is made to maintain a sterile environment throughout the entire process. Verbal contact is maintained with the surgeon so that follicular aspirates do not "stack up" while the eggs are being washed and transferred to culture dishes and also so that the surgeon knows exactly how many eggs have been recovered. A closed circuit viedo system eliminates most communication problems as the surgeon can monitor progress in the embryo culture laboratory directly.

Procedure:

1. Just prior to the first follicular aspiration, the FLUSHING medium is removed from the IVF incubator and given to the circulating nurse. The surgeon will use this medium to "rinse" the needle after aspirating the follicle or to irrigate the follicle if necessary.
2. Immediately after aspiration, the aspirate tube is labeled with the patient's name, follicle number and the ovary from which it was obtained. Also record if it was a direct aspirate, needle flush or irrigation.

3. Record the size of the follicle, as estimated by the surgeon, and the volume of the aspirated fluid. The latter can be measured readily by direct comparison with a calibrated tube.
4. Pour the aspirate into a sterile dish (Falcon 1007 or 3001 depending on the volume) on the stage of the dissecting microscope and look for the cumulus mass containing the egg. Often the mass can be seen with the unaided eye, usually as a clear to white fluffy aggregate, like a small piece of clear to white gelatin. Under the dissection microscope, this mass is clearly distinct from the darker, more dense granulosa sheets or plaques. When the straw colored follicular fluid is contaminated with blood, pick out for further examination all suspicious looking cellular particulates and transfer to a dish containing INSEMINATION I. Confirm the presence of an egg. If after looking through both the follicular aspirate and needle flush, no egg is found, inform the surgeon so that the follicle can be irrigated. Check the irrigated fluid as above, and repeat if necessary. If an oocyte is recovered from a bloody irrigant, be sure to wash in medium before transferring to the organ culture dish. Adherent blood clots or granulosa cell plaques can be removed from the cumulus with 26 gauge needles attached to tuberculin syringes.
5. Once the cumulus mass with an egg is identified, transfer the entire mass with the aid of a sterile pasteur pipette attached to a 5 ml pipettor to a 35 x 10 mm dish (Falcon 3001) containing INSEMINATION I. Comment: Usually, the egg-cumulus mass is identified immediately and transferred to the wash medium within 60 seconds. Minimize exposure to light. With regards to temperature control during these procedures, we are not concerned so much about maintaining 37° as we are about avoiding temperature shock.
6. Prepare an organ culture dish (Falcon 3037), labeled with the patient's name, follicle number and ovary by placing 0.9 ml of INSEMINATION II in the center well of the dish and 2.0 ml in the outer chamber. While the capacity of the center well is 1 ml, a smaller volume helps prevent any overflow when the dishes are moved to the incubator. Use a separate dish for each egg.
7. Carefully transfer the egg to the organ culture dish and place in the IVF incubator. Note: We do not overlay with paraffin or silicone oil in human IVF. When using cultures that are not covered with oil, it is imperative that the incubator is humidified and that the culture medium is changed in the dishes every 24 hours. Record notes on cumulus, corona, and egg quality.
8. Inform the surgeon to continue with additional follicular aspirations.

9. Incubate mature eggs for 5-6 hours in the IVF incubator with a humified atmosphere of $5\%CO_2$: $5\%O_2$: $90\%N_2$ before insemination. Any eggs classified as immature must be cultured for at least 24 hours before insemination (Veeck et al., 1983). For a detailed discussion of the appearance of a mature or immature oocyte, see Chapter 12.

INSEMINATION

Equipment required:

Dissecting microscope
Microscope; for sperm analysis
Micropipettor; capable of dispensing 1-100 µm.
Hemacytometer; for sperm count

Glassware-Plasticware required:

Pipettor tips; sterile, for dispensing 1-100 µm.

Comment:

It is important to classify the eggs as mature or immature before insemination. Take all factors into account when making this decision: follicle size; follicular fluid volume; size and appearance of the cumulus mass; and the density and organization of the corona. Mature eggs should be inseminated 5-6 hours after aspiration (Trounson et al., 1982). Immature eggs need to be cultured in the absence of sperm for an additional 24 hours before adding sperm (Veeck et al., 1983). Immature eggs apparently will not mature properly in the presence of sperm.

When immature eggs are cultured for insemination, a second semen sample is requested on the day of the insemination. The sperm is prepared exactly as the first sample.

Procedure:

1. Remove one of the sperm suspension tubes from the incubator and place it in a rack in a vertical position. This allows the immotile sperm and non-sperm cells to slough to the bottom of the tube. Three to 4 minutes is sufficient to allow the cells to settle out.
2. Remove an aliquot of the sperm suspension from the upper phase.
3. Determine the percent motility, progression and sperm concentration. Usually the percent motility and progression

scores are enhanced over the original semen analysis while the sperm concentration may be decreased by an order of magnitude.

4. Calculate the volume necessary to inseminate the egg with 50,000 progressively motile sperm. We are currently using 50,000 motile sperm to inseminate the eggs when the husband presents with a normal semen analysis. If the husband presents with a history of abnormal semen parameters, i.e., oligospermia, poor motility or progression, 500,000 motile sperm are used. See Chapter 12 for further explanation.
5. Remove the second sperm tube from the incubator and place it upright in the laminar flow hood. Allow the cells to settle as above.
6. Using a sterile pipette tip and an accurate pipettor, transfer the calculated volume of sperm suspension to each oocyte to be inseminated. If the volume necessary for insemination is larger than 50 μl, remove the same volume from the center well before insemination.
7. Check each dish for the presence of sperm and return it to the IVF incubator.
8. Record the time and the volume of sperm employed in each insemination.
9. If the dish contains an immature egg do not inseminate it immediately. Culture it for an additional 24 hours, transfer it to a new dish with fresh medium and inseminate it following the exact procedure described above.

ASSESSMENT OF OOCYTE FERTILIZATION AND SUBSEQUENT EMBRYONIC DEVELOPMENT

Chemicals Required:

GROWTH MEDIUM

Equipment Required:

Dissecting microscope
Forceps; sterile, fine tip
Disposable syringes; 1 ml
Pipettor; 5 ml capacity
Pipettor; 10 ml capacity
Burner

Glassware-Plasticware Required:

60 x 15 mm organ culture dish; sterile, disposable, tissue culture grade plastic.
Pasteur pipette; 5 3/4 inch, sterile, IVF washed.
Pasteur pipette; 9 inch, sterile, IVF washed
Pipette; 5 or 10 ml, sterile, disposable, tissue culture grade plastic.

Comment:

Egg observation and fertilization assessment should be done between 13 and 19 hours after insemination when pronuclei are visible. For a detailed discussion on embryonic development see Chapter 12.

Procedure:

1. Using a low flame, hand pull several sterilized 9 inch pasteur pipettes to fine, narrow tips. Place in laminar flow hood.
2. Transfer the insemination dish to the dissecting microscope under the hood and observe. Document the presence of motile sperm. At this point the cumulus mass should be dispersed and the egg with corona should be clearly visible. Dislodge the egg from the bottom of the dish by directing a stream of culture medium, from a fine pipette. Sometimes with clomiphene citrate and often when Pergonal is used in follicular recruitment, the egg, after insemination and cumulus dispersal, is entrapped in a "rubbery" mass. If this occurs, gently tease the mass away from its oocyte with the tips of 27 gauge needles being careful not to damage the egg.
3. Using sterile forceps, break back the tip of a drawn pipette until it is slightly larger than the egg-corona mass. Do not make the tip too small as egg distortion will result. Judge the correct size by placing the tip near the egg (Figure 2).
4. Attach the drawn pipette to a 5 ml pipettor, pre-rinse to be sure broken glass is gone and gently aspirate the egg-corona mass in and out until enough of the corona cells are dislodged to allow a clear view of the egg's cytoplasm.
5. Using high magnification (100 x) carefully observe the egg. At this point in time you should see 2 distinct pronuclei in the cytoplasm and one or two polar bodies in the perivitelline space.
6. Prepare a sterile organ culture dish by labelling with the patient's name, follicle number, and the ovary from which it was aspirated. Add 0.9 ml of GROWTH MEDIUM to the center well and 2.0 ml to the outer chamber.
7. Carefully transfer the egg to the culture dish using a standard bore sterilized pasteur pipette.
8. Return the fertilized egg to the IVF incubator.
9. Record the time of observation and appearance of the egg.
10. Repeat the process for each egg. We do not reinseminate if the egg fails to fertilize.
11. At forty hours post-insemination a second observation is made at which time the fertilized eggs (now embryos) range from the 2-cell to 4-cell stage.
12. Record the time of observation and appearance of the embryos.

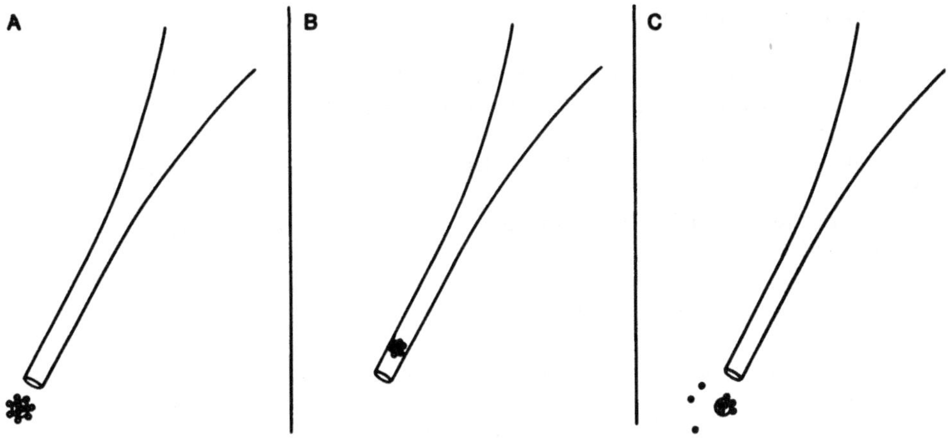

Figure 2

Mechanical removal of corona cells from human oocytes

A. Appearance of appropriately sized micropipette prior to oocyte aspiration.
B. Aspiration of oocyte - corona complex into the micropipette.
C. Expulsion of oocyte with dislodgement of corona cells.

The shearing force of corona cells against the walls of the micropipette is sufficient to dislodge them.

13. Arrange with the Clinical Coordinator for transfer of the embryos to the patient within 4-5 hours of the last observation.
    NOTE: Any immature eggs that were inseminated 24 hours later than the mature oocytes obtained at the same laparoscopy will be 24 hours out of synchrony and will be transferred at the pronuclear stage, with the cleaving embryos. In the absence of the latter, this pronuclear egg can be cultured for an additional 24 hours to document cleavage before transfer.

EMBRYO TRANSFER

Chemicals Required:

TRANSFER MEDIUM

Equipment Required:

Catheter (#20 Teflon tubing, i.d.: 0.86 mm, o.d.: 1.47 mm, length: 40 cm, plugged end with side opening), sterile.
Dissecting microscope
Introducer (#12 steel needle tubing, i.d.: 2.157 mm, curved tip), sterile.
Microsyringe; 1 ml, gas tight. Pipettor; 5 ml capacity. #19 Blunt Needle.

Glassware-Plasticware required:

35 x 10 mm petri dish; sterile, disposable, tissue culture grade plastic.
Pasteur pipettes; 5 3/4 inch, sterile, IVF washed.

Comment:

For a detailed description of the transfer catheter and introducer, see Chapter 15.

Procedure:

1. Fill a shallow sterile petri dish with TRANSFER MEDIUM. The top of a Falcon 3001 dish is adequate.
2. Assemble the Transfer aparatus (Chapter 15, Figure 1). Rinse the distal end of the catheter (approximately 5 cm) twice with TRANSFER MEDIUM.
3. Using a sterile pasteur pipette, transfer the cleaving embryos to the petri dish.
4. Pull the barrel of the syringe back approximately one quarter of the way.
5. Aspirate 10 μl of medium (approximately 1 cm) into the catheter followed by 10 μl of air.
6. While monitoring with the dissecting microscope, carefully aspirate all embryos into the catheter keeping the total volume to approximately 10-15 μl. Usually the medium is swirled slightly over the embryo to "float" the embryos allowing easy aspiration through the side opening of the catheter (Figure 3). After all the embryos have been loaded draw in 10 ul of air followed by 10 μl of TRANSFER MEDIUM.
8. Retract the catheter into the introducer and replace the entire unit into the sterile sleeve.
9. Transport the transfer unit to the physician.
10. Following the transfer of the embryos to the patient, carefully examine the catheter under the dissecting microscope to ensure that all embryos are gone. Pay special attention to the opening of the catheter; if the tip has an

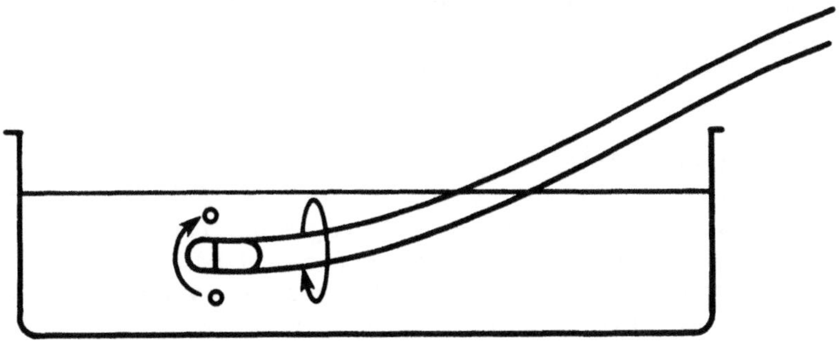

Figure 3

Loading embryos into the transfer catheter. The tip of the catheter is swirled sufficiently to float the embryos allowing easy aspiration through the side opening in the catheter tip.

accumulation of mucus the embryo can be trapped there. If this occurs, free the embryo and reload it into the catheter for a second attempt at transfer to the patient. Even if the catheter is mucus free and no embryo is seen it should be rinsed 2 to 3 times with TRANSFER MEDIUM to ensure that all embryos have been expelled.

BIOASSAY FOR EMBRYO CULTURE CONDITIONS: PREIMPLANTATION DEVELOPMENT OF TWO-CELL MOUSE EMBRYOS TO HATCHING BLASTOCYSTS

The adequacy of the in vitro culturing conditions for human eggs and embryos should be assessed by culturing mouse embryos from the two-cell to the hatching blastocyst stage. For a general description of mammalian embryo culturing techniques, refer to B. Mintz (1967). Embryos recovered from inbred rather than random bred animals usually support higher levels of preimplantation development. For our studies, Swiss Webster-CRL:CFW (SW) BR animals (7 to 8 week virgin females; Charles Rivers, Wilmington, MA) were employed.

Embryo Recovery:

Superovulation of animals is induced by the intraperitoneal injection of 10 IU of PMS on day 0 followed 48 hours later by 10 IU units of hCG. Following the hCG injection, two females are caged with one male (12 to 14 weeks old) by transferring the females to the male cage. Mating can be confirmed by checking for the presence of a vaginal plug; superovulated females that do not mate may be reinjected at a later time. We have averaged 30 eggs per superovulated animal. The timing of pronuclear formation, syngamy and cleavage has been studied in superovulated mice by Edwards and Gates (1959). Approximately 24 hours are required for a penetrated egg to complete fertilization and proceed to the two-cell stage. Hence, mated animals are sacrificed, by cervical dislocation, approximately 36 hours after hCG administration. The reproductive tract is exposed and the entire oviduct is excised, trimmed free of fatty tissue and placed in culture medium (Modified Ham's F-10, supplemented with 15% maternal serum: GROWTH MEDIUM) in a petri dish (Falcon 3001) under a layer of silicone oil (Dow Corning 200 fluid; Dow Corning Corp., Midland, MI). Embryos are flushed from the oviduct by inserting a blunt tipped 30 gauge needle attached to a 1 cc disposable syringe into the infundibulum (fimbriated end of the oviduct) and injecting approximately 100 microliters of culture medium. During flushing, the oviduct is held in place around the needle with fine forceps. Alternatively, the oviduct can be pinned to the dish with the 30 gauge needle. Two-cell embryos recovered by this technique are utilized for preimplantation development experiments only when at least 75% of the recovered eggs or embryos from an individual animal are at the two-cell stage. This precaution is taken since the use of high doses of PMS has been associated with the recovery of abnormal eggs (Mintz, 1967). Embryos are transferred with a micropipette to a fresh aliquot (1 ml) of culture medium in an organ culture dish (Falcon #3037) on a 37° warming block. Occasionally two-cell embryos are recovered with some cumulus still attached; cumulus dispersal can usually be completed by simply washing in a micropipette. After all oviducts have been flushed, pooled two-cell embryos are divided into dishes for culturing. Dr. Stanley Leibo of Rio Vista International in Castroville, Texas, has indicated that cryopreserved 2-cell embryos will be commercially available through his company.

Preimplantation Development *In Vitro*

The developmental sequence from the two-cell to the hatching blastocyst in the mouse shows considerable interstrain variation and, of course, is dependent upon the *in vitro* culturing conditions. Cleavages within any single embryo are not necessarily synchronous and it is therefore possible to observe all numbers of blastomeres during early development. The developmental sequence observed in our studies is depicted in Figure 4. Approximately 24 hours after embryo recovery, the predominant stage will be four-cell (Figure 4A); 48 hours after recovery, most embryos will be in the morula stage of development

(Figure 4B); 72 hours after recovery, embryos will be in the early blastocyst stage (Figure 4C); and by 96 hours post-recovery the predominant stage is the hatching blastocyst (Figure 4D). We have been using this assay to assess current culturing conditions for human IVF-ET as well as to screen the stocks of Hams F-10 in use at the time. The culture medium employed in preimplantation development is changed daily and typically 75-80% of the two-cell embryos develop to hatching blastocysts under these conditions; culturing in organ culture dishes, in a humidified incubator and a gas atmosphere of 5% oxygen, 5% CO_2 and 90% nitrogen. In addition to monitoring current culturing conditions, we have used

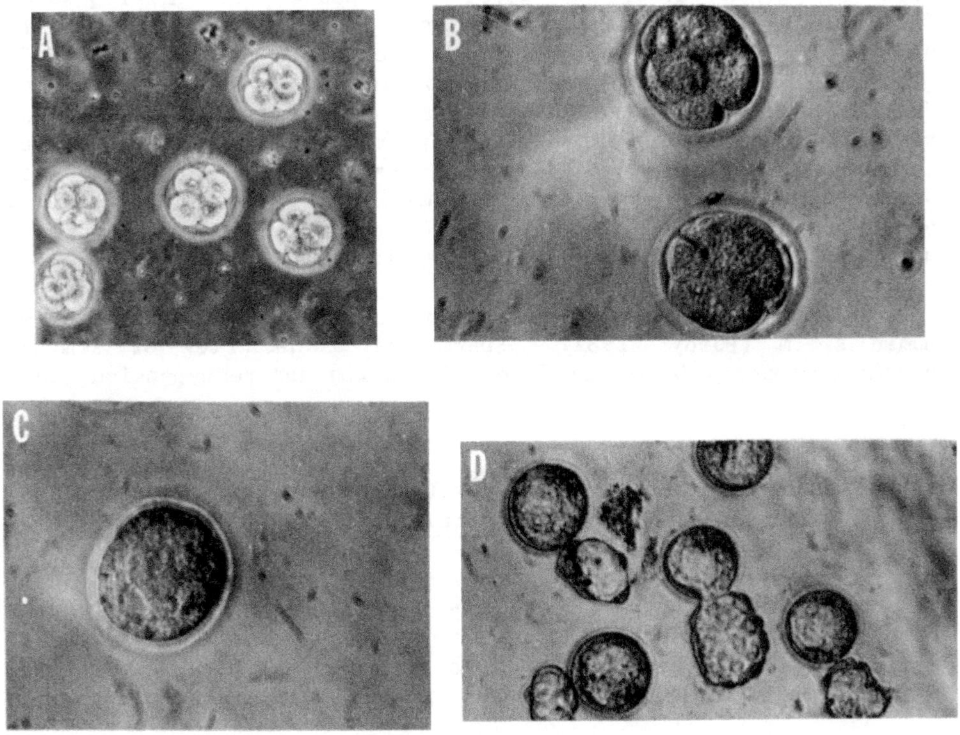

Figure 4

Micrographs depicting various stages of preimplantation development in the mouse.

A. 4-Cell
B. Morula
C. Early - cavitating blastocyst
D. Hatching blastocyst

mouse preimplantation development to assess how new conditions or equipment might influence the culturing of human embryos (Wolf and Dandekar, unpublished results). Examples of this approach include the comparison of the vessels used in culturing embryos: organ culture dishes (Falcon #3037) contrasted with petri dishes (Falcon #3001) or individual wells in microtest culture plates (Falcon #3034). In two separate experiments, the organ culture and tissue culture dishes supported similar preimplantation development rates, 85 and 84% respectively, while the culturing of 5 to 10 embryos in individual wells (15 ml) of microtest culture plates was inferior (61% development to hatching blastocyst $p < 0.01$). Similarly, we demonstrated that there were no significant differences in preimplantation development rates when cultures were overlaid with silicone oil or when culture media was prepared with 5X glass distilled water as opposed to Milli-Q-Water (Millipore) glass distilled once in a Corning mega-pure still. Several different culture media have been employed in human IVF-ET (Table 1) and we have conducted comparative studies contrasting Whittingham's T6, modified Whittens, and Hams F-10 media with regards to the ability to support mouse preimplantation development (Table 2). Although the overall percentages of development were somewhat lower than usual (42-76%), in three experiments involving several hundred embryos, these culture media were equally capable of supporting development.

A second bioassay for assessing culture conditions utilizes human sperm (Purdy, 1982). Sperm are washed free of seminal plasma components by repeated centrifugation and resuspension (see

Table 2. Mouse preimplantation development in three culture media employed for human *in vitro* fertilization

Embryos were harvested at the 2-cell stage and the percent developing to hatching blastocysts was recorded. Culture was in organ culture dishes and an atmosphere of 5% CO_2; 5% O_2; 90% N_2. All media contained 15% heat-treated maternal serum.

Experiment Number	Number of Embryos/Culture	Whittingham's T-6	Modified Whittens	Ham's F-10
1	50	76%	66%	70%
2	50	61%	72%	65%
3	12	50%	42%	57%

pgs above) and suspended in medium. Although concentrated suspensions are usually tested, the more sensitive approach may well involve sperm concentrations on the order of 50,000 to 100,000/ml. Motility and progression should be scored at least every 24 hours and decay curves can be established. Ideally, several proven fertile donors can be identified and used repeatedly in order to avoid donor variation.

REFERENCES

Edwards, R. G., and Gates, A. H., 1959, Timing of the stages of the maturation divisions, ovulation, fertilization and the first cleavage of eggs of adult mice treated with gonadotrophins, J. Endocr., 18:292.

Feichtinger, W., Kemeta, P., Szalay, S., and Janisch, H., 1983, Early hormone parameters and embryonic development in pregnancies established by in vitro fertilization and embryo transfer, in: "Fertilization of the Human Egg In Vitro," H. M. Beier and H. R. Linder, eds., Springer-Verlag, Berlin.

Hoppe, P.C., and Pitts, S., 1973, Fertilization in vitro and development of mouse ova, Biol. Reprod., 8:420.

Jones, H. W., Jr., Jones, G. S., Andrews, M. C., Acosta, A., Bundren, C., Garcia, J., Sandow, B., Veeck, L., Wilkens, C., Witmyer, J., Wortham, J. E., and Wright, G., 1983, The program for in vitro fertilization at Norfolk, Fertil. Steril., 38:14.

Kruse, P. F., and Patterson, M. K., 1973, "Tissue Culture Methods and Applications," Academic Press, New York.

Lopata, A., Johnston, I.W.H., Hoult, I. J., and Speirs, A. L., 1980, Pregnancy following intrauterine implantation of an embryo obtained by in vitro fertilization of a preovulatory egg, Fertil. Steril., 33:117

Mintz, B., 1967, Mammalian embryo culture, in: "Methods in Developmental Biology," F. M. Wilt, and N. K. Wessells, eds., Thomas Crowell Co, New York.

Purdy, J. M., 1982, Methods for fertilization and embryo culture in vitro, in: "Human Conception In Vitro," R. G. Edwards and J. M. Purdy, eds., Academic Press, London.

Quinn, P., Barros, C., and Whittingham, D. G., 1982, Preservation of hamster oocytes to assay the fetilizing capacity of human spermatozoa, J. Reprod. Fert., 66:161.

Testart, J., Lassalle, B., and Frydman, R., 1982, Success of in vitro fertilization in spontaneous or stimulated cycles and technical procedures used, in: "Proc. 4th R. de Graaf Symposium, Follicular Maturation and Ovulation, Nijmegan (Holland)," R. Rolland, E. V. Van Hall, S. G. Miller, K. P. McNatty and J. Schoemaker, eds., Excerpta Medica, Amsterdam.

Trounson, A, 1983, Factors controlling normal embryo development and implantation of human oocytes fertilized in vitro, in: "Fertilization of the Human Egg In Vitro," H. M. Beier and H. R. Lindner, eds., Springer-Verlag, Berlin.

Trounson, A., Mohr, L. R., Wood, C., and Leeton, J. F., 1982, Effect of delayed insemination on in vitro fertilization, culture and transfer of human embryos, J. Reprod. Fertil, 64:285.

Veeck, L. L., Wortham, J. W. E., Jr., Witmyer, J., Sandow, B. A., Acosta, A. A., Garcia, J. E., Jones, G. S., and Jones H. W., Jr., 1983, Maturation and fertilization of morphologically immature human oocytes in a program of in vitro fertilization, Fertil. Steril., 39:594.

14

FERTILITY POTENTIAL EVALUATION WITH THE ZONA-FREE HAMSTER EGG BIOASSAY

Don P. Wolf and Joseph E. Sokoloski

The evaluation of male fertility traditionally has centered on semen analysis describing semen volume, sperm density, morphology, motility and progression. Unfortunately, results from such analyses correlate poorly with fertility except in the extreme cases of azoospermia or asthenospermia. This poor correlation has forced attention to direct measurements of sperm function. Presently several bioassays are available for this purpose including _in vivo_ sperm penetration of cervical mucus (the post coital or Sims-Huhner test), the _in vitro_ capillary tube penetration test (with bovine or mid-cycle human cervical mucus) and sperm-egg interaction systems. At least two _in vitro_ sperm-egg interaction assays have been described in addition to the fertilization of human eggs. In one, sperm are incubated with non-living human oocytes and the ability of sperm to penetrate the zona pellucida is measured (Overstreet and Hembree, 1976). The other, the zona-free hamster egg bioassay, utilizes the living naked egg of the hamster and sperm-egg fusion is the measured parameter (Yanagamachi et al., 1976).

The feature of the hamster egg that is exploited in this bioassay is the apparent absence of any species specificity at the level of the egg plasma membrane. The hamster is unique in that zona-free eggs from the mouse, rat and guinea pig do not incorporate heterologous sperm as readily (Hanada and Chang, 1972; Quinn, 1979; Pavlok, 1979; Thadani, 1980). In addition, the hamster egg plasma membrane is unusual in its apparent inability to control its own penetration by sperm (Barros and Yanagimachi, 1972; Binor et al., 1982a), despite the documented release of cortical granules from the egg at fertilization (Austin, 1976).

Heterologous penetration by sperm from man (Yanagimachi et al., 1976), mouse, rat and rabbit (Hanada and Chang, 1972, 1976, 1978), guinea pig (Yanagimachi, 1972) goat (Kim et al., 1980), boar (Imai et al., 1977), bull and stallion (Brackett et al., 1982) has been reported illustrating the potential versatility of the bioassay in measuring fertility potential of mammalian sperm (Figure 1). This bioassay has also been applied to the karyotyping of human sperm (Rudak et al., 1978), to investigations of immunologic infertility (Menge and Black, 1979; Haas et al., 1980; Dor et al., 1981), to human epididymal sperm maturation (Hinrichsen and Blaquier, 1980) and, of course, carries potential for contraceptive development, for evaluating the effects of environmental factors on male fertility, and for basic fertilization research in humans as well as other mammals.

Several investigators have applied the hamster egg bioassay to the diagnosis of human male infertility (Rogers et al., 1979; Overstreet et al., 1980; Hall, 1981; Zausner-Guelman et al., 1981; Karp et al., 1981; Tyler et al., 1981; Martin and Taylor, 1982; Aitken et al., 1982a,b; Cohen et al., 1982). The premise for this application is that male factors are prevalent in couples under evaluation for primary infertility of unknown etiology and that such male factors are expressed in rather specific sperm dysfunction; namely, the inability of sperm to undergo the process of capacitation, an acrosome reaction and fusion with an oocyte. For a detailed discussion of sperm capacitation, see Chapter 11.

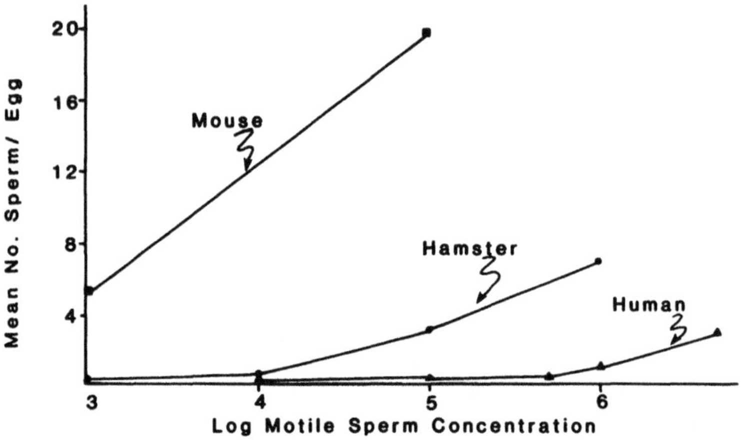

Figure 1

Sperm concentration dependence in the penetration of zona-free hamster eggs by mouse, hamster and human sperm.

Despite limiting factors, the consensus of many investigators is that the bioassay has application in the management of the infertile couple. Several different names have been used to describe the bioassay including SPA (Sperm Penetration Assay), the humster test and the heterologous or cross species penetration test. Unfortunately the experimental protocols associated with the diagnostic application of the bioassay are not standardized, despite the extensive efforts of several investigators to define critical variables (Tyler et al., 1981; Cohen et al., 1982; Martin and Taylor, 1982; Wolf and Sokoloski, 1982; Rogers et al., 1983a). While the recovery and preparation of zona-free eggs from superovulated hamsters is relatively uniform, the handling and preincubation of sperm is not. The bioassay as we currently conduct it is detailed below (Figure 2).

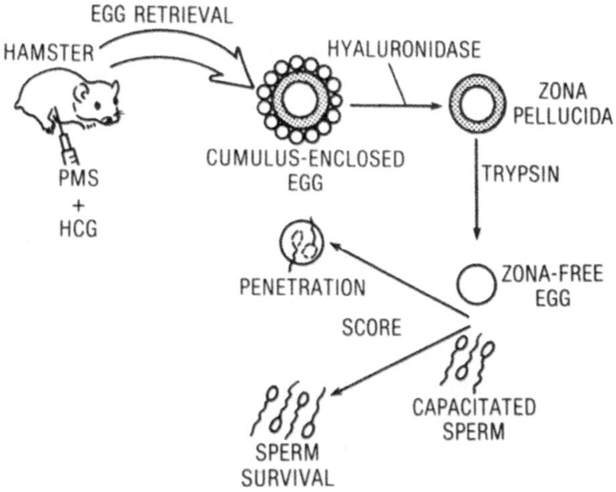

Figure 2

Schematic representation of the zona-free hamster egg bioassay. Modified from Haas et al., 1980.

BIOASSAY CONDITIONS

Egg Recovery and Handling

Follicular maturation and ovulation induction is controlled by the administration of PMS and hCG. Juvenile or mature golden Syrian hamsters (Charles River Breeding Labs, Inc., Wilmington, MA or Engle Lab Animals, Inc., Farmersburg, IN) are maintained on light/dark cycles of 10/14 or 12/12. Animals selected at random with regard to the estrous cycle are superovulated by the intraperitoneal injection of pregnant mare's serum gonadotrophin (PMS) (30 IU, Gestyl^R, Diosynth, Chicago, IL) followed 55 to 57 hours later by hCG (30 IU, Sigma, St. Louis, MO). Although a 48 to 52 hour PMS-hCG interval can be employed, the longer interval is associated with a higher degree of animal response and an increased yield of ovulated eggs (Wolf and Sokoloski, 1982). For the storage of PMS or hCG, we routinely prepare large batches at a concentration of 100 units per ml in PBS and store 1 ml aliquots frozen. Samples are then thawed immediately prior to use and any surplus is discarded. Animals are sacrificed by asphyxiation with carbon dioxide approximately 15 to 17 hours after hCG administration. After rinsing with 95% ethanol, the ventral body wall is opened and the reproductive tract is exposed. Oviducts are removed and placed in silicone oil (Dow Corning 200 dielectric fluid, Dow Corning Corp., Midland, MI) in a disposable plastic petri dish (Falcon #3001) at ambient temperature. The dish is transferred to the stage of a dissecting microscope at ambient temperature and the cumulus masses are released from the oviducts. Release is accomplished by puncturing the oviduct at the site of the cumulus mass with a 27 gauge needle attached to a 1 cc disposable tuberculin syringe (Figure 3). The cumulus mass is then teased free from the oviduct with two needles, one to manipulate the oviduct and the other the cumulus mass. Cumulus masses from all oviducts are accumulated as one mass and transferred together to a drop of culture medium under oil in a second petri dish on a 37^oC heating block. This transfer can be made with watchmakers forceps and does not require microscopic observation. All subsequent steps are conducted at 37^oC. Normally we transfer eggs in cumulus directly to culture medium containing hyaluronidase. The culture medium, BWW (Biggers et al., 1971, see Table 1) contains 3 milligrams per ml of human serum albumin (HSA; Sigma Chemical Co., Fraction V) at pH 7.5. Cumulus dispersal requires approximately 10 minutes exposure to 0.1% hyaluronidase (approximately 510 NF units per milligram, Sigma Chemical Co. St. Louis, MO) at 37° (Figure 4). Following the hyaluronidase treatment, the eggs must be treated individually. For this purpose hand drawn micropipettes are prepared by pulling out 5 3/4 inch pasteur pipettes using a 19 gauge syringe needle as a burner. The tip end

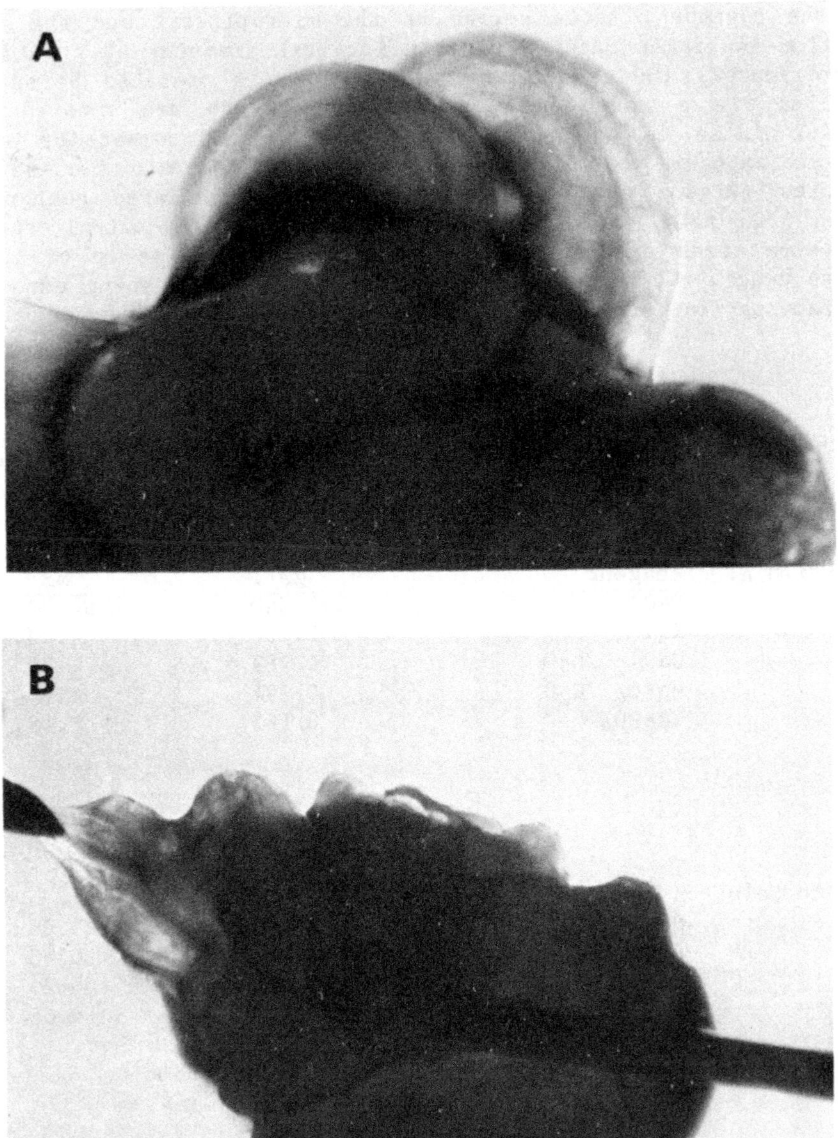

Figure 3

A) Excised oviduct of a superovulated hamster. The distended portion of the oviduct (containing the cumulus mass) is in the upper center of the micrograph. X 225. B) Low power micrograph of the oviduct during cumulus release with 27_g needles. X 138.

of the pasteur pipette serves as the micropipette and the drawn portion is broken back to give an internal diameter at the tip of approximately 100 to 125 um. The pipette is operated by suction applied via a mouth held rubber tube. Eggs are removed from hyaluronidase in batches of 25 to 50 and washed repeatedly in BWW before exposure to 0.1% bovine pancreatic trypsin for several minutes (Figure 5). In processing relatively large numbers of eggs (200-300), it is not always possible to control trypsin exposure times precisely. However, this appears to be of little consequence. We have contrasted 1 and 4 minute trypsin exposures on penetration scores and found comparable percentages of eggs

Table 1. Composition and Preparation of BWW Medium modified from Biggers et al (1971).

		Concentration	
Solution A:	Reagent	gm/l	mM
	NaCl	5.540	94.78
	KCl	0.356	4.77
	$CaCl_2$ $2H_2O$	0.189	1.29
	$MgSO_4$ $7H_2O$	0.294	1.19
	KH_2PO_4	0.162	1.19
Add to Solution A for Working Medium:			
	$NaHCO_3$	2.106	25.06
	Glucose	1.000	5.55
	Na Pyruvate	0.028	0.25
	Na Lactate (60% Syrup)	3.7 (ml)	19.65
	HSA	3.000	
	Penicillin G	100,000 Units	
	Streptomycin Sulfate	100,000 g	

Media Preparation:
The stock salt ingredients (Solution A above) are weighed out and added to 1.0 liter of distilled-deionized water. This stock can be kept stored at 4° for up to 1 month. The additional components, sufficient for 100 ml of medium, are weighed on the day of use and added to 100 ml of the stock salt solution. The pH is adjusted to 7.4-7.6 and the medium is passed through a 0.22 μm filter prior to use each day.

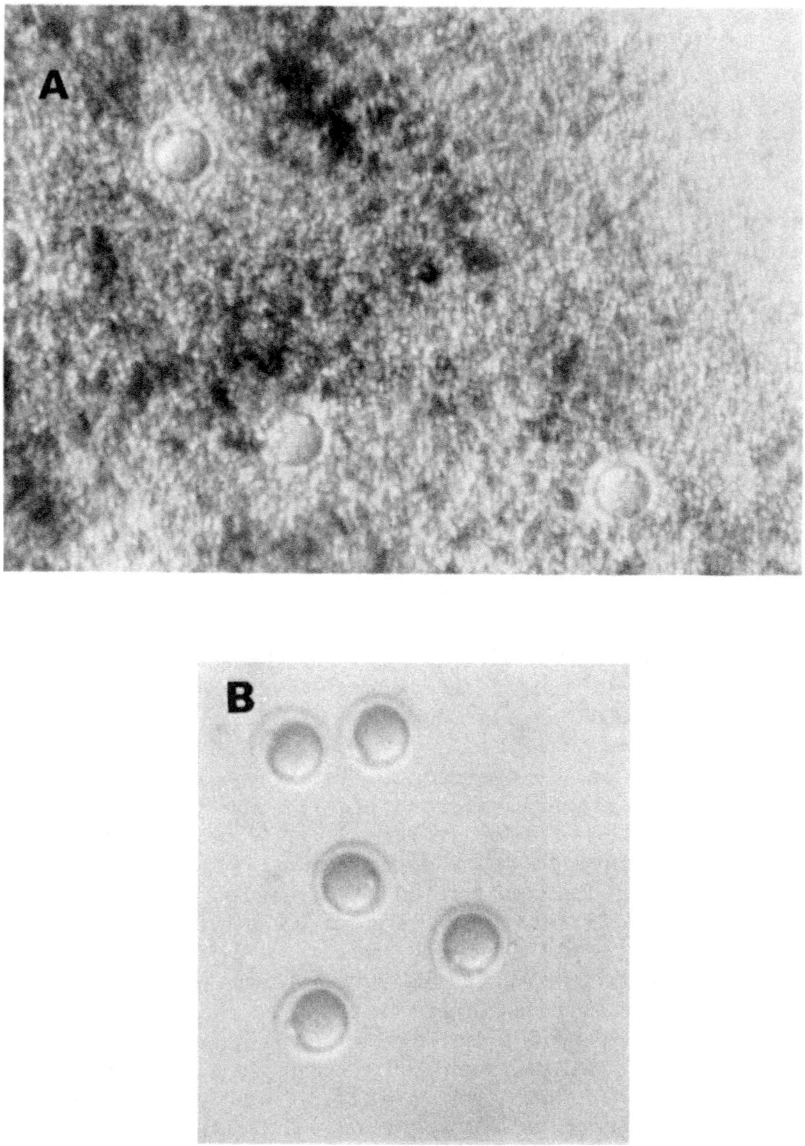

Figure 4

Light micrographs of hamster eggs following hyaluronidase dispersal of the cumulus. (A) Eggs are visible against a background of dispersed cumulus cells. X 300 (B) Zona-intact eggs after washing in culture media. X 300.

penetrated and mean numbers of sperm per egg. Incomplete zona removal can prevent sperm-egg interaction and often impacts on egg processing as partially digested zona material is gelatinous and can occlude micropipettes. Distortion of the egg commonly occurs during zona removal (Figure 5A). The zona-free state can be assessed visually by observing whether or not treated eggs are touching each other (Figure 5B). Zona-free eggs are removed from the trypsin suspension, 25-50 at a time and washed through 5 drops of BWW under oil and held for insemination. Gametes are held and inseminations are conducted in a 37°C incubator in 5% CO_2 in air or in a 100% air atmosphere. The estimated viable lifetime of the zona-free egg in vitro is limited and eggs should be inseminated within an hour of harvesting. Binor et al. (1982) defined this lifetime by recovering eggs from animals and inseminating at intervals over a 7 hour time course with different preparations of capacitated hamster sperm. High penetration levels were obtained for the initial three hours of insemination; however, after 5 hours of exposure to in vitro culture conditions a drastic decline in egg fertility was apparent.

Sperm Processing

Human semen samples are obtained by masturbation from healthy donors after a sexual abstinence time of 48 hours. Samples are allowed to liquify at 37°C. A 30-60 minute liquifaction time appears optimal as shorter or longer times are associated with decreased penetration levels (Sokoloski and Wolf, 1983; Rogers et al., 1983a). Sperm motility, as the percentage of swimming cells, and progression, as determined subjectively and reported on a scale of 0-4, are assessed microscopically and sperm concentration is quantitated with a hemocytometer. Two methods are commonly employed for separating sperm from seminal plasma. One involves repeated cycles of centrifugation-resuspension in culture medium (Rogers et al., 1979) while the second is a swim-up procedure in which semen is layered under the culture medium and motile cells are subsequently recovered in the supernatant (Overstreet et al., 1980). In our experience, sperm washed by the swim-up technique support higher levels of sperm-egg fusion; however, the yield of motile sperm in the swim-up procedure is considerably lower (approximately 10%) than that realized from the centrifugation technique (approximately 25% recovery of total sperm but nearly complete recovery of the motile population; Binor et al., 1980). If sperm are to be washed by centrifugation-resuspension, a measured portion of semen is diluted with three volumes of BWW containing 0.3% HSA and centrifuged at 600xg for 10 minutes at ambient temperature. This process is repeated two times and the final pellet is resuspended in a volume of BWW equivalent to the volume of semen washed. The final BWW contains 3.5% HSA. In the

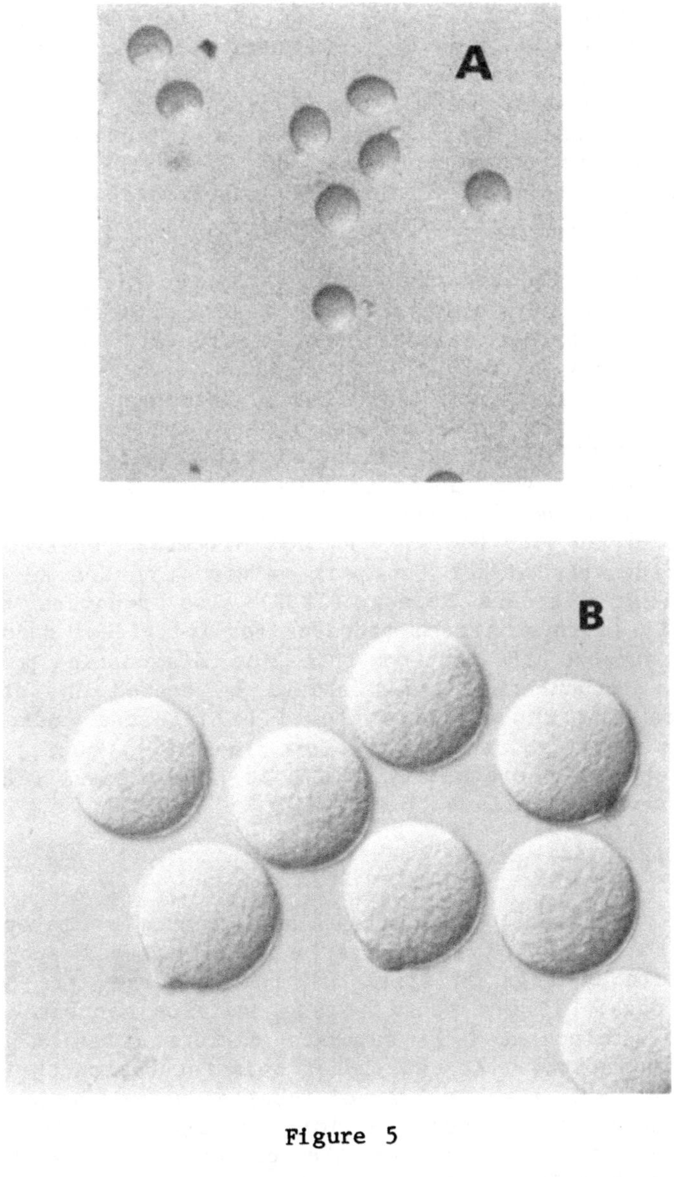

Figure 5

Light micrographs of hamster eggs during zona removal. Zonae are dispersed by exposure to trypsin. (A) Egg distortion that normally accompanies early phases of zonae removal is apparent in a few of these eggs. (X 168) (B) Zona-free eggs. Note that at least some of these eggs are touching each other indicating that the zona is completely removed. (X 365).

swim-up technique, an aliquot of semen (0.5 ml) is layered under a solution of BWW (2.0 ml) containing 0.3% serum albumin and the tube is incubated at an angle of 30° for one hour at 37°C. The supernatant is removed and sperm in the supernatant are collected by centrifugation and washed twice by centrifugation-resuspension. The final pellet is resuspended in BWW with 3.5% HSA. Sperm suspensions are incubated at 37° for 3 hours either in tubes at high (50-100 x 10^6 cells/ml) sperm concentrations or in petri dishes in insemination drops under oil at 5-10 x 10^6 motile cells/ml.

The time period and the concentration of albumin utilized for sperm preincubation represent two major parameters which vary substantially among laboratories. Moreover the kinetics of capacitation may be unique to each donor. As an example of how these parameters impact on bioassay outcome, our comparative studies on sperm from 6 donors are informative (Wolf and Sokoloski, 1982). The kinetics of capacitation were evaluated over 24 hours for each donor in both 0.3 and 3.5% albumin (Figure 6). In low albumin, maximum penetration was observed in sperm preincubated for 6.5 hours. In 3.5% albumin, penetration scores were considerably higher but peak values were not seen until 13 hours. Perreault and Rogers (1982) also reported substantial variability in capacitation patterns for individual donors. These findings support the notion that for diagnostic purposes two different preincubation times should be tested or, at the very least, men that score poorly should be retested under different conditions. At short capacitation times (1-3 hours) the "slow capacitator" may score poorly, while at longer times (18-24 hours) sperm survival may become limiting.

Insemination Reaction

Two different approaches are commonly taken in the insemination of zona-free hamster eggs with human sperm, namely, the addition of eggs to sperm and the converse, the addition of sperm to eggs. If the sperm to egg addition sequence is chosen, sperm are preincubated in separate culture tubes at relatively high concentrations. At the end of this incubation the population is sampled and the number of motile sperm present in the preparation is determined. A drop, usually 200 microliters of culture medium, is added to the center of a petri dish and overlaid with silicone oil. We prefer to add a portion of the culture media drop (approximately 100 µl) to the dish first to define drop size. Silicone oil is then added, with the balance of the culture media added last. Ten to 30 zona-free hamster eggs are added and the insemination is begun by the addition of a volume of sperm suspension calculated to provide a final motile sperm concentration of 5 to 10 x 10^6 cells per ml. Using this approach, the relationship between sperm penetration and the motile sperm concentration has been determined (Figure 7) (see also Overstreet et al., 1980; Tyler et al., 1981; Rogers et al., 1983a, Martin and Taylor, 1983). At concentrations of less than 10^6 motile cells per ml, penetration is limited while at higher concentrations a log linear relationship is established between these two parameters. At very high sperm concentrations ($\geq 10 \times 10^6$) a fall off in penetration may occur (Tyler et al., 1981). If an egg to sperm addition sequence is utilized, 200 microliter drops of culture medium are prepared and overlaid with silicone oil. Sperm at a final motile concentration of 5 to 10 x 10^6 per ml are added at the beginning of the sperm preincubation time. To initiate the insemination reaction, zona-free eggs are added to this preincubated sperm suspension. In our experience, (Wolf and Sokoloski, 1982; Dandekar and Wolf, 1982), the egg to sperm addition sequence supports higher levels of sperm-egg fusion. We presently suspect that a sperm derived factor, perhaps of seminal plasma origin, is mediating the higher levels of sperm-egg fusion seen in the egg to sperm addition sequence (Dandekar and Wolf, 1983). The insemination reaction is allowed to proceed at 37°C in 5% CO_2 in air or room air for several hours. While insemination times of as short as 1-2 hours have been reported (Barros et al., 1978; Cohen et al., 1982) longer times ($\geq$ 3 hrs) will probably result in higher penetration levels (Table 2) consistent with the estimated 3-5 hour viable life time of zona-free hamster eggs <u>in vitro</u> (Binor et al., 1982a). Longer insemination times can be employed, for instance, up to 6 hours, but overnight incubations are detrimental in that the resulting eggs are often granular and difficult to score. The insemination reaction is terminated by simply removing eggs from the inseminating drop and washing them through several drops of culture medium. During this washing procedure, which does not involve an oil overlay, eggs are aspirated in and out of finely drawn micropipettes to remove loosely adherent sperm on the egg surface. Upon completion of washing, eggs (5-10) are transferred in a small drop (approximately 10 microliters) to a glass slide (Figure 8). A cover slip is prepared with a small amount of a vaseline:paraffin (20:1) mixture added to each corner. The cover slip is centered over the drop of medium containing the eggs and depressed onto the vaseline-paraffin supports until the eggs are compressed. This is a delicate procedure for too little compression of the egg precludes an accurate assessment of the mean number of sperm per egg while too much compression results in egg lysis. Next a drop of 1% glutaraldehyde is added at the edge of the cover slip and coaxed to fill the area under the cover slip by very gentle compression of the cover slip. The slide is next transferred to a coplan jar containing 10% formalin in Dulbecco's PBS where it can be held indefinitely. When penetration is to be scored, slides are removed from the 10% formalin solution, rinsed

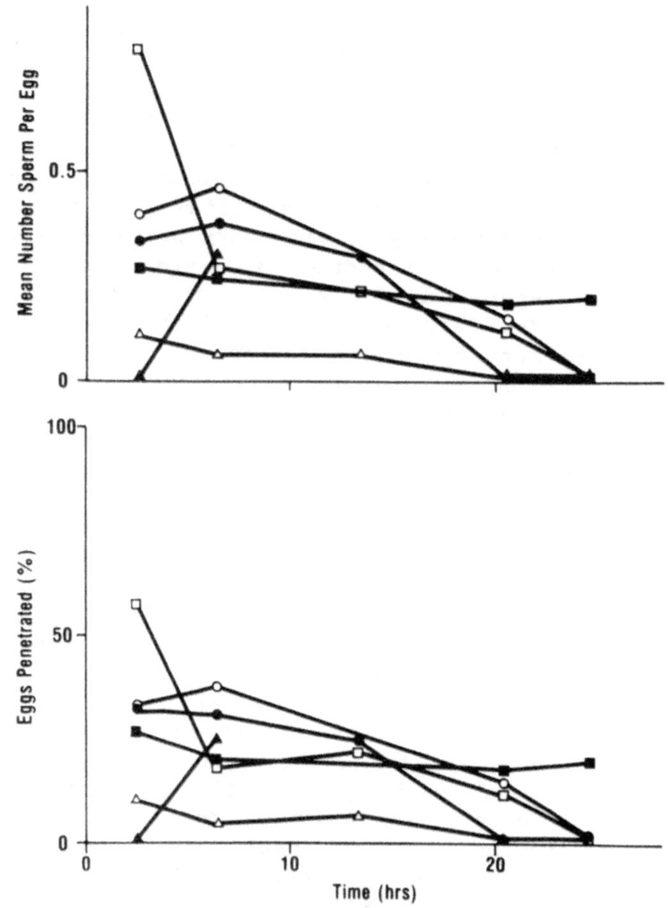

Figure 6A

Kinetics of human sperm capacitation in culture media containing 0.3% serum albumin. Single ejaculates from six donors were washed by the swim-up technique and incubated in BWW containing 0.3% HSA. At the indicated times eggs were recovered from superovulated hamsters, rendered zona-free and inseminated at $5x10^6$ motile sperm cells/ml. Five hours later, eggs were removed and processed for penetration scoring. The number of eggs in individual experiments varied from 9 to 23. Each symbol represents a different donor and applies to both 6A and 6B. From Wolf and Sokoloski, 1982.

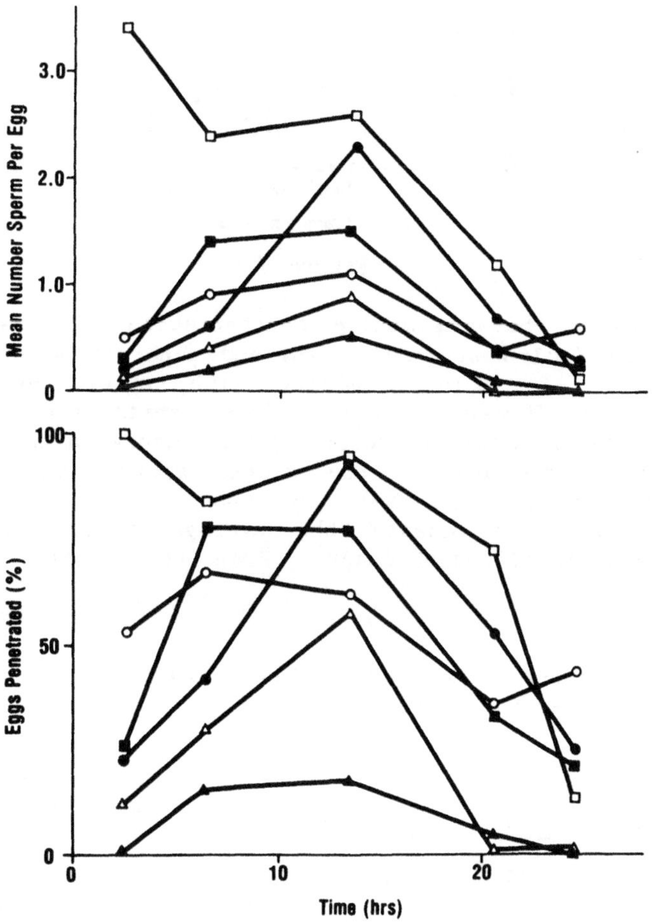

Figure 6B

Kinetics of human sperm capacitation in culture media containing 3.5% serum albumin. The number of eggs in individual experiments varied from 13 to 24 (see Figure 6A legend for experimental details). From Wolf and Sokoloski, 1982.

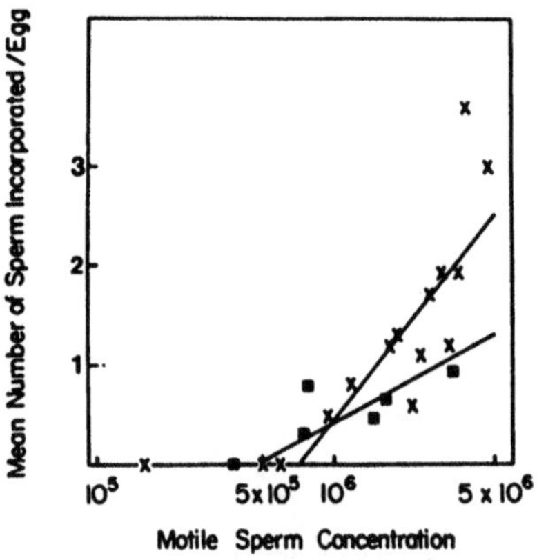

Figure 7

The relationship between motile concentration of fresh (X) and freeze-thawed (solid squares) sperm and penetration of zona-free hamster eggs. Eggs were inseminated with various concentrations of motile sperm (fresh and freeze-thawed sperm were preincubated for 4 hours and 2 hours, respectively) and scored after 8 hours of insemination. The log of the motile sperm concentration is plotted against the mean number of sperm incorporated per egg. Each data point represents the average value from several experiments using different donors. From Binor et al., 1980.

Table 2. Zona-free hamster egg test scores as a function of insemination time

Time (hrs.)							Reference
1	2	3	4	5	6	7	
	76	96	87	-	-	-	Rogers et al., 1983a
25	-	56	-	56	-	52	Berger et al., 1983
20	38	69	-	-	-	-	Yanagimachi et al., 1976

Results are expressed as the percentage of eggs penetrated.

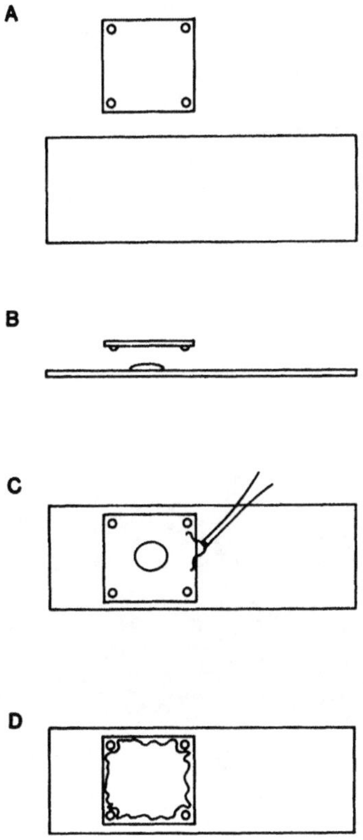

Figure 8

Schematic representation of the processing of zona-free hamster eggs for penetration scoring.

A) Glass microscope slide and cover slip with vaseline-paraffin column at each corner.

B) Placing the cover slip over the drop of medium containing the eggs.

C) The cover slip is depressed onto the vaseline-paraffin supports until the drop is contacted and flattened slightly. Glutaraldehyde is then added at the edge of the coverslip.

D) The fixative spreads under the cover slip fixing and compressing the eggs.

briefly in a stream of distilled water and transferred to a coplan jar containing 95% ethanol. Following dehydration, the slide is removed and stained with a 0.25% lacmoid in 45% acetic acid solution. The stain can conveniently be drawn under the cover slip by using a paper tissue as a wick. Stained eggs are located with the aid of a dissecting microscope, marked on the bottom of the slide with a felt tip pen, and scored with a phase contrast microscope at 200-400x. Eggs are considered penetrated when a swollen sperm head (or heads) or male pronucleus (or pronuclei) and a corresponding sperm tail(s) are found within the ooplasm (Figure 9). Results are recorded as the percentage of eggs penetrated and the mean number of penetrating sperm per inseminated

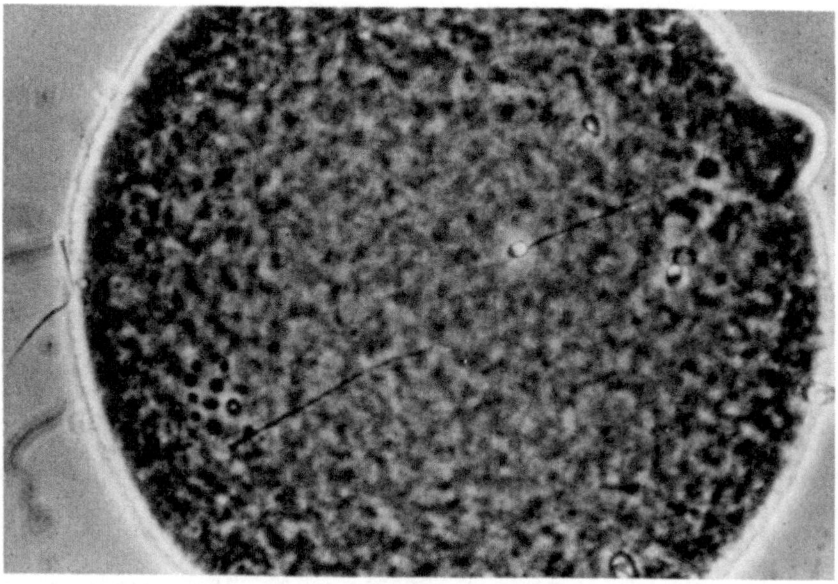

Figure 9

Light micrograph of penetrated zona-free hamster egg. Aceto lacmoid stained (X 400). Sperm were preincubated for 3 hours and cultured with eggs for 3 hours. Enlarged sperm head with a corresponding sperm tail is visible in the ooplasm as well as an intact sperm on the egg surface.

egg. The statistical significance of data can be treated by several techniques including the Students' t test (Snedecor and Cochran, 1967). For routine assessment of human sperm fertilizing ability, many investigators have used a simplified scoring method whereby swollen sperm heads in the egg cytoplasm are identified directly in living oocytes at x400 magnification (Yanagimachi et al., 1976; Rogers et al., 1979). In these cases results are usually recorded as simply the percentage of eggs penetrated without reference to the number of times each egg is penetrated (polyspermy level). However, since the zona-free hamster egg does not possess a block to polyspermy (Usui and Yanagimachi, 1976; Binor et al., 1982a) each fusion should be accorded equal weight. The value of this approach is especially obvious when differentiation of high scores is desired i.e., where percent penetration is no longer discriminating. For example, in our previous kinetic study of the performance of sperm from 6 different donors (Figure 6B) at the 13 hour time period in 3.5% HSA, the highest penetration scores varied between 60 and 90 percent (1.5 fold) while the mean number of sperm/egg varied from 0.9 to 2.6 or almost 3 fold.

EVALUATION OF BIOASSAY RESULTS

In considering the sperm penetration bioassay as a routine diagnostic test, variables which affect bioassay outcome must first be evaluated. Standard conditions should be established and tested with sperm from a single ejaculate. Interassay variability on the same specimen, as reported by virtually all laboratories is minimal, therefore, results from different technicians in the same laboratory should agree within a few percentage points. In contrast, within subject variation for bioassay results is often substantial. Examples of this phenomenon are widespread. For instance, Tyler et al. (1981) recorded penetration rates for six different semen samples collected over time from three subjects. Subject A showed a mean penetration of 42% with a range from 4 to 73%; Subject B a mean of 8.6% and a range from 3 to 22.7%; and Subject C a mean of 35.9% with a range from 15.6 to 61.9%. As a second example, Rogers et al. (1983a) tested 5 different semen samples collected over a period of 1 year from 27 men. These individuals were ranked according to the mean penetration levels and 15 of them fell in a variable catagory with ranges from less than 5% to as high as 99% penetration. If, as it presently appears, such variability in test results reflects real differences in the sperm from different ejaculates, implications to the diagnostic use of the test are profound.

CORRELATION OF ASSAY RESULTS WITH SEMEN PARAMETERS

As alluded to earlier in the chapter, although semen parameters have traditionally been employed diagnostically in the evaluation of male fertility, the accuracy of this approach is limited. Nevertheless early studies using the sperm penetration assay sought correlations between assay outcome and individual or combined parameters of the semen analysis. Rogers et al. (1979) saw no clear relationship between sperm density or motility in semen and the ability of the washed cells to fuse with hamster eggs. Similarily, Hall (1981) evaluated morphology in addition to density and motility and could not show a strong correlation with penetration results except when semen values were very low. Karp et al. (1981) in evaluating the diagnostic use of the penetration assay conducted extensive comparisons of sperm penetration outcome with seminal fluid analyses. The penetration assay was considered by those authors to be superior to semen analysis in predicting both fertility and infertility.

CORRELATION OF ASSAY RESULTS WITH MUCUS PENETRATION

Sperm passage through the cervix is a necessary prerequisite to successful fertilization, consequently an evaluation of sperm interaction with cervical mucus may be regarded as an integral component of any investigation of unexplained infertility. Although it seems inherently obvious that the sperm penetration assay measures different sperm properties than does a mucus interaction test, correlations between the two have been sought. Soules et al. (1982) reported a direct relationship between post-coital test results and the penetration assay but the correlation was not strong enough to allow the recommendation that either test be dropped from a routine infertility workup. In studies conducted with bovine mucus in capillary tubes _in vitro_ (Rogers et al., 1983b) the correlation between hamster egg penetration and mucus penetration was so low that the authors concluded that the two tests measure different sperm properties.

CORRELATION OF ASSAY RESULTS WITH DONOR STATUS

A significant body of information has accumulated over the past 6 to 7 years correlating results of the zona-free hamster egg bioassay with donor status. Bioassay results for males of proven fertility are summarized in Table 3. As can be seen in the table, the conditions employed for capacitation vary substantially between laboratories with regard to both preincubation time and

Table 3. Zona-free hamster egg test results for males of proven fertility

	Mean Penetration %	Range %	Number of Donors	Capacitation Time (Hrs)	Albumin %	Reference
	44	14-90	35	7	1.8	Aiken et al., 1982
	54	11-100	26	16-17	0.3	Cohen et al., 1982
	66	20-100	22	15-18	1.0	Hall, 1981
	-	15-96	25	18	0.4	Karp et al., 1981
	68	2-100	6	1	3.5	Overstreet et al., 1980
	56	14-100	21	18-20	0.3	Rogers et al., 1979
	54	19-100	8	6	1.8	Rudak, 1981
	60	24-89	15	18	0.3	Tyler et al., 1981
	81	15-100	9	2-3	3.5	Zausner-Guelman et al., 1981
Total Weighted Value	57%	2-100	167			-

Results are presented as the mean percentage of inseminated eggs penetrated. Sperm capacitation time and the albumin concentration employed are also itemized.

albumin concentration. The weighted mean penetration level for the results expressed in the table is 57% with a range in penetration from 2 to 100%. Note, however, that the range in penetration drops below 10% in only 1 of the 9 studies; the majority showing lower limits of approximately 15%. It must be pointed out that these results are surprisingly consistent in view of the lack of interlaboratory standardization, and it would appear that one can, at least within the confines of the conditions itemized in Table 3, compare penetration results (% penetrated but not necessarily polyspermy levels) from a laboratory using a short capacitation time with another using long capacitation times. It remains to be determined how much of an influence more exotic protein additives (egg yolk buffer or 50% heated serum, Binor et al., 1982b,c) will have on penetration results.

Another patient catagory which has been evaluated extensively with the penetration assay is the infertile couple. For convenience, couples can be subdivided further into those in which the wife shows evidence of infertility and those in which there is no clinical evidence of infertility in the wife and there may or may not be clinically recognized infertility in the husband. When wives showed clinical evidence of infertility, penetration test results for husbands were comparable to fertile donors with an average percent penetration of 52% (Table 4). The range in penetration for these patients was also comparable to that for proven fertile donors. In contrast, when there was no clinical evidence of infertility in the wife and/or the husband was clinically infertile, penetration scores were dramatically lower. The grand weighted mean for the 6 studies reported in Table 4 is 6% penetration and the range of penetration in 4 of the 6 studies was from 0 to 10%.

As attested to by the data included in Tables 3 and 4, then, there is not much controversy over whether or not the mean scores for the different donor groups differ. Rather, the major controversy concerns whether or not there is overlap in groups. In other words, is it appropriate to assign or define an arbitrary but absolute cutoff point that differentiates between the score of a proven fertile donor and that of a subfertile or clinically infertile male? The relatively high incidence of false negatives when a 10-15% cutoff is utilized indicates that fertility prognosis at the present time cannot be made solely on the basis of penetration scores. Thus, males of proven fertility do occassionally score poorly in repeated testing (Overstreet et al., 1980; Zausner-Guelman et al., 1981) and a subset of infertility patients who score poorly in the bioassay father children (Cohen et al., 1982; Binor et al., 1982c; Stenchever et al., 1982). In

Table 4. Zona-free hamster egg test results for infertility patients

Wife Showing Evidence of Infertility			No Chemical Evidence of Infertility in Wife: Some Husbands Clinically Infertile			
Mean % Penetration	% Range	Number of Patients	Mean % Penetration	% Range	Number of Patients	References
57.2	22.5–100	10	2.0	0–8.9	18	Rogers et al., 1979
52.1	11.6–98	16	2.6	0–10	30	Rudak, 1981
52	12–98	16	1.2	0–5	12	Aitken et al., 1982b
48	0–100	19	14	0–45	17	Zausner-Guelman et al., 1981
54	11–100	43	9	0–87	79	Cohen et al., 1981
-	-	-	1.7	0–9	24	Tyler et al., 1981
Total Weighted Value 52	0–100	104	6.0	0–45	180	-

fact, Stenchever et al. (1982) have proposed the existence of an "equivocal" group with scores between 11 and 14% that may truly represent a subfertile population. Perhaps the middle ground in this controversy over arbitrary cutoffs would simply be to take any penetration as a sign of fertility and a penetration score of less than 15% as a suggestion of subfertility which must be confirmed by repeat testing on a second ejaculate under the same conditions as well as under altered conditions of sperm capacitation.

CORRELATION WITH HUMAN IN VITRO FERTILIZATION

The availability of human in vitro fertilization embryo transfer programs provides a unique opportunity to assess further the accuracy of the zona-free hamster egg bioassay by comparing the results directly with observations of human sperm-human egg interaction in a controlled setting. A study of this nature has recently been undertaken (Wolf et al., 1983), where husband's sperm were used in inseminations of wives eggs and zona-free hamster eggs. In 16 of the 18 husbands (with normal semen parameters) who fertilized their wives eggs, a positive ($\geq$ 10%) penetration score was obtained with the zona-free hamster egg test. A false negative assessment i.e., a score of less than 10% penetration was obtained for 2 of these husbands. However, if the arbitrary value of 10% is ignored and we consider any penetration as an indicator of fertility, then all 18 husbands showed a positive fertility assessment (Table 5). This study indicates that in husbands with normal semen analyses, bioassay outcome is highly correlated with the fertilization of human eggs in vitro. In oligospermic husbands, however, the results are not as encouraging (Table 6). Over the past several months we have had occasion to treat 6 oligospermic males by IVF-ET, 5 of whom fertilized wives eggs (Table 6). A false negative penetration score was observed in 2 of these males and the patient who failed to fertilize his wife's eggs showed hamster egg penetration after 24 hours of sperm preincubation (false positive).

APPLICATION OF THE ASSAY TO THE INFERTILE COUPLE

Primarily because of the expense involved (approximately $200) and the scarcity of laboratories (limited to several major medical centers) conducting the test, use of the sperm penetration assay is limited at present. This situation holds despite reports on the cryopreservation of zona-free hamster eggs (Fleming et al., 1979; Quinn et al., 1982) and the use of cryopreserved human sperm (See Figure 7; Binor et al., 1980; Cohen et al., 1981). Clinically its application is warranted when a couple presents with persistent unexplained infertility despite normal semen parameters. Thus, it is considered an adjunct to a routine semen analysis and as such is reserved for selected cases (Tyler et al., 1981; Cohen et al., 1982; Stenchever et al., 1982). Its use has also been advocated before intensive, expensive or risky therapy for female factors are initiated or to assess the success of therapy for various male factors (Shy et al., 1982). Currently, we are interested in further characterization of sperm from donors or patients who score poorly in the assay with the ultimate objective of developing new treatment modalities for certain cases of male infertility. For instance, where capacitation and/or the acrosome reaction may be limiting, we would like to optimize capacitation in vitro with the sperm penetration assay, and treat the infertility by intrauterine insemination.

APPLICATION OF THE SPERM PENETRATION ASSAY TO IVF-ET

At the present time, based on our own experience, fertility assessment with the zona-free egg bioassay has little application to the normal fertile male participating in IVF-ET, i.e., a male of proven fertility or a male partner, with normal semen parameters, of an infertile couple in which the wife is clinically infertile. The situation reverts to that discussed in the previous section when we consider long standing idiopathic infertility with normal semen parameters and evidence of infertility in the wife. Although our experience with correlating penetration scores with IVF outcome from oligospermic men has not been encouraging (see above and Table 6), it is preliminary in nature and must be corroborated. Ideally, penetration test results would be used to preclude pointless oocyte recovery or alternatively to direct the infertile couple to donor insemination.

Table 5. Correlation between fertilization of human eggs and penetration of zona-free hamster eggs *in vitro*. Taken from Wolf et al., 1983.

Human In Vitro Fertilization			Fertility Asessment		
			Inseminating Motile Sperm Concentration	Penetration	
Subject No.	Eggs Inseminated	Eggs Fertilized		Percentage	Sperm/Egg
			x 10^6/ml		
1	1	1	10	82	1.2
2	2	1	3.9	95	3.8
3a	3	1	10.4	15	0.2
3b	3	2	19.8	100	3.5
4	3	2	4.8	6	0.1
5a	1	0	8.4	71	1.1
5b	4	2	3	13	0.1
6	2	1	10.4	100	2.4
7	2	2	8.5	40	0.4
			6.5	48	0.5
8	1	0	4.8	69	0.9
9a	3	3	13.2[a]	0	0
9b	3	2	6.3	0	0
			7.9[a]	7.7	0.1

10	2	1	6.8	33	0.3
11	1	0	14	38	0.4
12	4	4	22	88	2.1
13	1	0	11.7	40	0.4
14	2	2	23.8	100	3.7
			11.9	100	5.8
15	2	2	9	25	0.3
16	1	1	17.3	67	0.7
17	1	1	19.2	100	1.3
18	2	1	15.8	47	0.5
			7.9	19	0.2
			3.9	21	0.2
19	2	2	2.5	77	0.9
20	2	0	7.3	31	0.3
			3.6	12	0.1
21	1	0	9.5	13	0.1
			4.7	5	0.1
22	1	1	3.6	22	0.2
23	2	0	13.3	14	0.1
24	1	1	23.3	60	0.6

[a]Twenty-four-hour preincubation.

Table 6. Human IVF and hamster egg penetration results for Oligospermic men

Semen Parameters[a]	Human IVF[b] Eggs Fertilized / Eggs Inseminated	Hamster Egg Penetration[c] Sperm Preincubation time (hr.)	Eggs Penetrated (%)
$7x10^6$/42%/2+/ >60%	1/1	3	0
$12x10^6$/42%/3/50%	0/2	3	0
		24	6
$9.5x10^6$/67%/2+/>50%	2/2	3	0
		24	0
$14x10^6$/54%/3/ >60%	2/2	3	0
	3/4	24	50
$12x10^6$/63%/3+/ >60%	2/4	3	13
$17x10^6$/55%/3/ >60%	1/2	3	33

[a]count/motility/progression/morphology (% normal forms).

[b]Human eggs recovered from ≥ 20mm follicles and inseminated at 4-$5x10^5$ motile cells/ml.

[c]Zona-free hamster eggs (15-25) inseminated at 3-$15x10^6$ motile cells/ml in BWW containing 35 mg/ml BSA.

REFERENCES

Aitken, R. J., Best, F. S. M., Richardson, D. W., Djahanbakhch, O., and Lees, M. M., 1982a, The correlates of fertilizing capacity in normal fertile men, Fertil. Steril., 38:68.

Aitken, R. J., Best, F.S.M., Richardson, D. W., Djahanbakhch, O., Mortimer, D., Templeton, A. A. and Lees, M. M., 1982b, An analysis of sperm function in cases of unexplained infertility: conventional criteria, movement characteristics and fertilizing capacity, Fertil. Steril., 38:212.

Austin, C. R., 1976, Developmental anomalies arising from errors of fertilization and cleavage, Curr. Topics Path., 62:3.

Barros, C. and Yanagimachi, R., 1972, Polyspermy-preventing mechanisms in the golden hamster egg, J. Exp. Zool., 180:251.

Barros, C., Gonzales, J., Herrera, E. and Bustos-Oregon, E., 1978, Spermatozoa evaluated by actual penetration of foreign eggs, Contraception, 17:87.

Biggers, J. D., Whitten, W. K., and Whittingham, D. G., 1971, "Methods in Mammalian Embryology," Freeman, San Francisco.

Berger, T., Marrs, R. P., Saito, H., and Kletzky, O. A., 1983, Factors affecting human sperm penetration of zona-free hamster ova, Am. J. Obstet. Gynecol., 145:397.

Binor, Z., Sokoloski, J. E., and Wolf, D. P., 1980, Penetration of zona-free hamster eggs by human sperm, Fertil. Steril., 33:321.

Binor, Z., Sokoloski, J. E., and Wolf, D. P., 1982a, Sperm interaction with the zona-free hamster egg, J. Exp. Zool., 222:187.

Binor, Z., Ras, R., Ramaa, R., van der Ven, H., and Scommegna, A. 1982b, The effect of albumin gradients and human serum on the longevity and fertilizing capacity of human spermatozoa in the hamster ova penetration assay, Fertil. Steril., 38:222.

Binor, Z., Ramaa, R., and Scommegna, A., 1982c, Further studies on dysfunctional human spermatozoa using the zona-free hamster oocyte penetration assay, Fertil. Steril., 37:300

Brackett, B. G., Cofone, M. A., Boice, M. L., and Bousquet, D., 1982, Use of zona-free hamster ova to assess sperm fertilizing ability of bull and stallion, Gamete Res., 5:217.

Cohen, J., Felten, P., and Zeilmaker, G. H., 1981, In vitro fertilizing capacity of fresh and cryopreserved human spermatozoa: a comparative study of freezing and thawing procedures, Fertil. Steril., 36:356.

Cohen, J. Weber, R. F. A., van der Vijver, J. C. M., and Zeilmaker, G. H., 1982, In vitro fertilizing capacity of human spermatozoa with the use of zona-free hamster ova: interassay variation and prognostic value, Fertil. Steril., 37:565.

Dandekar, P. V., and Wolf, D. P., 1982, Evidence for a sperm derived factor that enhances human sperm penetration of zona free hamster eggs, J. Cell Biol., 95:162a.

Dandekar, P. V., and Wolf, D. P., 1983, Characteristics of a human sperm-associated factor that enhances sperm fusion with zona-free hamster eggs, presented at J. Cell Biol., In press.

Dor, J., Rudak, E. and Aitken, R. J., 1981, Antisperm antibodies: their effect on the processes of fertilization studied in vitro, Fertil. Steril., 35:535.

Fleming, A. D., Yanagimachi, R., and Yanagimachi, H., 1979, Fertilizability of cryopreserved zona-free hamster ova, Gamete Res., 2:357.

Haas, G.G., Jr., Sokoloski, J.E., and Wolf, D.P., 1980, The interfering effect of human IgG antisperm antibodies on human sperm penetration of zona-free hamster eggs, Am. J. Reprod. Immunol., 1:40.

Hall, J. L., 1981, Relationship between semen quality and human sperm penetration of zona-free hamster ova, Fertil. Steril., 35:457.

Hanada, A. and Chang, M. C., 1972, Penetration of zona-free eggs by spermatozoa of different species, Biol. Reprod., 6:300.

Hanada, A. and Chang, M. C., 1976, Penetration of hamster and rabbit zona-free eggs by rat and mouse spermatozoa with special reference to sperm capacitation, J. Reprod. Fertil., 46:239.

Hanada, A. and Chang, M. C., 1978, Penetration of the zona-free or intact eggs by foreign spermatozoa and the fertilization of deer mouse eggs in vitro, J. Exp. Zool., 203:277.

Hinrichsen, M. J. and Blaquier, J. A., 1980, Evidence supporting the existence of sperm maturation in the human epididymis, J. Reprod. Fertil., 60:291.

Imai, H., Niwa, K. and Iritani, A., 1977, Penetration in vitro of zona-free hamster eggs by ejaculated boar spermatozoa, J. Reprod. Fertil., 54:379.

Karp, L. E., Williamson, R. A., Moore, D. E., Shy, K. K., Plymate, S. R. and Smith, W. D., 1981, Sperm penetration assay: useful test in evaluation of male fertility, Obstet. Gynecol., 57:620.

Kim, C. I., Niwa, K., Imai, H. and Iritani, A., 1980, Penetration of zona-free hamster eggs in vitro by goat spermatozoa preincubated in the reproductive tract isolated from a maturing gilt, J. Exp. Zool., 213:181.

Martin, R.H. and Taylor, P.J., 1983, Effect of sperm concentration in the zona-free hamster ova penetration assay, Fertil. Steril., 39:379.

Menge, A. C. and Black, C. S., 1979, Effects of antisera on human sperm penetration of zona-free hamster ova, Fertil. Steril., 32:214.

Overstreet, J. W. and Hembree, W. C., 1976, Penetration of the zona pellucida of non-living human oocytes by human spermatozoa in vitro, Fertil. Steril., 27:815.

Overstreet, J. W., Yanagimachi, R., Katz, D. F., Hayashi, K. and Hanson, E. W., 1980, Penetration of human spermatozoa into the human zona pellucida and the zona-free hamster egg: A study of fertile donors and infertile patients, Fertil. Steril., 33:534.

Pavlok, A., 1979, Interspecies interaction of zona-free ova with spermatozoa in mouse, rat, and hamster, Animal Reprod. Sci., 2:395

Perreault, S. D. and Rogers, B. J., 1982, Capacitation pattern of human spermatozoa, Fertil. Steril., 38:258.

Quinn, P., 1979, Failure of human spermatozoa to penetrate zona-free mouse and rat ova in vitro, J. Exp. Zool., 210:497.

Quinn, P., Barros, C., and Whittingham, D. G., 1982, Preservation of hamster oocytes to assay the fertilizing capacity of human spermatozoa, J. Reprod. Fertil., 66:161.

Rogers, B. J., Van Campen, H., Ueno, M., Lambert, H., Bronson, R. and Hale, R., 1979, Analysis of human spermatozoa fertilizing ability using zona-free ova, Fertil. Steril., 32:664.

Rogers, B. J., Perreault, S. D., Bentwood, B. J., McCarville, C., Hale, R. W., and Soderdahl, D. W., 1983a, Variability in the human-hamster in vitro assay for fertility evaluation, Fertil. Steril., 39:204.

Rogers, B. J., Takemoto, F., Wiltbank, M., and Hale, R. W., 1983b, Comparison of the penetration ability of human spermatozoa into bovine cervical mucus and zona-free hamster eggs, Fertil. Steril., 39:437.

Rudak, E., 1981, Interspecific fertilization, in: "Bioregulators of Reproduction," G. Jagiello and H.J. Vogel, eds., London Academic Press.

Rudak, E., Jacobs, P. A., and Yanagimachi, R., 1978, Direct analysis of the chromosome constitution of human spermatozoa, Nature (London), 274:911.

Shy, K.K. Soules, M.R., and Karp, L.E., 1982, The SPA - a new test of male fertility, Contemp. Ob/Gyn., 19:20.

Snedecor, G. W., and Cochran, W. G., 1967, Statistical methods, Iowa State University Press, Ames.

Sokoloski, J. E., and Wolf, D. P., 1983, Effect of Seminal Plasma on human sperm fertility assessment, Abst. presented at the Annual Meeting of the Amer. Soc. of Androl., Philadelphia, PA.

Soules, M.R., Moore, D.E., Spadoni, L.R., and Stenchever, M.A., 1982, The relationship between the postcoital test and the sperm penetration assay, Fertil. Steril., 38:384.

Stenchever, M. A., Spadoni, L. R., Smith, W. D., Karp, L. E., Shy, K. K., Moore, D. E., and Berger, R., 1982, Benefits of the sperm (hamster ova) penetration assay in the evaluation of the infertile couple, Am. J. Obstet. Gynecol., 143:91.

Thadani, V. M., 1980, A study of hetero-specific sperm-egg interactions in the rat, mouse, and deer mouse using in vitro fertilization and sperm injection. J. Exp. Zool., 212:435.

Tyler, J. P. P., Pryor, J. P., and Collins, W. P., 1981, Heterologous ovum penetration by human spermatozoa, J. Reprod. Fert., 63:499.

Usui, N., and Yanagimachi, R., 1976, Behavior of hamster sperm nuclei incorporated into eggs at various stages of maturation, fertilization and early development, J. Ultrastruct. Res., 57:276.

Wolf, D. P., and Sokoloski, J. E., 1982, Characterization of the sperm penetration bioassay, J. Androl. 3:445.

Wolf, D. P., Sokoloski, J. E., and Quigley, M. M., 1983, Correlation of human in vitro fertilization with the hamster egg bioassay, Fertil. Steril., 40:53.

Yanagimachi, R., 1972, Penetration of guinea pig spermatozoa into hamster eggs in vitro, J. Reprod. Fertil., 28:477.

Yanagimachi, R., Yanagimachi, H and Rogers, B. J., 1976, The use of zona-free ova as a test system for the assessment of the fertilizing capacity of human spermatozoa, Biol. Reprod., 15:471.

Zausner-Guelman, B., Blasco, L. and Wolf, D. P., 1981, Zona-free hamster eggs and human sperm penetration capacity: a comparative study of proven fertile donors and infertility patients, Fertil. Steril., 36:771.

15

TECHNIQUES OF EMBRYO TRANSFER

Cecilia L. Schmidt

In vitro fertilization and embryo transfer (IVF-ET) has approximated the tubal functions of oocyte retrieval, housing of fertilization and transport of the embryo to the uterine environment in patients lacking functioning fallopian tubes. However, normal appearance following cleavage of concepti at the time of transfer has not improved the low success rate in terms of pregnancies per embryo transferred (Wood et al., 1981).

In an effort to eliminate faulty technique of embryo transfer as a factor limiting pregnancies, the least traumatic method of embryo transfer should be utilized to mimic "natural transfer" from the fallopian tube to the uterus in women. In choosing our technique, we have endeavored to benefit from both animal experimentation and previous human experience.

ANIMAL STUDIES OF EMBRYO TRANSFER

When Walter Heape performed the first animal embryo transfers at the end of the last century, he did not foresee that human embryo transfers would follow within the ensuing 100 years. Heape utilized a spear-headed needle to transport fertilized rabbit ova to a "uterine foster mother" (Heape, 1891). As detailed in an historical review of animal embryo transfers by Betteridge (1981), these early methods led to a variety of non-surgical techniques, both transvaginal and transrectal.

Three main factors contributing to the success of embryo transfer in lower mammals, principally rabbits, mice and cattle, are the stage of the embryo at transfer (age of the conceptus), the time interval between ovulation in the recipient and the donor (age of the uterus) and the method of transfer.

Although pregnancies have been established in mammals after uterine or tubal transfer of embryos ranging in age from the one-cell (Marston et al., 1977; Craft et al., 1982) to the blastocyst stage (Schneider et al., 1980; Wright, 1981; Buster et al., 1983), a species-specific developmental stage seems to guarantee maximal success. Of 2286 non-surgical embryo transfers in cows, pregnancies occurred in 44% of morula transfers versus 65% of blastocyst transfers (Wright, 1981). Although not as dramatically, Schneider et al. (1980) noted a similar trend. Pregnancies resulted from 61% of early morula compared to 67% of late morula and 71% of late blastocyst embryo transfers in cows. Statistical analysis confirmed that the differences between pregnancy rates after morula and blastocyst transfers were not solely related to a higher proportion of poorer embryos (grades 2 and 3) in the morula stage. Perhaps these differences in optimal developmental stages reflect species variations in the ability of the uterine cavity to support early cleavage (See Chapter 16). Although the normal entry time of rabbit embryos into the uterus is 78 to 84 hours post-coital at the blastocyst stage (Hodgson and Pauerstein, 1976), implantation has occurred with transfers as early as 48 hours after ovulation. Attempts to further accelerate entry time of donor ova inseminated in vivo to a recipient pseudopregnant rabbit uteri to within 24 to 48 hours of ovulation have resulted in failure of pregnancy secondary to uterine expulsion (Chang, 1950; Adams, 1979). Transfers of rabbit fertilized ova between 48 and 72 hours after ovulation have resulted in term births in 22% (Chang, 1950) to 27% (Adams, 1979) of transfers.

The most dramatic acceleration of ovum transport is achieved by transplanting an ovary into the uterine cavity. This operation was first employed in women to achieve pregnancies and was popularized as the "Estes procedure" at the turn of the century. W. L. Estes, Sr., performed bilateral salpingectomies and a unilateral oophorectomy, implanting the remaining ovary into a uterine window at the cornual-isthmic stump. Of 270 cases collected from the literature by Adams (1979), 29 women had become pregnant. Adams calculated that the odds of conceiving after an Estes procedure were 6.78 pregnancies/100 women years. Furthermore, Craft et al. (1982) achieved continuing pregnancies in 2 of 31 women after transfer of oocytes and sperm into the uterus. The oocytes were aspirated from ovarian follicles, pre-incubated for 6 hours, then incubated in the presence of sperm for an additional hour. Twenty μl of medium containing the oocytes and 10,000 to 20,000 sperm were then transferred. Estes Jr., and Heitmeyer (1934) failed to produce pregnancies with ovarian transplantation to the uteri of 18 rabbits despite their concurrent success with this operation in women. Adams (1979) was similarly unsuccessful in applying this procedure to rabbits and guinea pigs. Marston et al. (1977) recovered fertilized eggs from the oviducts of 13 naturally mated rhesus monkeys. Eight pregnancies resulted from transfers to the contralateral oviduct of 9 one-to-six-cell concepti. However, pregnancies were not established after a similar tubal transfer of a 22-cell morula or after singleton transfers to the uterus of one 5-cell or of two 7-to-8-cell embryos. Hence, disparities exist between the early uterine exposure of ova and pregnancy establishment in lower animals, in sub-human primates and in women.

In determining the optimal embryological age at which to perform embryo transfers, the effect of in vitro culture upon the developing conceptus must be considered. Ultrastructural comparisons of fertilized rabbit ova maintained in vitro with those developing in vivo suggest deficiencies in vitro after 5 days (Van Blerkom et al., 1973). In comparing in vitro and in vivo cleavage rates of monkey embryos, Kreitmann and Hodgen (1981) noted a progressive failure to sustain normal rates of cleavage beyond 24 hours in vitro. Animal studies focussed upon the age of the uterus have demonstrated that a certain degree of asynchrony between the cycles of the donor and the recipient can be tolerated (Whittingham, 1979). This latitude is greatest in species where implantation is somewhat delayed after the embryo enters the uterus. In cattle and sheep, pregnancies can occur when recipients are as much as ± 2 days out of synchrony with the donor (Whittingham, 1979). Although implantation in man occurs approximately 6 days after ovulation (Boving and Larsen, 1980), the degree of asynchrony between recipient and donor that can be tolerated has yet to be determined. Since only one report of a successful transfer of a donated human oocyte fertilized in vitro has appeared (Trounson et al., 1983), the relationship between animal studies and human experience remains undefined. However, continuing attempts at human embryo freezing (Trounson et al., 1981b) with embryo transfers scheduled for alternate cycles and, possibly, for "foster uteri" will eventually address this subject. Finally, the establishment of pregnancies in 2 infertile women after the transfer of in vivo-fertilized donated ova at the blastocyst stage has been described (Buster et al., 1983). These authors reported that the recipients had ovulated 2 days before the donor.

Early animal transfer methods used a surgical, transfundal approach to the uterus under anesthesia. Brand and Drost (1977) admitted that the surgical maneuver avoids creation of a cervical mucus tract for escape of the embryo but has the disadvantages of requiring anesthesia and possibly introducing blood into the uterus. Initial non-surgical transcervical attempts at embryo transfer evidenced low success rates of between 2 and 4% in both goats (Otsuki and Soma, 1964) and pigs (Polge and Day, 1968). However, as noted by Seidel (1981), refinement of cervical transfer methods in cattle has resulted in pregnancy rates (30 to 60%) only slightly inferior to those of surgical, transfundal transfers (50 to 70%). Furthermore, animal experiments employing sham embryo transfers have shown that the potential deleterious effects of entry into the uterus through the cervix do not constitute major problems. Passage of the cervical catheter into the uterus was not associated with either trauma to the endometrium, introduction of microorganisms, or injection of embryos into the uterine muscle or fallopian tubes (Seidel et al., 1975). In contrast, similar sham transfers into surgically removed human uteri revealed that all types of catheters disrupted the surface endometrium (Johnston, 1982). It is somewhat surprising, then, that profound effects upon pregnancy rates in cattle have been attributed to differences among various technicians (Schneider et al., 1980; Seidel, 1981). The degree of skill of diverse technicians both in quickly and atraumatically passing the catheter (Tervit et al., 1980) and in depositing the embryo at the proper site (Seidel, 1981) may explain the contrasting pregnancy rates.

TRANSCERVICAL TRANSFERS OF HUMAN EMBRYOS

Almost all human embryo transfers have been performed via a transcervical route to the uterus at stages of development between 2 and 16 cells. Edwards et al. (1980) described 4 pregnancies resulting from 32 singleton embryo transfers at the 8-to-16-cell stage. Two pregnancies resulted from 14 embryo transfers at the 8-cell stage in another series (Lopata et al., 1980). Trounson et al. (1981a) found that of 45 embryos transferred to 34 patients, 8 women had elevated -hCG levels between 7 and 16 days after laparoscopy, but only 4 pregnancies were documented. In a follow-up report by the Monash Research Group (Trounson and Wood, 1981) 9 of 112 women undergoing laparoscopies had embryo transfers which produced pregnancies continuing beyond 12 weeks. Jones et al. (1983) reported the transcervical transfer of 3-to-6-cell embryos at 44 hours after insemination using a teflon catheter through a stainless steel catheter guide. Transfer was accomplished with ease 93 out of 94 times and resulted in 21 pregnancies.

A controversy continues about the ideal developmental stage for human embryos at the time of transfer. Human embryos have not been recovered from the uterus before the 12-to-16-cell stage (Boving and Larsen, 1980; Biggers, 1978). Successful embryo transfers before the 2-cell stage, within the first 24 hours after aspiration of the oocyte, have only been reported in the human. Most dramatically, as already described, the Estes operation has resulted in occasional pregnancies after an oocyte was presumably ovulated directly into the uterus and fertilized there. Hence, unlike rabbit ova (Estes, Jr., and Heitmeyer, 1934), prolonged human oocyte exposure to the tubal environment does not seem mandatory for pregnancy establishment. This observation is further supported by the pregnancies established after transfer of incubated human oocytes and sperm to the uterus (Craft et al., 1982) as already described. Furthermore, Veeck et al. (1983) reported successful _in vitro_ maturation of 64 of 74 immature oocytes. Eight pregnancies resulted from the subsequent transfer to 30 women of 44 concepti at pronuclear to 8-cell stages. However, none of these pregnancies could be attributed solely to a pronuclear stage conceptus. A final argument for early embryo transfer is that limiting the _in vitro_ exposure of the conceptus may decrease chances of inadvertent physical damage to the developing embryo. Furthermore, as detected in monkey embryos cultured _in vitro_ (Kreitmann and Hodgen, 1981), progession of embryonic development may be retarded by _in vitro_ culture beyond 24 hours.

The arguments for embryo transfer beyond the 16-cell stage point to the possibility that follicular aspiration and laparoscopic manipulation may disturb ovarian and uterine physiology. By delaying the transfer beyond 48 hours, the conceptus may be delivered into a more receptive endometrial cavity. The technology required to mature fertilized human ova to the fully developed blastocyst stage _in vitro_ has been demonstrated in 2 of 6 retrieved oocytes studied (Steptoe et al., 1971). Similarly, Trounson et al. (1982) noted that 50 to 60% of regularly cleaving embryos will continue to develop to at least the morula stage. Furthermore, Buster et al. (1983) have recently reported two pregnancies by transcervical transfer of husband-fertilized donor blastocysts to two infertile recipients who had ovulated two days before the donors. These successes sharply contrast with the ectopic implantation of a blastocyst reported by Steptoe and Edwards (1976). Obviously, the most auspicious stage of human embryo development for embryo transfer has not been determined.

The use of only a small volume of transfer medium in single-catheter transcervical embryo transfers is optimal as shown by both human experience and animal experimentation. Most IVF-ET programs deliver a total of less than 100 μl, usually ranging between 20 and 50 μl, of transfer medium to the uterus with the embryo (Trounson and Wood, 1981; Jones et al., 1983; Smith et al., 1983 and Trotnow et al., 1983). Liedholm et al. (1980) found that

125- µm microspheres transferred transcervically through 2mm plastic catheters in 25 to 50 µl of Ham's F-10 medium lodged in uterine fundi within 1cm of the estimated sites of transfer. Hence, this volume of transfer fluid allowed adequate delivery of the microspheres without permitting outflow into the fallopian tubes.

THE TECHNIQUE OF TRANSCERVICAL EMBRYO TRANSFER AT HOUSTON

In essence, our technique involves the single transfer of all normally cleaving embryos or fertilized immature oocytes (previously matured in vitro) into the donor's uterus between 48 and 56 hours after follicular aspiration. At the time of transfer, embryos from mature oocytes are at the 2-to-8-cell stage. When only immature oocytes have been retrieved, transfers have been done either at the pronuclear stage (16 hours post-insemination, 48 to 56 hours post-recovery) or following cleavage (40 hours post-insemination, 72 to 80 hours post-recovery).

As described in detail in Chapter 13, inseminated mature oocytes are first examined at 16 hours after insemination following removal of the corona cells. The oocytes are then inspected for pronuclei. A finding of 2 pronuclei constitutes presumptive evidence of fertilization. After transfer from inseminating medium (containing 7.5% heat-inactivated patient's serum) to growth medium (containing 15% heat-inactivated patient's serum), the fertilized oocyte is next examined 24 hours later. Arrangements are made for embryo transfer if cleavage to the 2-to-4-cell stage has taken place. Our recent success with fertilization of immature oocytes following in vitro maturation has fostered replacement into the uterus of embryos as early as the pronuclear stage.

Early in the development of the IVF-ET program at Houston, several types of catheters were evaluated. All the transfer catheters were connected to an air-tight Hamilton syringe (Gastight #1001 - Hamilton Company, Reno, NV). The "Tomcat" catheter (Monoject, St. Louis, MO) is 11.5cm in length with a 0.3mm opening at the bullet-shaped tip (Kerin et al., 1981). Several different open-ended, single and double teflon catheters (Penn-tube Plastics, Clifton Heights, PA) were tried before choosing our present apparatus. In the double-catheter apparatus, the outer tube was inserted into the cervical canal to the level of the internal os and the inner catheter was advanced to the uterine fundus. Our current catheter, as previously described by Jones et al. (1983), is composed of American Wire Gauge #20 Teflon tubing of thin-wall thickness and is manufactured by the William Kelly Instrument Company (Baltimore, MD). We utilize a 40cm length of this catheter with an internal diameter of 0.86mm and an outside diameter of 1.47mm. The closed tip is sealed without cement by a bullet-shaped nylon plug (Figure 1). A side opening equal to the internal diameter of the tubing allows fluid emission at a 45° angle to the long axis. The advantages of the side opening include reducing the chances of blood or mucus either plugging the aperture or entangling the conceptus. However, this side opening makes embryo loading somewhat more difficult. The base of the transfer catheter is attached to a #19 gauge blunt needle connected to an air-tight Hamilton syringe with a one ml total volume. The rigid carrying tube with a curved tip is composed of #12 steel needle tubing with an internal diameter of

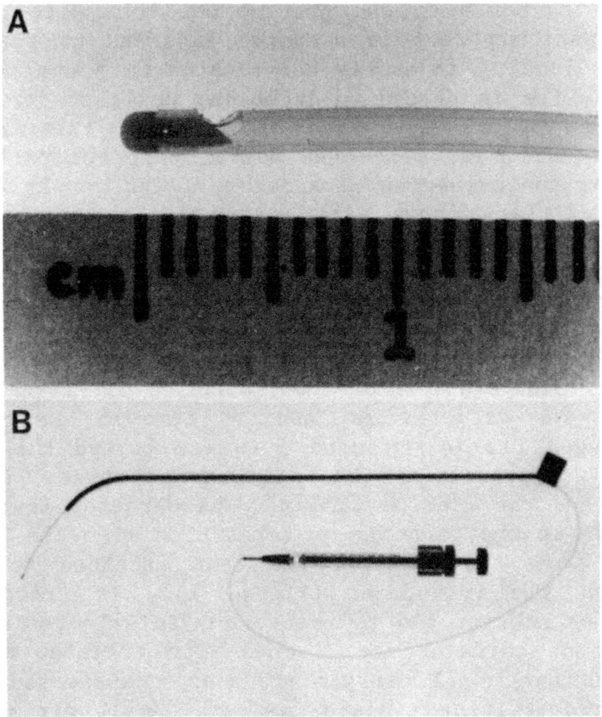

Figure 1

Close-up view of the plugged tip of the side-opening Teflon catheter (A). The assembled apparatus consists of the teflon catheter guided through the rigid stainless steel holder and attached to an air-tight Hamilton Syringe (B). Tape on the catheter allows estimation of the extent of advancement into the uterine cavity.

2.16mm. Our use of the rigid loader has replaced awkward manipulation of a flexible catheter with ring forceps. Figure 1 illustrates a close-up view of the catheter tip as well as the catheter-syringe set-up guided through the metal holder as assembled sterilely just prior to loading the embryo(s). The first 4 pregnancies resulted from embryo transfers using growth media, i.e., 15% heat-inactivated patient's serum in modified Ham's F-10. However, all subsequent pregnancies involved transfer in "high serum" (75 to 90% heat-inactivated patient's serum in modified Ham's F-10, Feichtinger et al., 1983). The transfer medium is prepared concomitantly with media for insemination and growth (Chapter 13).

Once the decision to transfer the embryo(s) has been made, the patient is admitted to the hospital. Ten mg of diazepam is administered by mouth to the patient one hour prior to transfer. Since the operating room is situated adjacent to the laboratory, the catheter loading is easily coordinated with the preparation of the patient. She is placed in lithotomy position for insertion of the bivalved vaginal speculum. A bimanual examination is not performed at this time since the position of the patient's uterus is known from the screening laparoscopy. The cervix is cleaned of mucus and cellular debris with cotton balls attached to a ring forceps. Unlike other protocols (Trotnow et al., 1983), we do not grasp the cervix with a tenaculum since the rigid guide allows alteration of the angle of the transfer catheter (Figure 2).

As soon as patient preparation is completed, the procedure of loading the embryo(s) into the catheter is commenced in the laboratory. The catheter is inserted through the carrying tube and the plugged tip is extended 5 to 6cm beyond the rigid guide. This length approximates the distance between the external cervical os and the uterine fundus. The catheter is marked with a piece of tape at the point in juxtaposition with the carrying tube to indicate when the catheter has been extended to the desired distance past the introducer (Figure 1). In order to prevent desiccation of embryos and to remove any soluble contaminants, the initial 30cm of catheter are flushed with transfer medium to wet the inner surface. All embryos are then transferred to a single culture dish containing transfer medium. Ample air is drawn into the first portion of the Hamilton syringe. The catheter is loaded in sequence with approximately 10 μl of transfer medium, a 10 μl air bubble, 10 to 15 μl of transfer medium containing all embryos, a second 10 μl air bubble and a final 10 μl of transfer medium.

The apparatus containing the embryo(s) is carried in a sterile envelope to the operating room. The catheter guide is not passed into the cervical canal unless difficulty is encountered in passing the internal os (Figure 2a). Only the plugged tip of the catheter is advanced beyond the metal guide into the external

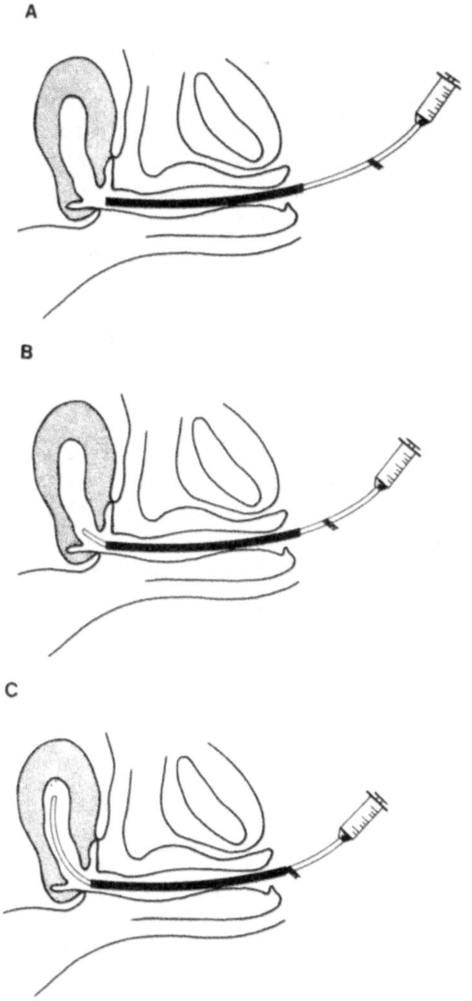

Figure 2

Sequential transcervical advancement of the teflon catheter into the uterine cavity for embryo transfer. Note that the rigid guide never traverses the cervical canal.

cervical os and into the cervical canal (Figure 2b). The catheter tip is gently advanced to the fundus as estimated by the tape demarcation. By manipulating the angle of the rigid guide, the flexible catheter can be moved along the contour of the uterine cavity. The entire column of air in the Hamilton syringe is forced into the catheter to expel the embryo(s) (Figure 2c). Following embryo transfer, the catheter is gently withdrawn and returned to the laboratory where it is carefully examined for retained embryos. Any mucus and/or blood present on the catheter tip is teased away with tuberculin needles from the tip. Finally, the distal end of the catheter is rinsed with culture medium. If the embryo(s) has not been retained in the catheter, the speculum is removed from the patient's vagina and she is returned to her hospital room. If an embryo(s) is retained in the catheter, the procedure of embryo transfer is repeated.

Our patients are placed at complete bedrest for the 18 to 24 hours following embryo transfer. The patient receives 12.5 mg of progesterone in oil IM daily for 5 days beginning at transfer. Earlier attempts to administer progesterone beginnning on the day of laparoscopy were associated with difficult transfers secondary to a relative narrowing of the cervical os. Our patients are advised to refrain from intercourse until menses ensues or pregnancy is detected. As described in Chapter 6, no evidence of luteal phase defects has been found in these patients receiving the 50 mg-clomiphene citrate regimen.

From May 1982 to June 1983, 58 embryo transfers have been performed in women treated with 50 mg clomiphene citrate daily on days 5 through 9 (See Chapter 6). Ten clinical pregnancies have resulted. All 10 successful embryo transfers were marked by a single, atraumatic transcervical passage of the plug-tipped, side-opening teflon catheter. After removal of the catheter, slight bleeding was noted in only 1 of these 10 patients and mild cramping was reported by another. These results agree with earlier statistics. Trounson and Wood (1981) commented that in 9 patients who achieved pregnancies, embryo transfer was performed quickly and without difficulty. The catheter contained mucus or blood in only 2 of 9 patients. A similar number of patients noted a brown discharge 24 hours later.

Our experience with multiple-embryo transfers agrees with the notion that there is an advantage in transferring 2 embryos to the uterus compared to transferring one (Edwards et al., 1980; Trounson, 1983; Jones et al., 1983; Kerin et al., 1983) but the numbers are too small to establish any advantage to the transfer of 3 or more concepti (Table 1). In contrast to other reports, neither ectopic pregnancies nor twin gestations have occurred in this treatment population. Kerin et al. (1983) reported multiple gestations in 7 of 20 pregnancies with a trend toward multiple pregnancies when 4 or more embryos were transferred. Eight of our 10 pregnancies resulted from the transfer of 1 or 2 embryos. Although 5 of these 10 pregnancies have occurred after transfer of 2 embryos, larger numbers of pregnancies need to be studied before determining the optimal number of embryos for transfer.

In summary, we have employed a simple, painless method of transcervical embryo transfer to establish 10 pregnancies in our IVF-ET program. Utilizing an ultrasound-monitored, 50 mg-clomiphene citrate regimen to foster follicular development, retrieved oocytes have been fertilized and matured in vitro to the 2-to-6-cell stage within 48 hours. Embryo transfers of 1 to 5 embryos at this stage of development using this relatively atraumatic method have resulted in singleton pregnancies (Table 1). At the time of writing, 7 healthy babies have been born while the remaining 3 gestations are progressing normally between 11 and 30 weeks of intrauterine development.

Several questions remain to be answered about optimal embryo transfer concerning the number of embryos transferred, the time of transfer and the feasibility of routine embryo freezing. It is undoubtedly the resolution of these fundamental issues, rather than further refinement of the actual technique of embryo transfer, that will profoundly improve the success rates of IVF-ET programs.

Table 1. Comparison between the number of pregnancies established and the number of embryos transferred in 58 embryo transfers in women treated with the 50 mg clomiphene citrate regimen.

Number of Embryos Transferred	Number of Patients	Clinical Pregnancies Established	
		#	%
1	36	3	8.3%
2	15	5	33.3%
3	4	0	0%
4	2	1	50.0%
5	1	1	100.0%

REFERENCES

Adams, C.E., 1979, Consequences of accelerated ovum transport, including a re-evaluation of Estes' operation, J. Reprod. Fert., 55:239.

Betteridge, K.J., 1981, An historical look at embryo transfer, J. Reprod. Fert., 62:1.

Biggers, J.D., 1978, Fertilization and blastocyst formation, presented at: Symposium on Animal Models for Contraceptive and Fertility Research, National Academy of Sciences, Washington, D.C.

Brand, A., and Drost, M., 1977, Embryo transfer by non-surgical methods, in:"Embryo Transfer in Farm Animals". A Review of Techniques and Applications, K.J. Betteridge, ed., Monograph #16, Canada Department of Agriculture, Ottawa.

Boving, B.G., and Larson, J.F., 1980, Implantation, in: "Human Reproduction, Conception and Contraception", E.S.E. Hafez, ed., Harper and Harper, Cambridge.

Buster, J.E., Bustillo, M., Thorneycroft, I.H., Simon, J.A., Boyers, S.P., Marshall, J.R., Louw, J.A., Seed, R.W., and Seed, R.G., 1983, Non-surgical transfer of in vivo fertilized donated ova to five infertile women: report of two pregnancies, Lancet, 2:223.

Chang, M.C., 1950, Development and fate of transferred rabbit ova or blastocyst in relation to the ovulation time of recipients, J. Exp. Zool., 114:197.

Craft, I., McLeod, F., Green, S., Djahanbakhch, O., Bernard, A., and Twigg, H., 1982, Human pregnancy following oocyte and sperm transfer to the uterus, Lancet, 1:1031.

Edwards, R.G., Steptoe, P.C., and Purdy, J.M., 1980, Establishing full-term human pregnancies using cleaving embryos grown in vitro, Br. J. Obstet. Gynaecol., 87:737.

Estes, W.L., Jr., and Heitmeyer, P.L., 1934, Incidence of pregnancy following ovarian implantation, Am. J. Surg., 24:563.

Feichtinger, W., Kemeter, P., Szalay, S., Janisch, H., 1983, Early hormone parameters and embryonic development in pregnancies established by in vitro fertilization and embryo transfer, in: "Fertilization of the Human Egg In Vitro", H.M. Beier and H.R. Lindner, eds., Springer-Verlag, Berlin.

Heape, W., 1891, Preliminary note on the transplantation and growth of mammalian ova within a uterine foster-mother, Proc. R. Soc., 48:457.

Hodgson, B.J., and Pauerstein, C.J., 1976, Comparison of oviductal transport of fertilized and unfertilized ova after hCG or coitus-induced ovulation in rabbits, Biol. Reprod., 14:377.

Jones, H.W., Acosta, A.A., Garcia, J.E., Sandow, B.A., Veeck, L., 1983, On the transfer of conceptuses from oocytes fertilized in vitro, Fertil. Steril., 39:241.

Johnston, I.W.H., 1982, The luteal uterus: cellular interactions with blastocysts, and the damaging effects of catheters in: "Human Conception In Vitro", R. G. Edwards and J.M. Purdy, eds., Academic Press, London.

Kerin, J.F.P., Warnes, G.M., Jeffrey, R., Cox, L.W., and Broom, T.J., 1981, A simple technique for human embryo transfer into the uterus, Lancet 2:726.

Kerin, J.F., Warnes, G.M., Quinn, P.J., Jeffrey, R., Kirby, C., Matthews, C.D., Seamark, R.P., and Cox, L.W., 1983, Incidence of multiple pregnancy following human in vitro fertilization and embryo transfer, Lancet, 2:537.

Kreitmann, O., and Hodgen, G.D., 1981, Retarded cleavage rates of preimplantation monkey embryos in vitro, J.A.M.A., 246:627.

Liedholm, P., Sundstrom, P., and Wramsby, H., 1980, A model for experimental studies on human egg transfer, Arch. Androl., 5:92.

Lopata, A., Johnston, I.W.H., Hoult, I.J., and Speirs, A.I., 1980, Pregnancy following intrauterine implantation of an embryo obtained by in vitro fertilization of a preovulatory egg, Fertil. Steril., 33:117.

Marston, J.H., Penn, R., and Sivelle, P.C., 1977, Successful autotransfer of tubal eggs in the rhesus monkey (Macaca mulatta), J. Reprod. Fert., 49:175.

Otsuki, K., and Soma, T., 1964, Transfer of fertilized ova through the cervix in goats, Bull. Nat. Inst. Anim. Ind., 6:27.

Polge, C.E., and Day, B.N., 1968, Pregnancy following non-surgical egg transfer in pigs, Vet. Rec., 82:712.

Schneider, H.J., Jr., Castleberry, R.S., and Griffin, J.L., 1980, Commercial aspects of bovine embryo transfer, Theriogenology 13:73.

Seidel, G.E., Jr., 1981, Critical review of embryo transfer procedures with cattle, in : "Fertilization and Embryonic Development In Vitro", L. Mastroianni, Jr., and J.D. Biggers, eds., Plenum Press, New York.

Seidel, G.E., Jr., Bowen, J.M., Homan, N.R., and Okun, N.E., 1975, Fertility of heifers with sham embryo transfer through the cervix, Vet. Rec., 97:307.

Smith, D.H., Picker, R.H., Sinosich, M.J., Saunders, D.M., and Grudzinskas, J.G., 1983, Effects of clomiphene administration on ovarian function as measured by estradiol and ultrasound, Obstet. Gynecol., 61:695.

Steptoe, P.C., and Edwards, R.G., 1976, Reimplantation of a human embryo with subsequent tubal pregnancy, Lancet, 1:880.

Steptoe, P.C., Edwards, R.G., and Purdy, J.M., 1971, Human blastocysts grown in culture, Nature, 229:132.

Tervit, H.R., Cooper, M.W., Goold, P.G., and Haszard, G.M., 1980, Non-surgical embryo transfer in cattle, Theriogenology 13:63.

Trotnow, S., Al-Hasani, S., Kniewald, T., Becker, H., and Hunlich, T., 1983, Transfer of human embryos at early cleavage stages, in: "Fertilization of the Human Egg In Vitro", H.M. Beier and H.R. Lindner, eds., Springer-Verlag, Berlin.

Trounson, A., 1983, Factors controlling normal embryo development and implantation of human oocytes fertilized in vitro, in: "Fertilization of the Human Egg In Vitro," H.M. Beier and H.R. Lindner, eds., Springer-Verlag, Berlin.

Trounson, A., Leeton, J.F., Besanko, M., Wood, C., and Conti, A., 1983, Pregnancy established in an infertile patient after transfer of a donated embryo fertilised in vitro, Br. Med. J., 286:835.

Trounson, A.O., Leeton, J.F., Wood, C., Webb, J., and Wood, J., 1981a, Pregnancies in humans by fertilization in vitro and embryo transfer in the controlled ovulatory cycle, Science, 212:681.

Trounson, A.O, Mohr, L.R., Pugh, P.A., Leeton, J.F., Wood, C., 1981b, The deep-freezing of human embryos, in: "Proceedings of Third World Congress of Human Reproduction," Berlin, Excerpta Medica, Amsterdam.

Trounson, A.O, Mohr, L.R., Wood, C., and Leeton, J.F., 1982, Effect of delayed insemination of in vitro fertilization, culture and transfer of human embryos, J. Reprod. Fert., 64:285.

Trounson, A., and Wood, C., 1981, Extracorporeal fertilization and embryo transfer, Clin. Obstet. Gynaecol., 8:681.

Van Blerkom, J., Manes, C., and Daniel, J.C., Jr., 1973, Development of preimplantation rabbit embryos in vivo and in vitro, Devel. Biol., 35:262.

Veeck, L.T., Wortham, J.W.E., Witmyer, J., Sandow, B.A., Acosta, A.A., Garcia, J.E., Jones, G.S., and Jones, H.W., 1983, Maturation and fertilization of morphologically immature human oocytes in a program of in vitro fertilization, Fertil. Steril., 39:594.

Whittingham, D.G., 1979, In-vitro fertilization, embryo transfer and storage, Br. Med. Bull., 35:105.

Wood, C. Trounson, A., Leeton, J., Talbot, J.M., Buttery, B., Webb, J., Wood, J., and Jessup, D., 1981, A clinical assessment of nine pregnancies obtained by in vitro fertilization and embryo transfer, Fertil. Steril., 35:502.

Wright, J.M., 1981, Non-surgical embryo transfer in cattle embryo-recipient interactions, Theriogenology, 15:43.

16

IMPLANTATION

Paul D. Webb and Stanley R. Glasser

Studies from several countries over the last two centuries have shown that the chances of a fertile couple producing viable offspring in any one menstrual cycle is about 25% (Vessey et al., 1976; Short, 1979). Unfortunately little data is available on what percentage of the failure is due to ovulatory, fertilization, implantation, or developmental dysfunction. In farm animals there is a high incidence of early embryonic loss; in the case of the pig as large as 30-40%. This also appears to be the situation in the human where it has been estimated that such losses may be as high as 50% of presumed conceptions (Leridon, 1977; Short, 1979). The majority of these spontaneously aborted embryos are either genetically or morphologically abnormal. Laboratory and domestic species exhibit a behavioral period (estrus) during their reproductive cycles when females will accept males and copulate. Although the human reproductive cycle has a similar hormonal basis, acceptance of the male is not restricted to an exclusive period of behavior. It is of interest therefore that in comparison with domestic species, fecundity in humans is low. To date, the success rates achieved by IVF-ET protocols are, at 15-20%, only marginally below the accepted norm. However, this success rate is disconcerting when it is considered that patients undergoing IVF-ET have single or multiple embryos transferred; these embryos represent a selected surviving population which has satisfied existing criteria for transfer. Of the losses that follow attempts to establish pregnancies by IVF-ET, most can be attributed to implantation failure (Edwards et al., 1980); (Figure 1). Since errors in implantation appear to be the largest single cause of failure, it is appropriate to analyze the implantation period to better understand the contributing factors.

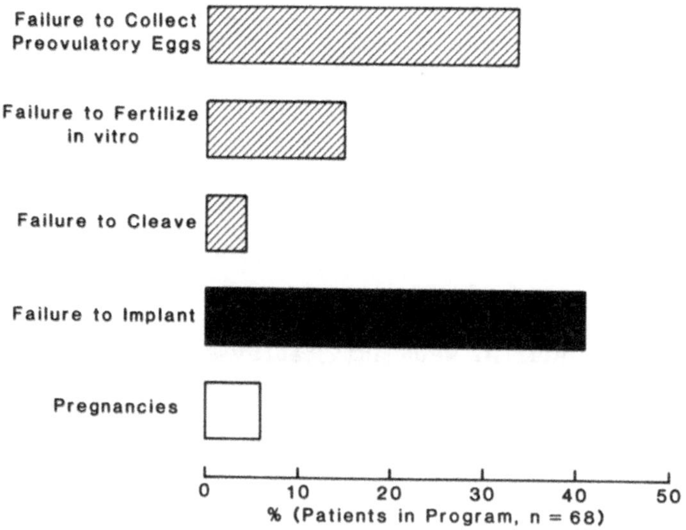

Figure 1

Illustration of the relative proportion of unsuccessful stages in an early *in vitro* fertilization treatment program. This chart is prepared from data which reported the clinical outcome of 79 women in a treatment group which resulted in the first successful human *in vitro* fertilization pregnancy (Edwards et al., 1980). Of the 79 women monitored during the course of spontaneous menstrual cycles, 68 underwent laparoscopy for attempted oocyte retrival resulting in the delivery at term of two normal infants.

Our understanding of human implantation is impaired by the absence of prospective experimentation; ethical and legal restrictions obviate this approach. Thus, a great deal of our knowledge is derived from comparative reproductive biology. The subjects available for study represent surviving examples of a divergent evolution of the mammalian reproductive system and as such are imperfect analogies of human reproduction. Nevertheless, comparative analysis has proven productive and common mechanisms seem to characterize the implantation process.

SYNCHRONY

One of the keystones of the technology of embryo transfer is the concept of synchrony. Synchrony suggests that an ordered integration of the developmental programs proceeding independently in both the embryo and endometrium, sometimes over relatively great distances, is required for the embryo to interact with the endometrium, i.e., implant, at a species specified time. Simply stated, with respect to a species specific implantation day, the greatest success, as assessed by development to term, is achieved if the transferred donor embryo is the same age, or one day older, than the recipient uterus (Noyes et al., 1963; Beier and Mootz, 1979). Younger embryos of laboratory species find the uterus hostile to survival or non-receptive to implantation (Figure 2).

The prevailing concept of preimplantation biology is that in response to ovarian hormones, the uterus matures from a hostile (lethal to the embryo, no implantation) to a non-receptive (not

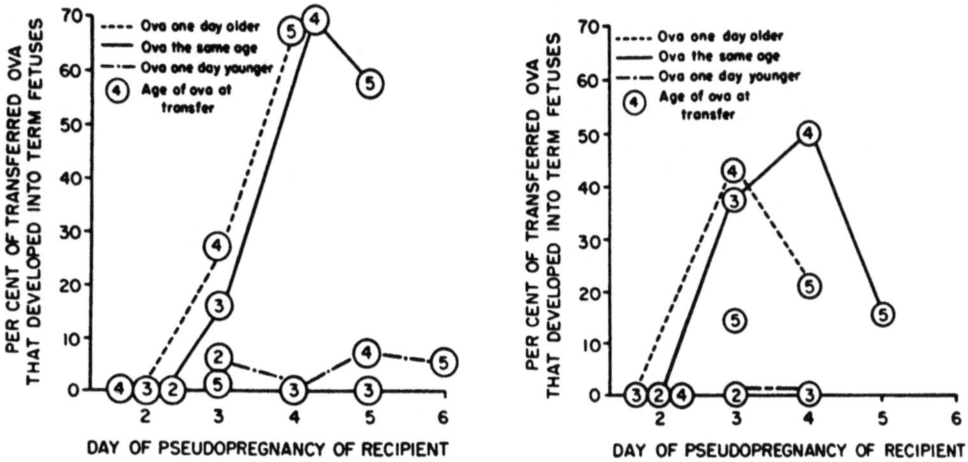

Figure 2

(Left panel) The percentage of rat ova that developed to term fetuses following transfer of 885 ova into 60 pseudo-pregnant recipients. Synchronous transfers (4 - 4) resulted in the highest success rate as did day 5 ova - day 4 uterus. Other transfers, particularly asynchronous transfers where ova were 1 day less developed than the uterus (3 - 4) were less successful. (Right panel) Data from mice are qualitatively similar. Day 3 is the day of implantation so synchronous transfers are 3 - 3. There were 1247 ova and 124 pseudo-pregnant recipients used (Noyes et al., 1963).

immediately lethal, no implantation) and finally, to an environment receptive to the blastocyst and that implantation is a property of the receptive uterus. This hypothesis is confirmed by physiological data (Psychoyos, 1973; Glasser and Clark, 1975) and supported by morphological (Potts, 1966; Nilsson, 1970; Sherman and Wudl, 1976) and biochemical correlates (Glasser, 1972; O'Grady and Bell, 1977; Glasser and McCormack, 1979a). The concept of synchrony was experimentally developed before sophisticated methods of hormone assay and molecular endocrinology were available. Nevertheless it has proven of considerable predictive value in the study of implantation. Methods derived from embryo transfer in laboratory animals have been extended to domestic animals to the point of being commercially feasible. For a variety of reasons synchrony has not received much attention as a strategy for human embryo transfer. In part, this reflects the report that ET in primates functions independently of synchrony (Marston et al., 1977). The limited, perhaps even fortuitous, success with human cleavage embryos indicates that the synchrony between the human uterus and the developing embryo is not as controlled as are the implantation events in other species. It is suggested that the early preimplantation human uterus may not be as hostile to the embryo; certainly a number do survive and develop <u>in vitro</u> until and beyond the time of implantation.

Concerns about possible developmental abnormalities occurring during longer embryo culture periods are appropriate but misplaced. The database on <u>in vitro</u> development is essentially free of evidence suggesting abnormalities. Human ova recovered by laparoscopic aspiration and fertilized <u>in vitro</u> could be maintained in culture through at least the blastocyst stage without risk. Transferred at that time, these blastocysts might yield pregnancies with greater success. Support for this strategy derives from very preliminary reports on "ovum transfer" of embryos obtained by flushing the lower reproductive tract of surrogate donors (Buster et al., 1983).

IMPLANTATION

Implantation, the unique interaction of the developing embryo and the endometrial cells of the maternal host, is best understood as a continuous process. In its narrowest sense, it includes the specific phases which occur following entry of the blastocyst into a receptive uterus, i.e., hatching, apposition, attachment/adhesion and migration/invasion. In a broader sense, implantation should include the complex set of integrated morphological, physiological and biochemical correlates which describe the preimplantation period during which the uterus is transformed to a receptive environment for the embryo. It is now recognized that these changes are synchronized by the action of varying ratios of progestrone and estrogen and that the endpoint of this program is the implantation process. It is advantageous to consider the specific events which comprise implantation in terms of cell-cell interactions, i.e., recognition, communication, adhesion.

Preimplantation Changes: Uterine Morphology

During an optimized human 28-day menstrual cycle, ovulation occurs on day 14 in response to mid-cycle peaks of FSH and LH secretion. Based on limited morphological material available from the human (Falk-Larsen, 1980) implantation occurs about days 20-21. Transport of the egg (fertilized or unfertilized) through the oviduct takes on the order of 2 to 3 days (Hertig et al., 1954; Croxatto et al., 1972). During the cycle, both the uterus and developing embryo undergo morphological and biochemical changes that prepare them for implantation. The uterus is transformed into an environment receptive to blastocyst survival and implantation. These changes, primarily those of the endometrium, are regulated by the ovarian steroids progesterone and estrogen.

The most obvious feature of the human reproductive cycle is the periodic flow of hemorrhagic debris from the uterus. In the absence of a behavioral phase, endometrial shedding is used as an event marker and thus, the terminology menstrual cycle. The loss of superficial endometrium leaves a basal region that is hormonally non-responsive and which undergoes few morphological changes during the cycle. However it is the basis for successive regeneration of the endometrium.

Even before menstruation has ceased, the epithelial cells lining the remains of the glands embedded in the basal stroma start to grow and resurface the endothelium. This repopulation is under the influence of increasing plasma concentrations of estrogens and marks the beginning of the proliferative phase. Peculiar to the human is the increased mitotic activity observed in the glandular epithelium and stroma. Stromal mitoses do not occur concurrently with epithelial proliferation in rats or mice (Tachi et al., 1972; Martin et al., 1973a, 1976).

In contrast to most laboratory animals, the human endometrium, following ovulation, enters a fully developed secretory phase regulated by luteal production of both progesterone and estrogens. The first half of the preimplantation phase is characterized primarily by changes in the glandular epithelium (Nilsson, 1972). The glandular cells initially vacuolate, with the contents eventually being emptied into the lumen of the gland. Secretion reaches a peak around the time of possible implantation; days 20-21. At this time edema within the stroma becomes evident. These changes characterize the predecidual stromal cells which, to date, have only been described in human endometrium (Noyes et al., 1950). During the secretory phase, the endometrium continues to develop and the spiral arteries convolute further and move closer to the endometrial lining.

Comparison of the human endometrial cycle with cyclic changes occurring in the rat or mouse uterus is instructive because experimental approaches not yet applied to the human are possible. The reproductive cycle in rats and mice is condensed in time, with a true secretory endometrium (representative of a functional corpus luteum), not being observed in the absence of a fertilized ovum. Following ovulation, only the epithelial cells proliferate (Finn and Martin, 1967). They undergo two mitotic cycles in response to the elevated concentrations of estrogen of the preceeding proestrus. There are no attendant changes in stroma and there is no decidualization. Should fertilization ensue, the corpus luteum is rescued and becomes morphologically and functionally competent. Progesterone secretion serves to redirect the mitogenic action of estrogen to the stromal cells. These cells proliferate in response to rising plasma titers of both progesterone and estrogen of the preimplantation period. Decidualization of these stroma cells does not occur until stimulated by the implanting blastocyst.

From animal studies, it has also become evident that the uterus is comprised of many individual cell types, i.e., luminal and glandular epithelium (McCormack and Glasser, 1980), a mixed population of 10-12 fixed and migratory stromal cells (Glasser and McCormack, 1980, 1981) and myometrium. In studies of separated endometrial cells, it has been recorded that each homogeneous cell type responds separately and individually to the different steroid hormones. Separated endometrial cell types, by their receptor mediated responses, can each distinguish between progesterone, estrogens and importantly, relative to the current protocols for human IVF-ET, antiestrogens (Markaverich et al., 1981).

While studies of steroid hormone receptors abound, relatively few have applied the current model for steroid hormone action to an analysis of cyclic and preimplantation changes of the endometrium. Individual studies attempt to explain the differences, in terms of steroid hormone receptors, between the cell cycle kinetics of luminal epithelium, glandular epithelium and stroma. Others characterize the divergent responses of preimplantation epithelia and stroma (Glasser and McCormack, 1980) and the differences in the growth of the uterus in response to estradiol vs clomiphene. Contradictory reports surround the observation that increased numbers of progesterone receptors are localized at the site of blastocyst attachment at the time of implantation (Sartor, 1980; Martel and Psychoyos, 1980). The methodology of molecular endocrinology remains to be applied systematically to the analysis of human endometrial cell types.

The histological changes occurring in the endometrium following ovulation are some of the morphological correlates of the process by which the uterus becomes receptive to the developing embryo. In spite of limitations, morphological methods prove very useful in the analysis of the implantation process because of the relative paucity of data from biochemical studies.

Preimplantation Changes: Uterine Secretions

Early morphological studies suggested that uterine secretions might serve as biochemical correlates of the development of receptivity. The quality and quantity of secretions which accumulate under the influence of ovarian steroids within the uterine lumen during various phases of the reproductive cycle have been studied in several species. Investigations were designed to identify phase specific or hormone specific secretory products that might be correlated with some unique facet of implantation. Few attempts have been made to assess critically if the synthesis of these proteins was induced de novo, or whether the appearance of such markers represents synthesis of some constitutive protein which was selectively stimulated. In rats and mice, high concentrations of estrogen elicit intrauterine secretions, particularly of proteins, while high concentrations of progesterone tend to reverse this effect (Armstrong, 1968; Surani, 1975; Aitken, 1977; Pratt, 1977; Fishel, 1979). Individual reports describe unique uterine secretory proteins, one appearing between 18-20 hours after estrogen injection (Surani, 1975). This time interval corresponds with that normally found in cycling rats between the pulse of ovarian estrogen that is released late on the morning of day three (estrogen "surge", prenidatory estrogen) and the early phases of implantation (day 4). Whether the appearance of such unique proteins is coincidental or correlative remains to be resolved, and the relationship of such putatively induced proteins to a specific key embryonic or endometrial function is unproven. These are critical and difficult proofs but necessary because intrauterine proteins could be serum transudates or metabolic or degradation products unrelated to the specific steps being studied.

The balance between estrogens and progestins is of particular importance in altering the nature and amount of uterine secretions and is best demonstrated by studies of uteroglobin. This protein, found in the flushings of the preimplantation uterus, was originally thought to be specific to the rabbit uterus. The protein is detectable by day three post-coitum, peaks between days 4-6 (implantation) and then declines rapidly to non-detectable concentrations by day nine. Secretion of uteroglobin was shown, in both intact pregnant and progesterone-treated, castrate rabbits, to be under the control of progesterone (Bullock et al., 1981). Down regulation of uteroglobin secretion was thought to be directed by estrogen.

At its peak, uteroglobin comprises 25-50% of total uterine proteins (Bullock et al., 1981). The abundance of this protein recommended it as an ideal subject to analyze, for the first time, the molecular control of a hormonally induced mammalian protein of the reproductive tract. The close physiologic correlation between progesterone peak, uteroglobin secretion and the day of implantation promised that such analyses would provide insights into the complexities of implantation. Molecular studies demonstrate that uteroglobin synthesis by endometrial cells is regulated by progesterone (Atger et al., 1980). It has also been shown that regulation at the molecular level is more complex than originally hypothesized and that the protein is neither exclusive to the rabbit nor to its uterus. Both a steroid-binding and a proteinase inhibitory activity have been ascribed to the protein. The balance between blastocyst proteinases and proteinase inhibitors has been suggested as being critical to the implantation process in rabbits (Denker, 1980). Significantly, in spite of extensive and sophisticated research done with this protein, a specific role for uteroglobin in the preimplantation biology of the uterus or blastocyst either by virtue of its proteinase inhibitory activity or steroid binding capacity, remains to be identified.

Analysis of human endometrial washings have not revealed large concentrations of a specific protein such as is observed in the rabbit. Indeed most studies have found that the secretions consist mainly of proteins common to sera (Wolf and Mastroianni, 1975; Roberts et al., 1976; Hirsch et al., 1977). However the transudation of serum proteins appears to be selective, though altering, throughout the cycle (Beier and Beier-Hellwig, 1973). Electrophoretic analysis and more recent radiolabeling studies have noted specific proteins not found in sera. These range from low molecular weight components, possibly glycoprotein in nature, to proteins of 60 to 67,000 Daltons (Wolf and Mastroianni, 1975; Sylvan et al., 1981; MacLaughlin and Richardson, 1983). Furthermore, several of these proteins appear to be specific to the secretory phase of the endometrial cycle. Interestingly, immunochemical studies on human uterine washings have occasionally shown cross-reactivity against rabbit anti-uteroglobin. However the presence of a uteroglobin-like antigen is variable and studies have yet to isolate a protein with the characteristics of uteroglobin (Beier, 1980).

The same ambiguity surrounds other proteins of the uterine lumen. In uterine washings various enzymes have been found whose secretion is elevated above serum concentrations, for example glycosidases and antitrypsin (Casslen and Ohlsson, 1981; Roberts et al., 1976) and the fibrolytic activity of human uterine fluid varies with the endometrial cycle. It has been stated that these enzymes are involved in the implantation process (Casslen and Astedt, 1981).

Maathuis and Aitken (1978) have shown that proteins are not only secreted throughout the proliferative and secretory phases of the cycle but that the total concentrations are lower following ovulation. This is in accord with the findings of lower fluid volume in the 'secretory' phase (Clemetson et al., 1973). Obviously this does not preclude the fact that during this period specific proteins are secreted into the uterine lumen. Associated with the lower volume is an increased potassium ion concentration which is particularily marked around the time of implantation. Other non-protein components have also been shown to undergo changes throughout the cycle. The concentrations of fructose, a preferred metabolite of sperm, appear to increase around the mid-secretory phase while the concentration of glucose changes little in relation to the cycle (Douglas et al., 1970; Maathuis and Aitken, 1978).

Many studies have examined the role uterine secretions may play in early embryo development and implantation. Because they comprise the uterine environment, they probably help regulate the blastocyst while awaiting implantation. It is not known if this regulation is direct, i.e., secretions serve as informational signal proteins to the blastocyst or adhesive proteins which enhance cell-cell communication, indirect, i.e., secretory proteins serve as nutrients or modulators of pH or isotonicity of the uterine environment or passive in that secreted proteins contribute to the maintenance of the endometrial cell types or the pharmacodynamics of the myometrium. The opportunity for such proteins to influence the success of implantation exists even for species with short preimplantation periods where the blastocyst is free in the uterine environment for only 18-24 hours. In comparison, the human blastocyst remains in uterine luminal secretions approximately 72h in preparation for attachment (Hertig and Rock, 1945; Croxatto et al., 1972, 1978).

Steroids and the Developing Embryo

The role of progesterone and estrogen in the regulation of uterine receptivity is secure (Psychoyos, 1973; Glasser and Clark, 1975; Glasser and McCormack 1979a;) although the exact mechanisms of steroid hormone action in this system remain to be defined. A direct obligatory role for steroid hormones in the development of mammalian embryos is questioned by data from in vitro culture experiments. Conclusions drawn from in vivo experiments i.e. blastocyst implanting ectopically at extrauterine sites or under in vitro culture conditions, do not seem to be constrained by hormone dependency, quality and nature of the implantation substrate or time restrictions (Sherman and Salomon, 1975; Sherman and Wudl, 1976). For this reason the characteristic of autoregulation has been assigned to the blastocyst. The possibility that the blastocyst is both directly and indirectly interactive with its environment should not be discounted. Further refinements of in vitro culture conditions, which should include three dimensional matrices, may prove that the developing embryo has a great propensity for self-regulation but is not autoregulatory in the strict sense.

The evidence for a role of estrogen in the in utero behavior of the blastocyst has been obtained from species exhibiting embryonic diapause. This is a delay in the time required for the blastocyst to implant after its entry into the uterus. Implantation can be delayed because of seasonal effects (Sharman, 1963), post-partum lactation (Weichert, 1942) or experimentally by removing the ovary before the release of prenidatory estrogen and maintaining the animals on progesterone alone (Mayer, 1963). In the latter case, the program for implantation and subsequent development is resumed by the injection of a small dose of estrogen (Psychoyos, 1973). Implantation occurs within 24 hours of the estrogen injection.

Whether embryonic diapause is a direct response to hormone withdrawal or is influenced indirectly via an associated decrease or change in endometrial secretory activity remains an open question (Sherman and Wudl, 1976; Aitken, 1977). During the period of diapause, the blastocyst lies free, metabolically inert and unattached within the uterine lumen. Psychoyos (1973) attributes this to the presence, in the altered uterine environment, of a progesterone induced protein that inhibits the final stages of blastocyst/endometrial interaction. In the rat, the injection of a small dose of estrogen interrupts the progesterone sequence and activates the blastocyst. It also affects the secretory activity of the uterus by depressing the secretion of implantation inhibitor (Psychoyos and Casimiri, 1980) and altering the composition of uterine fluids so that the environment is compatible with implantation. Again, whether the reactivation of the blastocyst is a direct expression of steriod action (Sherman and Wudl, 1976) or results indirectly via changes in uterine secretions or both, is not settled.

These studies on the role of estrogen in the activation of diapaused blastocysts have been extended to species which require estrogen as a nidatory stimulus/signal during the normal reproductive cycle (rats, mice). The proposal has been made that while ovarian estrogen may have some role in nidation, it is the preimplantation embryo itself that synthesizes and secretes the estrogen that serves as the finite signal for attachment between the blastocyst and the receptive endometrium. Such a role for estrogen has been proposed for the rat, which requires estrogen, and the rabbit which does not (Dickmann et al., 1976). These data are controversial and have not been confirmed (Heap et al., 1981). However, there is good evidence that the trophectoderm of sheep and pig synthesizes and metabolizes steroid hormones prior to implantation (Heap et al., 1979; Flint et al., 1979). This property may be unique to species with extended (12-16 days) preimplantation periods. A specific role for preimplantation embryonic steroids has not been identified but it is suggested that these hormones subserve some function imposed by the prolonged period of living free in the uterus while continuing to develop.

It is known that human trophectoderm produces chorionic gonadotropin but of interest is the question whether hCG is secreted before (Saxena et al., 1974) or immediately after implantation (Catt et al., 1975). If this hormone is secreted after implantation, it could not function as a tropic hormone in regulating preimplantation events but would be limited to its recognized role in regulating the progesterone secretion by the fully differentiated corpus luteum to maintain pregnancy. Other factors hypothetically implicated in the implantation process include histamine, cyclic nucleotides and a variety of prostaglandins. There is valid evidence that trophoblast of the post-implantation blastocyst synthesizes and secretes both steroid and peptide hormones (Glasser and McCormack, 1979b) but there is reasonable doubt in many species including human, that the preimplantation embryo is endocrinologically competent.

STAGES OF IMPLANTATION

As a consequence of synchronized events the fertilized ovum enters the uterus as a blastocyst at a species specific time. The interval between entry and attachment of the blastocyst to the luminal epithelium is also species specific. The *in utero* stages of implantation which follow entry are hatching, apposition, attachment/adhesion and migration/invasion.

Hatching

Mammalian embryos hatch from their zonae pellucidae before attachment. Although blastocysts, free-living in the uterus, seem able to shed their zonae in the absence of any specific oviductal or uterine regulatory signal, a zona lytic factor, directly or indirectly controlled by ovarian steroids (presumably an estrogen) is believed to be at least partially responsible for hatching *in vivo* (Pinsker et al., 1974).

In rhesus monkeys (Heuser and Streeter, 1941) and humans (Falk-Larsen, 1980), the zona appears to be shed prior to attachment and adhesion. Whether a zona lysin is required for hatching in primates as has been proposed for rats, mice and rabbits (Pinsker et al., 1974; Denker, 1980) is not known. The guinea pig is unique because trophoblast processes penetrate the intact zona to establish contact with the endometrium.

Apposition

The human blastocyst spends approximately three days free in the uterus during which time it hatches from its zona pellucida, positions itself appropriately and attaches. Attachment, 6-7 days after fertilization, is at the embryonic pole of the blastocyst and antimesometrial with respect to the uterus (Hertig et al., 1956). Orientation of the blastocyst and the position of attachment is species specific and it is possible that errors in positioning could contribute to early embryonic death (Wimsatt, 1975). During the apposition phase the trophectoderm cells of the blastocyst appear quiescent but they are undergoing giant cell formation. They become flattened and can cover 8-10 epithelial cells. At this time, the luminal epithelial cells are characterized by large numbers of microvilli. This is presumptive evidence of the secretory activity of these cells (Sherman and Wudl, 1976).

Attachment/Adhesion

Hatched and in position, the blastocyst attaches and adheres to the receptive endometrium. This interaction between two genetically dissimilar cell populations represents a unique immunobiological adaptation. The embryo, sometimes considered a homograft, seems to have solved the problem of histocompatibility.

Attempts to analyze this special cell recognition process are long standing and have not been eminently productive. The analysis of developmental expression of antigens on the surface of the blastocyst has yielded trophectoderm specific monoclonal antibodies but it is not certain how the antigens they represent behave in the recognition process associated with nidation.

The ability to attach seems restricted to blastocysts and limited to a specific hormonally defined period of time. These constraints suggest the transient occurrence of morphological and functional features which are required for blastocyst-endometrial interaction. Morphologically, there are no notable changes in the surface of the trophectoderm but major changes, observable at the ultrastructural level, can be noted in the luminal epithelium. Microvilli disappear to be replaced by small regular projections. The plasma membrane of the luminal epithelium produces a smooth undulating border which flattens against the smooth trophectoderm surface membranes. These changes have been interpreted as representative of an increase in adhesiveness of the uterine surface. There has been essentially no work done on the cell biology or biochemistry of this adhesive phase of implantation.

Attachment and adhesion are aided by a decrease in the volume of the uterine cavity. The closure process obliterates the uterine lumen (Finn and Hinchcliffe, 1965) and brings the apposing epithelial walls into contact (Enders and Hendrickx, 1980; Figure 3). The formation of this "crypt" may involve endocytosis of uterine fluid by endometrial cells (Parr, 1980).

Coincident with the adhesive phase, the late blastocyst exhibits a reorganization of trophectoderm cytoskeleton (Jackson et al., 1980) and surface glycoprotein receptors (Brownell, 1977). These observations affirm the previously noted morphological changes that appear to enhance cell surface adhesiveness. There is evidence that cell surface adhesiveness of the mouse blastocyst increases in a programmatic manner independent of external stimuli (Sherman et al., 1979; Sherman and Matthai, 1980). There is some question (Atienza-Samols et al., 1980) about the validity of experiments that suggested that adhesiveness is the property of cell surface glycoproteins and that the addition of tunicamycin, a drug which specifically interferes with glycosylation of proteins, will predictably interfere with implantation (Surani, 1979). Adhesion related proteins of the trophoectoderm have yet to be identified and characterized but it is known that trophectoderm does not synthesize fibronectin (Zetter et al., 1978) which has been implicated in the attachment and adhesive process of many cells.

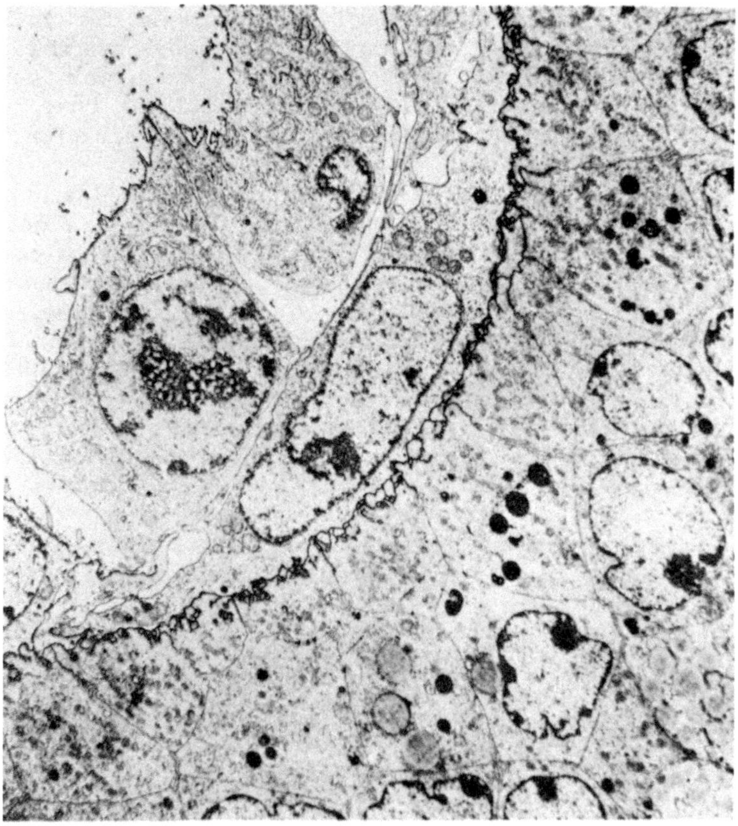

Figure 3

The border defining blastocyst-epithelium interaction in the uterus of a mouse in which blastocyst activation and initiation of implantation were stimulated (24 hr. previously) by an injection of estrogen. The border between the two tissues is observed as a dark irregularly running line. Trophoblast is right. Magnification 4000x (Nilsson, 1982).

At this time there is no reportable evidence of a regulative role of the endometrial epithelium in the adhesive phase of implantation. This also is a neglected area of study.

Migration/Invasion

Attachment of the blastocyst to the epithelium initiates stromal cell transformation to decidual cells. The interrelationship between epithelial and stromal cells as they influence adhesion and subsequent decidualization as well as the role of the decidual cell per se, particularly in the human uterus, remains obscure (Glasser and McCormack, 1980). Current thinking considers decidual cells to be a special cellular matrix that serves, in some manner, to regulate trophoblast invasion. Following attachment, the trophectoderm cells extend processes that serve to dislodge plaques of luminal epithelial cells from the basement lamina. This change from an adhesive cell to a migratory (invasive) cell is accompanied by another reorganization of the cytoskeleton (Sherman and Matthai, 1980) and signals changes in trophoblast cell surface biochemistry and initiates a detailed program of trophoblast differentiation (cessation of cell division, polyploidy, endoreduplication, steroid and peptide hormone production, synthesis and secretion of tissue remodeling enzymes). These are all correlates of interstitial implantation and establishment of the hemochorial placenta (Figure 4).

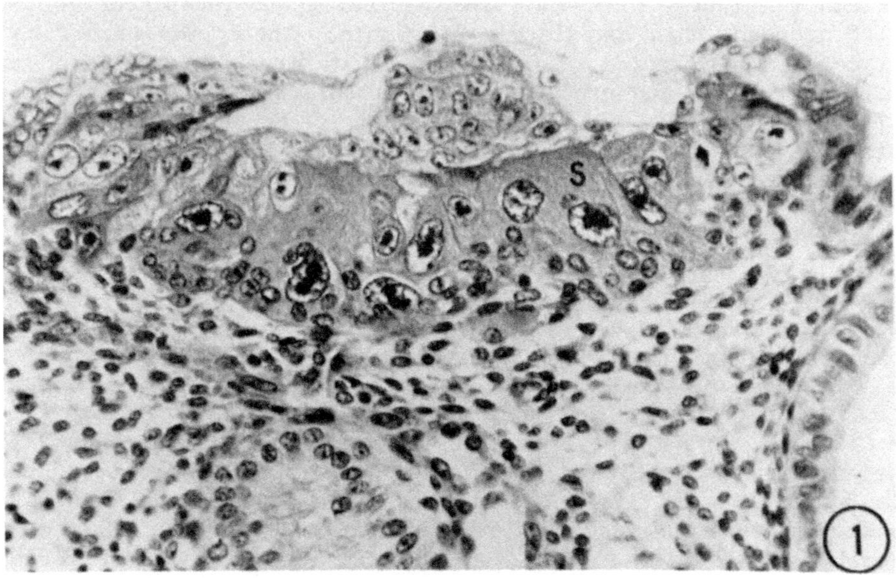

Figure 4

An early human implantation site, illustrating apparent syncytial trophoblast at the invasive front of the blastocyst on the endometrium. Stage 5, No. 8020 in the collection of the Carnegie Institution, Department of Embryology, Davis Division (Enders and Hendrickx, 1980.).

The attachment and invasive phases of implantation have been attributed to the action of trophectoderm proteolytic enzymes (Sherman and Salomon, 1975; Denker, 1980). The course of subsequent invasion of the decidua has been correlated with the programmed developmental secretion of similar types of enzymes as represented by plasminogen activator (Strickland et al., 1976). Not every laboratory confirms these data (Glass et al., 1979; Glasser and McCormack, 1979b). It has been proposed that contact withdrawal might be responsible, in part, for trophoblast penetration. No evidence for lytic penetration or a primary role of plasminogen activator was noted during implantation by mouse blastocysts on three dimensional matrices in cultures (Glass et al., 1983). Additional support derives from the studies of Tickle et al. (1978) which suggest that cells metastasize initially by contact inhibition and secondarily by enzymatic remodeling of space.

DECIDUALIZATION

Decidualization is a unique structural and presumably functional transformation of fibroblast-like cells of the uterine stroma to giant, polygonal, multinucleate, endoreduplicative cells with abundant thin cytoplasmic filaments. These cells are rich in glycogen and lipids. Specific alterations in nucleic acid (Glasser, 1975) and protein synthesis (Glasser, 1972; Glasser and Clark, 1975; Bell, 1979) are believed to be associated with the process. The decidual cell response can be induced in uteri after apporpriate hormonal preparation by blastocysts or, in laboratory animals, by a variety of artificial stimuli (Glasser, 1972). Decidualization is a progesterone dependent process (Glasser and Clark, 1975) and its response to the blastocyst signals that the uterus has matured from a hostile, non-receptive environment to a status receptive to the developing embryo.

The role of decidual tissue remains to be defined. Any number of functions have been ascribed to these cells (Glasser and McCormack, 1980). The idea that decidualization is a conservative mechanism by which invasion of the endometrium by the trophoblast is controlled and limited during establishment of the hemochorial placenta survives as the most tenable hypothesis (Bryce and Teacher, 1908). Whatever its function, decidualization reflects an informed change in the synchronized endometrial substrate which follows upon attachment. This alteration of endometrial cell expression is ordered by a precise program of hormone specific synthesis of informational proteins (Glasser and Clark, 1975). Rudimentary evidence now suggests that the decidual cells possess endocrine functions (Riddick and Daly, 1982a). If true, this would insert the decidual cell into the equation which regulates the endometrial response to the trophoblast. If this endocrine capability extends to the human predecidual cell a further provocative possibility presents itself, e.g., that the preimplantation endometrial stroma could play a role in the intricate modulation of those preparatory processes required for implantation.

The most interesting evidence for an endocrine function of decidual tissue follows the demonstration that human prolactin (hPRL) exists as a separate hormone discrete from growth hormone and that amniotic fluid contains extremely high concentrations of immunoreactive hPRL. Specific functions of PRL in the female are recognized on the mammary gland at post-partum lactation, in the regulation of the reproductive cycle, in the maintenance of pregnancy and in fetal (embryonic) growth and development. PRL in amniotic fluid is purportedly involved in the osmoregulation of the fetus. In seeking the source of PRL, neither primary maternal nor a fetal circulatory origin for amniotic fluid hPRL could be identified. Suppression of maternal pituitary PRL during pregnancy without affecting amniotic fluid concentrations suggested an extrapituitary site of production. After discounting the placenta and fetal membranes it was determined that the decidualized endometrium of pregnancy was the source of amniotic fluid PRL. Subsequently immunoreactive PRL was shown to be an in vitro culture product of decidua from the late luteal phase of the menstrual cycle (day 23 on) through term (Daly et al., 1983a).

More provocative is the report that proliferative human endometrium cultured in the presence of progesterone, with or without estrogen, produced immunoreactive PRL (Daly et al., 1983b). The amount of PRL produced was a function of the extent of "decidual differentation" and was progesterone dependent. Production of PRL by proliferative endometrium after six days in culture with progestrone and in the absence of a blastocyst suggests that PRL synthesis and secretion could be produced, in vivo, by early luteal endometrium which would include the "predecidual" cell. If this were indeed the case, it would infer that maturation of the uterus to a receptive environment might occur earlier in the human than anticipated, providing a possible endocrine basis for the success that early cleavage stage embryos enjoy following ET.

SUMMARY AND CONCLUSIONS

At the end of 1982, the combined efforts of 10 IVF-ET clinics had resulted in the birth of 100 infants (Lopata, 1983). Ten additional clinics had begun operations and it was predicted that the end of 1983 would find 50 successful clinics and over 300 children born to infertile couples as a result of IVF-ET procedures. This increased clinical activity has been accompanied by an enhanced interest in altering existing protocols to improve the success rate of these procedures. However, because the physiology of the preimplantation period is multifactorial, relatively simple modification of IVF-ET protocols which would result in predictable gains is difficult. Nevertheless, gains have resulted over the time period 1980-1982 as evidenced by the experience of Lopata and coworkers where the success rate of ongoing pregnancy has been raised to 38% of embryo recipients when multiple embryos are transferred (Lopata, 1983). Restructuring of IVF-ET protocols has, in the main, been directed towards achieving normal synchronization of follicular and oocyte maturation rather than to synchronization of the embryo with the endometrium.

While new procedures have resulted in increased recovery and fertilization rates and increased numbers of patients undergoing ET, the pregnancy rate has not improved substantially for single embryo transfers. Certainly, a strong correlation between success rates and the number of embryos transferred has been established (see Chapter 12).

To a certain extent, manipulation of oocyte maturation has contributed to improving the quality of transferred embryos. However, the absence of a correlation between the number of eggs recovered and pregnancy rates suggests that until methods become available to define the quality of the increased number of oocytes produced by various changes in protocol, this avenue is limited. The questions posed by this discussion of synchrony between blastocyst and endometrium become more relevant.

The 10-12% success rate achieved with ET of 8-cell embryos suggests that the conditions defining the onset of ovoreceptivity in the human are not as rigid as they appear to be in laboratory animals (Noyes et al., 1963). Perhaps the putative endocrine function of the predecidual cells of the human uterus render that environment less hostile so that the early stage embryos transferred can survive until at least 10-12% become blastocysts, capable of implantation.

Since it does not appear necessary to achieve the full spectrum of obligatory conditions of synchrony, it is probably not necessary in the human to extend _in vitro_ culture for the full period necessary to obtain implantation blastocysts. Yet extending _in vitro_ culture by shorter periods compatible with cost and risk may serve to selectively discriminate between the populations of cleavage stage embryos available for ET so that the establishment and maintenance of pregnancy is predictably enhanced.

REFERENCES

Aitken, R.J., 1977, Changes in the protein content of mouse uterine flushings during normal pregnancy and delayed implantation, and after ovariectomy and oestradiol administration, J. Reprod. Fertil., 50:29.

Armstrong, D.T., 1968, Hormonal control of uterine lumen fluid retention in the rat, Am. J. Physiol., 214:764.

Atger, M., Mornon, J.P., Savouret, J.P., Loosfelt, H., Fridlansky, F. and Milgrom, E., 1980, Uteroglobin: A model for the study of the mechanism of action of steroid hormones, in: "Steroid Induced Uterine Proteins," M. Beato, ed., Elsevier North-Holland, Amsterdam.

Atienza-Samols, S.B., Pine, P.R. and Sherman, M.I., 1980, Effects of tunicamycin upon glycoprotein synthesis and development of early mouse embryos, Dev. Biol., 79:19.

Beier, H.M. and Beier-Hellwig, K., 1973, Specific secretory proteins of the female genital tract, Acta Endcrinol. Suppl., 180:404.

Beier, H.M., 1980, The role of uterine proteins in the establishment of receptivity of the uterus, Prog. Reprod. Biol., 7:158.

Bell, S.C., 1979, Protein synthesis during deciduoma morphogenesis in the rat, Biol. Reprod., 20:811.

Brownell, A.G., 1977, Cell surface carbohydrates of preimplantation embryos as assessed by lectin binding, J. Supramol. Struct., 7:223.

Bryce, T.H. and Teacher, J.H., 1908, Contributions to the study of early development and imbedding of the human ovum, MacLehose Glasgow.

Bullock, D.W., Kao, L.W.L. and Young, C.E., 1981, Mechanisms of induction of uterine protein synthesis: Hormonal regulation of uteroglobin, in: "Cellular and Molecular Aspects of Implantation," S.R. Glasser and D. W. Bullock, eds., Plenum Press, New York.

Buster, J.E., Bustillo, M., Thorneycroft, I.H., Simon, J.A., Boyers, S.P., Marshall, J.R., Louw, J.A., Seed, R.W., and Seed, R.G., 1983, Non-surgical transfer of in vivo fertilized donated ova to five infertile women: Report of two pregnancies, Lancet, 2:223.

Casslen, B. and Ohlsson, K., 1981, Alpha$_1$-antitrypsin-complexation and inactivation in the uterine fluid of IUD-users, Acta. Obstet. Gynecol. Scand., 60:103.

Catt, K.J., Dufau, M.L. and Vaitukaitis, J.L., 1975, Appearance of hCG in pregnancy plasma following the initiation of implantation of the blastocyst, J. Clin. Endocrinol. Metab., 40:537.

Clemetson, C.A.B., Kim, J.D., De Jesus, T.P.S., Mallikarjuneswara, V.R. and Wilds, J.H., 1973, Human uterine fluid potassium and the menstrual cycle, J. Ob. Gyn. Brit. Comm., 80:553.

Croxatto, H.B., Ortiz, M.E., Diaz, S., Hess, R., Balmaceda, J., and Croxatto, H.D., 1978, Studies on the duration of egg transport by the human oviduct. II. Ovum location at various intervals following luteinizing hormone peak, Am. J. Obstet. Gynecol., 132:629.

Daly, D.C., Maslar, I.A. and Riddick, D.H., 1983a, Prolactin production during in vitro decidualization of proliferative endometrium, Am. J. Obs. Gyn., 145:672.

Daly, D.C., Maslar, I.A. and Riddick, D.H., 1983b, Term decidua response to estradiol and progesterone, Am. J. Obstet. Gynecol., 145:679.

Denker, H.W., 1980, Role of proteinases in implantation, Prog. Reprod. Biol., 7:28.

Dickmann, Z., Dey, S.K. and Sen Gupta, J., 1976, A new concept: Control of early pregnancy by steroid hormones originating in the preimplantation embryo, Vitam. Horm., 34:215.

Douglass, C.P., Garrow, J.S. and Pugh, E.W., 1970, Investigations into the sugar content of endometrial secretions, J. Ob. Gyn. Brit. Comm., 77:891.

Edwards, R.G., Steptoe, P.C. and Purdy, J.M., 1980, Establishing full-term human pregnancies using cleaving embryos grown in vitro, Br. J. Obstet. Gyn., 87:737.

Enders, A.C. and Hendrickx, A.G., 1980, Morphological basis of implantation in the rhesus monkey, Prog. Reprod. Biol., 7:270.

Falk-Larson, J., 1980, Human implantation and clinical aspects, Prog. Reprod. Biol., 7:284.

Finn, C.A. and Hinchcliffe, J.R., 1965, Histological and histochemical analysis of implantation chambers in the mouse uterus, J. Reprod. Fert., 9:301.

Finn, C.A. and Martin, L., 1967, Patterns of cell division in the mouse uterus during pregnancy, J. Endocrinol., 39:593.

Fishel, S.B., 1979, Analysis of mouse uterine proteins at pro-oestrus during early pregnancy and after administration of exogenous steroids, J. Reprod. Fert., 55:91.

Flint, A.P.F., Burton, R.D., Gadsby, J.E., Saunders, P.T.K. and Heap, R.B., 1979, Blastocyst oestrogen synthesis and the maternal recognition of pregnancy, in: "Maternal Recognition of Pregnancy," R.B. Heap and J. Whelan, eds., Ciba Foundation Symposium 64 (new series) Excerpta Medica, Amsterdam.

Glass, R.H., Spindle, A. and Pedersen, R.A., 1979, Mouse embryo attachment to substratum and interaction of trophoblast with cultured cells, J. Exp. Zool., 208:327.

Glass, R.H., Aggeler, J., Spindle, A., Pedersen, R.A. and Werb, Z., 1983, Degradation of extracellular matrix by mouse trophoblast outgrowths: A model for implantation, J. Cell Biol., 96:1108.
Glasser, S.R., 1972, The uterine environment in decidualization and implantation, in: "Reproductive Biology," H. Balen and S.R. Glasser, eds., Excerpta Medica, Amsterdam.
Glasser, S.R. and Clark, J.H., 1975, A determinant role for progesterone in the development of uterine sensitivity to decidualization and ovoimplantation, in: "The Developmental Biology of Reproduction," C. Markert and J. Papaconstantinou, eds., Academic Press, New York.
Glasser, S.R., 1975, A molecular bioassay for progesterone and related compounds, in: "Methods in Enzymology," Vol. 36, B. W. O'Malley and J. Hardman, eds., Academic Press, New York.
Glasser, S.R. and McCormack, S.A., 1979a, Estrogen modulated uterine gene transcription and relation to decidualization, Endocrinology, 104:1112.
Glasser, S.R. and McCormack, S.A., 1979b, Functional development of rat trophoblast and decidual cells during establishment of the hemochoreal placenta, Adv. Biosciences, 25:165.
Glasser, S.R. and McCormack, S.A., 1980, Role of stromal cell diversity in altering endometrial cell responses, in: "Blastocyst-Endometrium Relationships," F. Leroy, C.A. Finn, A Psychoyos, P.O. Hubinont, eds., Vol. 7, Karger, Basel.
Glasser, S.R. and McCormack, S.A., 1981, Separated cell types as analytical tools in the study of decidualization and implantation, in: "Cellular and Molecular Aspects of Implantation," S.R. Glasser and D.W. Bullock, eds., Plenum Press, New York.
Heap, R.B., Flint, A.P.F. and Gadsby, J.E., 1979, Role of embryonic signals in the establishment of pregnancy, Br. Med. Bull., 35:129.
Heap, R.B., Flint, A.P.F. and Gadsby, J.E., 1981, Embryonic signals and maternal recognition, in: "Cellular and Molecular Aspects of Implantation," S.R. Glasser and D.W. Bullock, eds., Plenum Press, New York.
Hertig, A.T. and Rock, J., 1945, Two human ova of the pre-villous stage having a developmental age of about seven and nine days respectively, Contrib. Embryol., 31:65.
Hertig, A.T., Rock, J., Adams, E.C. and Mulligan, W.J., 1954, On the preimplantation stages of the human ovum, Contrib. Embryol., 35:199.
Hertig, A.T., Rock, J. and Adams, E.C., 1956, A description of thirty-four human ova within the first seventeen days of development, Am. J. Anat., 98:435.
Heuser, C.H. and Streeter, G.L., 1941, Development of the macaque embryo, Contrib. Embryol., 29:15.

Hirsh, P.J., Fergusson, I.L.C. and King, R.J.B., 1977, Protein composition of human endometrium and its secretion at different states of the menstrual cycle, Ann. N.Y. Acad. Sci., 286:233.

Jackson, B.W., Grund, C., Schmid, E., Burki, K., Franke, W.W. and Illmensee, K., 1980, Formation of cytoskeletal elements during mouse embryogenesis, Differentiation, 17:161.

Leridon, H., 1977, "Human Fertility: The Basic Components," University of Chicago Press, Chicago.

Lopata, A., 1983, Concepts in human in vitro fertilization and embryo transfer, Fertil. Steril., 40:289.

Maathuis, J.B. and Aitken, R.J., 1978, Cyclic variation in concentrations of protein and hexose in human uterine flushings collected by an improved technique, J. Reprod. Fert., 52:289.

MacLaughlin, D.T. and Richardson, G.S., 1983, Analysis of human uterine luminal fluid proteins following radiolabeling by reductive methylation: Comparison of proliferative and secretory phase samples, Biol. Reprod., 29:733

Markaverich, B.M., Upchurch, S., McCormack, S.A., Glasser, S.R. and Clark, J.H., 1981, Differential stimulation of uterine cells by nafoxidine and clomiphene: Relationship between nuclear estrogen receptors and type II estrogen binding sites and cellular growth, Biol. Reprod., 24:171.

Marston, J.H., Penn, R. and Sivelle, P.C., 1977, Successful autotransfer of tubal eggs in the rhesus monkey (Macaca mulatta), J. Reprod. Fert., 49:175.

Martel, D. and Psychoyos, A., 1980, Behavior of uterine steroid receptors at implantation, Prog. Reprod. Biol., 7:216-233.

Martin, L., Das, R.M. and Finn, C.A., 1973, The inhibition by progesterone of uterine cell proliferation in the mouse, J. Endocrinol., 57:549.

Martin, L., Pollard, J.W. and Fagg, B., 1976, Oestriol, Oestradrol-17β and the proliferation and death of uterine cells, J. Endocrinol., 69:103.

Mayer, G., 1963, Delayed nidation in rats: A method of exploring the mechanisms of ovo-implantation, in: "Delayed Implantation," A.C. Enders, ed., University of Chicago Press, Chicago.

McCormack, S.A. and Glasser, S.R., 1980, Differential response of individual uterine cell types from immature rats treated with estradiol, Endocrinology, 106:1634.

Nilsson, O., 1970, Some ultrastructural aspects of ovo-implantation, in: "Ovo-implantation, Human Gondotrophins and Prolactin," P.O. Hubinont, F. Leroy, C. Robyn and Leleux, eds., Karger, Basel.

Nilsson, O., 1972, Ultrastructure of the process of secretion in the rat uterine epithelium at preimplantation, J. Ultrastruct. Res., 40:572.

Noyes, R.W., Dickmann, Z., Doyle, L.L. and Gates, A.H., 1963, Ovum transfers, synchronous and asynchronous, in the study of implantation, in: "Delayed Implantation," A.C. Enders, ed., University of Chicago Press, Chicago.

O'Grady, J.E. and Bell, S.C., 1977, The role of the endometrium in blastocyst implantation, in: "Development in Mammals," M.H. Johnson, ed., Vol. 1, North-Holland, Amsterdam.

Parr, M.B., 1980, Endocytosis in the uterine epithelium during early pregnancy, Prog. Reprod. Biol., 7:81.

Pinsker, M.C., Sacco, A.G. and Mintz, B., 1974, Implantation-associated proteinase in mouse uterine fluids, Dev. Biol., 38:285.

Potts, M., 1966, The ultrastructure of egg implantation, Am. J. Obstet. Gynec., 96:1122.

Pratt, H.P.M., 1977, Uterine proteins and the activation of embryos from mice during delayed implantation, J. Reprod. Fert., 50:1.

Psychoyos, A., 1973, Hormonal control of ovo-implantation, Vitam. Horm., 31:201.

Psychoyos, A. and Casimiri, V., 1980, Uterine blastotoxic factors, in: "Cellular and Molecular Aspects of Implantation," S.R. Glasser and D.W. Bullock, eds., Plenum Press, New York.

Riddick, D.H. and Daly, D.C., 1982, Decidual prolactin production in human gestation, Seminars in Preinatology, 6:229.

Roberts, G.P., Parker, J.M., and Henderson, J.R., 1976, Proteins in human uterine fluid, J. Reprod. Fertil., 48:153-157.

Sartor, P., 1980, Cell proliferation and decidual morphogenesis, Prog. Reprod. Biol., 7:115.

Saxena, B.B., Hasan, S.H., Haour, F. and Schmidt-Golloitzer, M., 1974, Radioreceptor assay of hCG: Detection of early pregnancy, Science, 184:793.

Sharman, G.B., 1963, Delayed implantation in marsupeals, in: "Delayed Implantation," A.C. Enders, ed., University of Chicago Press, Chicago.

Sherman, M.I. and Salomon, D.S., 1975, The relationships between the early mouse embryo and its environment, in: "The Developmental Biology of Reproduction," C.L. Markert and J. Papaconstantinou, eds., Academic Press, New York.

Sherman, M.E. and Wudl, L.R., 1976, The implanting blastocyst, in: "Cell Surface Interactions in Embryo Genesis," G. Poste and G.A. Nicholson, eds., North-Holland, Amsterdam.

Sherman, M.I., Shalgi, R., Rizzino, A., Sellens, M.H., Gay, S., and Gary, R., 1979, Changes in the surface of the mouse blastocyst at implantation, in: "Maternal Recognition of Pregnancy," Ciba Foundation Symposium 64 (new series) Excerpta Medica, Amsterdam.

Sherman, M.I. and Matthai, 1980, Factors involved in implantation-related events in vitro, Prog. Reprod. Biol., 7:43.

Short, R.V., 1979, When conception fails to become a pregnancy, in: "Maternal Recognition of Pregnancy," Ciba Foundation Symposium 64 (new series) Excerpta Medica, Amsterdam.

Strickland, S., Reich, E. and Sherman, M.I., 1976, Plasminogen activator in early embryo genesis: Enzyme production by trophoblast and parietal endoderm, Cell, 9:231.

Surani, M.A.H., 1975, Hormonal regulation of proteins in the uterine secretion of ovarectomized rats and the implications of implantation and embryonic diapause, J. Reprod. Fert., 43:411.

Surani, M.A.H., 1979, Glycoprotein synthesis and inhibition of protein glycosylation by tunicamycin in preimplantation mouse embryos: compaction and trophoblast adhesion, Cell, 18:217.

Sylvan, P.E., MacLaughlin, D.T., Richardson, G.S., Scully, R.E. and Nikrui, N., 1981, Human uterine fluid proteins associated with secretory phase endometrium: Progesterone-induced proteins? Biol. Reprod., 24:423.

Tachi, C., Tachi, S. and Lindner, H.R., 1972, Modification by progestrone of oestradrol-induced cell proliferation, RNA synthesis and estradol synthesis in the rat uterus, J. Reprod. Fertil., 31:59.

Tickle, C., Crawley, A. and Goodman, M., 1978, Mechanism of invasiveness of epithelial tumors, J. Cell Sci., 33:133.

Vessey, M., Doll, R., Peto, R., Johnson, B. and Wiggins, P., 1976, A long term follow up study of women using different methods of contraception-an interim report, J. Biosocs. Sci., 8:373.

Weichert, C.K., 1942, The experimental control of prolonged pregnancy in the lactating rat by means of oestrogen, Anat. Rec. 83:1.

Wimsatt, W.A., 1975, Some comparative aspects of implantation, Biol. Reprod., 12:1.

Wolf, D.P. and Mastroianni, S., 1975, Protein composition of human uterine flüid, Fertil. Steril., 26:240.

Zetter, B.R., Martin, G.R., Birdwell, C.R. and Gospodarowicz, D., 1978, Role of the high molecular weight glycoprotein, Ann. New York Acad. Sci., 312:299.

17

PREGNANCY MANAGEMENT FOLLOWING *IN VITRO* FERTILIZATION AND EMBRYO TRANSFER

Bernard Gonik

ARE PREGNANCIES RESULTING FROM IVF-ET HIGH RISK?

Once pregnancy is established following *in vitro* fertilization and embryo transfer (IVF-ET), the need for continued intensive supervision seems warranted. Although earlier animal studies and recent human experiences suggest that these pregnancies are similar to the spontaneous event, if a failure develops, the opportunities for further attempts at pregnancy are clearly limited. Given the "preciousness" of a pregnancy following *in vitro* fertilization, one should proceed under the assumption that high-risk antenatal care be available if needed with access to appropriate perinatal expertise. In addition, these patients do have certain special considerations given their generally older age (with increase in associated conditions such as hypertension), and newness of the procedure.

PRE - IVF-ET EVALUATION

Prior to initiating attempts at IVF-ET, a basic infertility evaluation is necessary. This investigation should include screening for underlying chronic illness, sources of teratogenic potential, and genetic alterations. Information concerning disease states such as diabetes mellitus, thyroid disease, connective tissue disorders, and hypertension should be ascertained so that proper control of these disorders during the pre-conception period may then be accomplished. Patient counseling with regard to dietary habits, smoking, and alcohol consumption are all related to successful pregnancy outcomes and should be discussed with both patient and husband.

Genetic screening and counseling prior to attempting IVF-ET should be considered for each parenting unit. Since many of these patients may fall into the older reproductive age group, care should be taken to fully inform them of the increased risks of an offspring with a chromosomal abnormality such as Down's syndrome. In addition, certain inheritable disorders can be excluded prior to the onset of pregnancy by pedigree charting and chromosomal karyotyping if indicated. Carrier testing for disease states such as Tay-Sachs and sickle cell anemia can also be accomplished prior to initiating the IVF-ET process.

EARLY DIAGNOSIS AND GESTATIONAL DATING

During uncomplicated early pregnancies, patients most often present to their physician after a missed menstrual period or when signs and symptoms of pregnancy develop. Confirmation of the gestational event is usually made by careful physical examination and urinary human chorionic gonadotropin assay. In the case of the *in vitro* fertilization patient, the time of pregnancy initiation can be precisely documented. In our institution, we begin specific testing for the beta subunit of hCG 10 days following the administration of a post-clomiphene hCG injection. By this time, most of the exogenously-administered hCG should have cleared and therefore, rising levels suggest at least a pre-clinical pregnancy. Commercially available serum pregnancy tests may not become consistently positive before 14 days following embryo transfer (Speroff et al., 1983). Estimating the date of confinement should follow the same parameters as those related to a normal spontaneous pregnancy. Since the timing of the IVF-ET treatment cycles corresponds to those in a spontaneous cycle, the last menstrual period represents a reliable reference point to calculate the weeks of gestation and the patient's date of confinement. More precise dating would appear to have no clinical relevance.

ULTRASOUND EVALUATION

Ultrasonography following the *in vitro* fertilization process has proven extremely valuable. When using this technique to confirm an established pregnancy one should await identification of the fetal pole within the gestational sac. This can be seen starting at 5 - 6 weeks after the last menstrual period (Figure 1). Occasionally, the diagnosis of a viable pregnancy is incorrectly made when only a gestational sac is seen (Figure 2). Serial ultrasound determinations may be necessary early on to accurately document single or multiple intrauterine pregnancies, especially if more than one fertilized ova is transferred (Figure 3). Care must be taken to search for an ectopic pregnancy if hCG determinations are suggestive of implantation and no gestational sac is visualized within the uterine cavity by the sixth week. Fetal cardiac function can first be observed during the eighth week of gestation.

The need for sequential ultrasonographic studies later in pregnancy is controversial. To date, there is no evidence to suggest that once a viable pregnancy is established, it differs from the same spontaneous event. However, given the newness of the IVF-ET process, prudent scrutiny of the pregnancy by this screening technique seems clinically appropriate.

With the use of pharmacologic stimulators for ovulation induction such as Pergonal, one may occasionally observe ultrasonographic evidence of ovarian enlargement with multiple

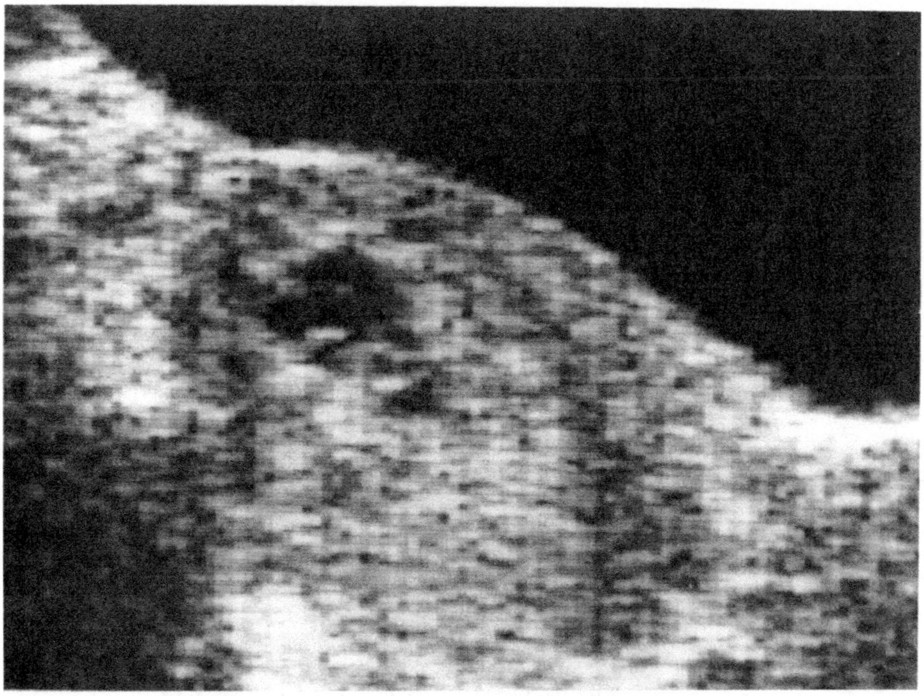

Figure 1

Ultrasonographic evidence of viable intrauterine pregnancy following IVF-ET at 6 - 7 weeks gestation. Fetal pole can easily be seen within the gestational sac. (Ultrasound photographs courtesy of Nabil F. Maklad, M.D., Ph.D., The University of Texas Medical School at Houston.)

cystic compartments (Figure 4). These may be followed expectantly since gradual resolution of the ovarian hyperstimulation event is the rule.

AMNIOCENTESIS - INDICATIONS, RISKS, BENEFITS

Accepted indications for amniocentesis include advanced maternal age, history of neural tube defects, previous delivery of a chromosomally-abnormal child, inheritable chromosomal or metabolic conditions, and certain sex-linked carrier states. Although the risk for a Down's syndrome child is approximately 1:2000 when the mother is in her 20s, by age 35 the risk increases to 1:350. If a previous child had a neural tube defect, the subse-

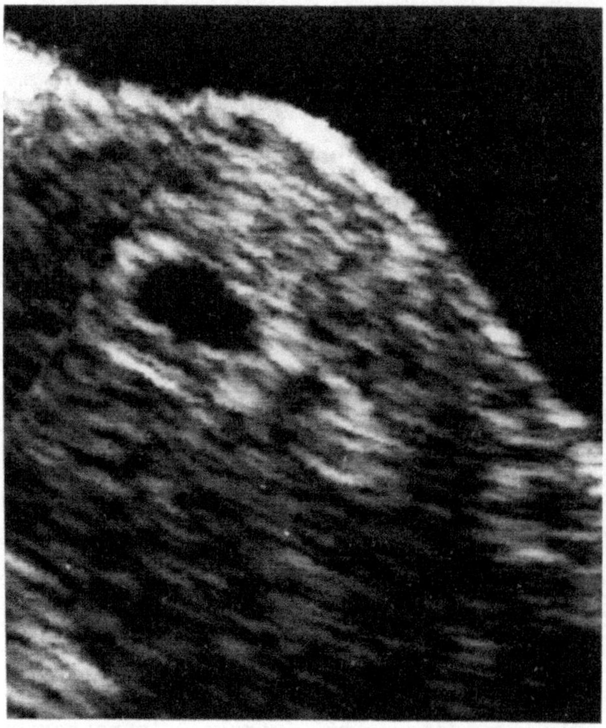

Figure 2

Gestational sac without identifiable fetal pole. This may represent a very early pregnancy (4 weeks' gestation) or a "blighted ovum" at a later gestational age.

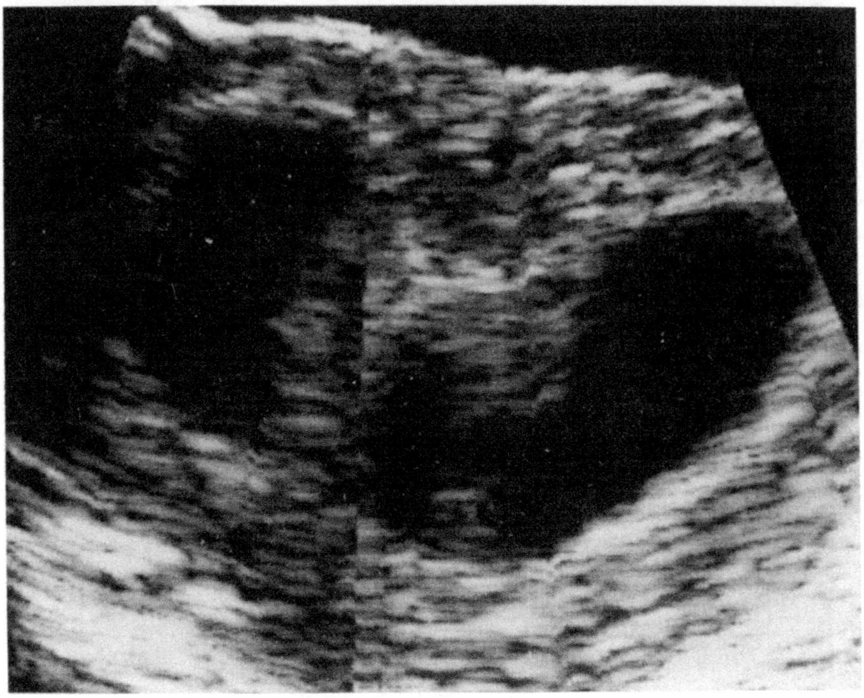

Figure 3

Viable twin gestation at 6 - 7 weeks' gestation following IVF-ET.

quent pregnancy carries an approximate 4% risk for a second abnormal child (Simpson et al., 1982). Carrier states and inheritable chromosomal anomalies require preconceptual testing in addition to antenatal evaluation as mentioned earlier. At the present time, IVF-ET alone is not an established indication for amniocentesis.

The decision to perform an amniocentesis following successful establishment of pregnancy in the IVF-ET patient is particularly difficult. On the one hand, the desire for progeny does not necessarily mean accepting a handicapped child. On the other hand, should diagnostic amniocentesis lead to inadvertent miscarriage of a normal fetus, the loss would be especially burdensome. Two cases of spontaneous abortions have already been reported following complications occurring as a result of amniocentesis in IVF-ET patients (Wood et al., 1982). Clearly, after appropriate informed consent with regard to risks and benefits of the procedure, the decision must be that of the parents.

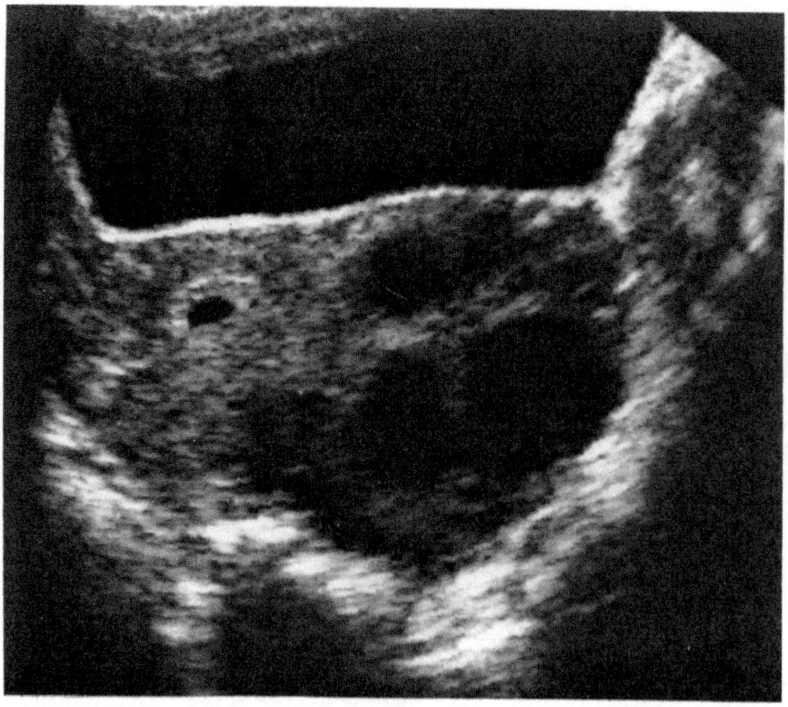

Figure 4

Multiloculated cystic structures within the left ovary following Pergonal and hCG administration. Note the early gestational sac seen in the adjacent uterus.

Whether IVF-ET per se increases the risk of anomalies has not yet been conclusively determined although limited human data suggests that it does not. Schlesselman (1979) points out how difficult it will be to assess the risks of abnormalities specifically related to the IVF-ET process by using extrapolated data from animal experiences and from information obtained regarding chromosomal anomalies in spontaneously aborted pregnancies. Proponents for amniocentesis point out that neither the sperm nor ova used in in vitro fertilization are capable of being tested for normality and, therefore, it is inevitable that a certain proportion of chromosomally abnormal embryos will be transferred to the uterus inadvertently. There is convincing evidence, however, to suggest that abnormal embryos are capable of being efficiently eliminated prior to live birth by spontaneous abortion or fetal death (Schlesselman, 1979).

Certain factors specifically related to the technique of *in vitro* fertilization and embryo transfer may theoretically increase the risk of birth defects. Several investigators have identified a higher rate of chromosomal aberrations occurring with superovulation in experimental animals (Boue and Boue, 1973; Fujimoto et al., 1974). From a technical standpoint, the ova recovered are exposed to higher concentrations of spermatozoa, perhaps making polyspermic fertilization occur more readily (Fraser and Maudlin, 1978). In this regard, fertilized ova with three pronuclei (most resulting from dispermic fertilization) can be easily identified 12 - 18 hours following insemination and should not be transferred (see Chapter 12). Normally, during passage through the female genital tract, there is evidence to suggest that abnormal sperm forms are selectively eliminated (Ahlgren, 1975; Krzanowska, 1974; Overstreet and Katz, 1977). Since this route is bypassed by the *in vitro* fertilization process, some have suggested an increased risk of fertilization with genetically imperfect spermatozoa (Biggers, 1981). Physical and chemical manipulation of the fertilized egg has as yet an undetermined effect. The stabilizing factor here is that the early embryo is relatively resistant to environmental effects.

PRENATAL CARE

Following successful IVF-ET, the patient should be referred to her attending obstetrician after documentation of a viable intrauterine pregnancy. Included in the *in vitro* fertilization team should be a perinatologist who can subsequently take charge of these patients or be available for consultation when the patient returns to her local physician. During the first antenatal visit, a complete physical examination should be performed, including a pelvic examination, to document the size of the uterus, presence of adnexal masses, and classic physical exam findings suggestive of pregnancy. Routine antenatal laboratory testing should be performed; obviously there is no need to reconfirm the diagnosis of pregnancy by a urine pregnancy test. Instructions with regard to nutrition and physical activity should be undertaken during this first antenatal visit. Weight gain during the pregnancy should be individualized for each patient with instructions to maintain a regular and balanced diet. Because of increased erythropoiesis in pregnancy, supplementation with iron and folic acid is indicated. As during the pre-conception counseling period, patients should be instructed on limiting their smoking and alcohol intake throughout the pregnancy.

The degree of physical and sexual activity recommended by the physician during spontaneous and *in vitro* fertilization pregnancies should differ minimally, if at all. Although there is a paucity of information on sexual intercourse following embryo transfer, at this point it is our recommendation that patients maintain pelvic rest until the diagnosis of pregnancy is confirmed. We encourage all of our patients to register for childbirth preparation classes although this seldom needs to be stressed. Follow-up prenatal visits should be dictated by clinical situations arising during the antenatal period and should be similar to those pregnancies which occur spontaneously. Fetal heart tones can be auscultated by Doppler technique at approximately 10 - 12 weeks of gestation. Fetal heart tones can later be documented by fetoscopic examination at 18 - 20 weeks of gestation. If a multiple gestation is identified, closer supervision of the pregnancy is needed. This includes more frequent visits to the office, serial ultrasound examinations to rule out discordance, and bed rest later in the gestation.

If amniocentesis is to be performed, this is best accomplished at 16 weeks following the last menstrual period. Ultrasound examination should always accompany the amniocentesis attempt. If the patient is known to be Rh negative, Rh(D) Immune Globulin should be administered at this time to prevent sensitization. The overall risk of complications resulting from amniocentesis including spontaneous abortion is estimated to be 0.5-1.5% in singleton pregnancies (Simpson et al., 1982).

The mode of delivery for *in vitro* fertilization pregnancies should be dictated by the antenatal and intrapartum courses. There is no evidence suggesting that a Cesarean section needs to be performed in order to obtain a favorable outcome. Standard indications for Cesarean section are well-documented in the various obstetrical textbooks and therefore will not be reviewed here. With trends toward a more "natural" form of intrapartum care, many patients are opting for birthing room experiences. As long as adequate monitoring can be accomplished, this option should be made available to those patients who request it.

THE STATE OF THE ART

In vitro fertilization programs in this country as well as throughout the world have been expanding rapidly. In the United States, the number of operational units currently stands at 44, with many more programs in the planning stages. The result of this is an expanding pool of successful *in vitro* established pregnancies. Current estimates place the number of live-born infants delivered following *in vitro* fertilization to be between 150 and 200. Included in this group are at least three sets of twins and one set of triplets. Cardiac anomalies have been identified in two of these sets of twins conceived in this manner. What must be appreciated is that the above data has been collected on an anecdotal basis only. No centralized organization exists thus far to tabulate this information in an ongoing fashion. For this reason, the National Institute of Child Health and Human Development has begun considering methods of data collection and analysis for pregnancies following in vitro fertilization and embryo transfer.

REFERENCES

Ahlgren, M., 1975, Sperm transport to and survival in the human fallopian tube, Gynecol. Invest., 6:206.

Biggers, J. D., 1981, In vitro fertilization and embryo transfer in human beings, N. Engl. J. Med., 304:336.

Boue, J. G., and Boué, A., 1973, Increased frequency of chromosomal anomalies in abortions after induced ovulation, Lancet, 1:679.

Fujimoto, S., Pahlavan, N., and Dukelow, W. R., 1974, Chromosome abnormalities in rabbit preimplantation blastocysts induced by superovulation, J. Reprod. Fertil., 40:177.

Fraser, L. R., and Maudlin, I., 1978, Relationship between sperm concentration and the incidence of polyspermy in mouse embryos fertilized in vitro, J. Reprod. Fertil., 52:103.

Krzanowska, H., 1974, The passage of abnormal spermatozoa through the uterotubal junction of the mouse, J. Reprod. Fertil, 38:81.

Overstreet, J. W., and Katz, D. F., 1977, Sperm transport and selection in the female genital tract, in: "Development in Mammals," M. H. Johnson, ed., North-Holland, Amsterdam.

Simpson, J. L., Golbus, M. S., Martin, A. O., and Sarto, G. E., 1982, Prenatal genetic diagnosis, in: "Genetics in Obstetrics and Gynecology," Grune & Stratton, New York.

Schlesselman, J. J., 1979, How does one assess the risk of abnormalities from human in vitro fertilization?, Am. J. Obstet. Gynecol., 135:135.

Speroff, L., Glass, R. H., and Kase, N. G., 1983, Clinical assays, in: "Clinical Gynecologic Endocrinology and Infertility," Williams & Wilkins, Baltimore.

Wood, C., Trounson, A., Leeton, J. F., Renou, P. M., Walters, W. A. W., Buttery, B. W., Grimwade, J. C., Spensley, J. C., and Yu, V. Y. H., 1982, Clinical features of eight pregnancies resulting from in vitro fertilization and embryo transfer, Fertil. Steril., 38:22.

18

THE CLINICAL COORDINATOR IN AN *IN VITRO* FERTILIZATION AND EMBRYO TRANSFER PROGRAM

Sylvia Pace-Owens

Treatment of infertile couples by *in vitro* fertilization and embryo transfer is unique in medicine in that it requires close coordination and cooperation from both basic scientists and clinicians, both of whom are actively involved in the patients' treatments. In addition, during an active treatment cycle, information is generated on a daily basis from the ultrasound department and/or radioimmunoassay laboratory concerning ovarian follicular development. All this information must be organized and provided to the clinicians and laboratory scientists in a timely fashion, so they can plan the actual events of oocyte recovery, fertilization and embryo transfer.

The *in vitro* fertilization treatment cycle is a stressful experience for the participating couple. They have often come a considerable distance and are strangers to the treatment facility. They are engaged in a new treatment modality, and usually have only a limited comprehension of the actual details of a treatment cycle. The availability of one individual, who is responsible for the day-to-day coordination of the various events involved in a treatment cycle, and is in constant contact with the patient/couples for their education, instruction, and reassurance substantially alleviates these potentially serious problems.

Although there are no absolute job requirements for this position, the individual who is best suited as a clinical coordinator has clinical nursing experience, preferably as a certified nurse-practitioner, in addition to administrative experience.

The clinical coordinator must become thoroughly familiar with all facets of the *in vitro* fertilization treatment cycle. This allows him/her to appreciate the information essential to each of the team members, and at which stage of the cycle. More importantly, this allows the clinical coordinator to instruct and guide the couple through the treatment protocol. Through each phase of the treatment cycle the coordinator must interpret the findings (for example, ultrasonographic follicular measurements) to the couple and explain their significance.

DUTIES OF THE CLINICAL COORDINATOR DURING A TREATMENT CYCLE

Follicular Recruitment Phase

Couples have previously been instructed to contact the clincal coordinator at the onset of the menstrual period. At that time they are informed as to the details of the drug regimen selected for follicular recruitment. The particular drug regimen may be clomiphene alone, human menopausal gonadotropins (Pergonal) alone, or some fixed combination of the two. If the couple is from out of the immediate area they are given the option of beginning the drug therapy at home. If the couple selects that option, the coordinator must be sure that the couple has access to the necessary drugs and that there is someone available in their local area who is willing to administer any injectable medications and draw blood samples as required. In either situation, the wife is instructed when and where the actual monitoring of follicular development, usually with ultrasonography, will begin.

The clinical coordinator meets with the couple at the time of their first ultrasound examination, usually on cycle day 10. At this time he/she has the opportunity to discuss the success rate of the various aspects of the program including oocyte retrieval, fertilization and cleavage rates and the overall chances of establishing a pregnancy. After this visit an instructional video tape which describes and illustrates each phase of the treatment cycle is shown to the couple*. Following this viewing, the clinical coordinator is available to answer any questions the couple may have regarding details of the treatment program.

A major responsibility of the clinical coordinator is data management. The coordinator is the only individual in daily contact with the couple and each of the various areas which interact to complete the treatment cycle. This program utilizes a

*Videotape entitled "Human *In Vitro* Fertilization: A Documentary" is available through The University of Texas Health Science Center's Media Relations Department, (713) 792-4226.

series of data collection forms (see Figures 5 to 11 in Chapter 19) which are distributed to the various laboratories and departments involved in the program. The clinical coordinator is responsible for seeing that each area receives the forms necessary for each patient's treatment and that the completed information is returned and entered into the computer system.

Ultrasound Monitoring

The clinical coordinator schedules the daily ultrasonographic examinations for each patient. At the time of the first visit he/she provides the ultrasonographer with the patient's relevant medical history, including information on the number and accessibility of ovaries and any known pelvic pathology, such as a hydrosalpinx, that may be confused with an ovarian follicle.

The clinical coordinator also ensures that daily blood samples are obtained, appropriately labeled and transported to the radioimmunoassay laboratories for analysis.

A daily summary of the ultrasonographic follicular measurements is provided to the clinicians. When the follicular diameters reach a predetermined diameter, the clinicians are informed, and a time for follicular aspiration is selected. The patient and her husband are instructed in the administration of human chorionic gonadotropins (hCG) and a time for its administration is set. In general, hCG is administered later that evening at a time 36 hours prior to the scheduled follicular aspiration.

At this point, the clinical coordinator is responsible for scheduling and arranging for the upcoming follicular aspiration. First, he/she draws blood which is used for supplementing the culture media. The whole blood is allowed to clot overnight at 4° and the separated serum is employed in all culture media. The embryo laboratory is informed of the time of the scheduled aspiration. The husband is provided with a sterile specimen container for obtaining a semen sample and is instructed when and where to deliver the sample. In this program, the semen sample is usually obtained one to two hours prior to laparoscopy. We have found that it is less stressful for the husband to obtain the semen sample prior to his wife's laparoscopy. The operating room is notified of the time of the aspiration and the name of the operating surgeon. If the laparoscopic aspiration falls on a week-day the patient's admission to the Day Surgery Unit is scheduled. If the aspiration is on Saturday or Sunday, arrangements are made for the patient to be admitted to the hospital the evening before the laparoscopy. Finally, all of the above arrangements are confirmed with the operating surgeon.

Laparoscopic Follicular Aspiration

The clinical coordinator meets with the patient and her husband in the hospital room or Day Surgery Unit prior to the time of laparoscopy. At that point, the *In Vitro* Fertilization Informed Consent (see Appendix B) is signed in triplicate with one copy given to the patient, one copy placed in hospital records, and one copy retained in the *in vitro* fertilization office. He/she ensures that the semen sample has been submitted, and answers any questions the couple may have.

The husband is encouraged to accompany his wife to the operating room. During the aspiration he may wait adjacent to the operating room where he can watch a closed circuit television system monitoring the microscopic observations in the embryo laboratory.

The clinical coordinator visits the couple prior to discharge and reviews their postoperative routine. In the event of successful oocyte recovery he/she makes arrangements to contact the couple the next two mornings with information as to whether or not fertilization and cleavage have occurred.

Embryo Transfer

On the second morning following laparoscopy, the clinical coordinator is informed by the embryo laboratory whether or not embryo transfer is to take place. If there is to be an embryo transfer, the couple is contacted and told when to report to the hospital. The admissions office is notified and the nursing unit is advised of the patient's arrival and of any premedication (usually 10 mg of diazepam orally one hour prior to transfer). The nursing unit is instructed to transport the patient to the operating room on a stretcher prior to the time of embryo transfer.

The husband is encouraged to be present with his wife at the time of embryo transfer. When the patient is in the operating room, the embryo laboratory is signalled to begin loading the catheter. The clinical coordinator assists the surgeon in positioning the patient for transfer and prepares a sterile field for the transfer equipment.

The clinical coordinator then transports the loaded transfer catheter from the laboratory, hands it to the clinician, and following the transfer, returns it to the embryo laboratory for examination.

When it has been confirmed that the transfer is completed, the coordinator administers the first dose of progesterone (12.5 mg of progesterone-in-oil intramuscularly).

Following transfer he/she confirms the instructions for the patient in the hospital. Prior to the patient's discharge from the hospital, he/she provides the patient with any injectable medication (such as progesterone) and, if necessary, instructs the husband in its administration. The couple is also provided with written instructions concerning the procurement of blood samples and given directions for delivering the blood samples to the laboratory. Finally, arrangements are made for the patient to have a serum pregnancy test performed approximately 18 days following hCG administration.

SEQUENCE OF ACTIVITIES ON AN AVERAGE DAY

1. Review the day's schedule as prepared yesterday. Collect any equipment that will be needed (blood tubes, Pergonal, tissue culture tubes for blood for culture media, etc.)
2. Accept/return calls from patients who have started menses and wish to come in for a treatment cycle.
   a) Explain the planned IVF-ET treatment protocol.
   b) Order clomiphene citrate for the patient (50 mg, days 5 through 9).
   c) Send Pergonal ampules with instructions by mail or plan the patient's appointments for injections.
   d) Arrange the ultrasound appointment for cycle day 10. Give the patient instructions to drink fluid and to have a full bladder prior to the ultrasound appointment.
   e) Refer patient to the financial counselor.
   f) Have the patient review the planned drug regimen, as well as the time, place and instructions for the ultrasound examination to ensure that she understands her schedule.
   g) Prepare patient data collection forms for the IVF-ET team.
3. Go to the Day Surgery Unit to check on patients who are scheduled for follicular aspiration.
   a) Make sure the signed Consent Form is placed in chart.
   b) Check that the sperm specimen has been taken to lab.
   c) Draw blood if required.
   d) Answer any questions that patient/couple might have. Plan to meet couple in the surgery area to show husband where he can sit during the laparoscopy to view the TV monitor attached to the embryo microscope.
4. Return to the office to obtain report of fertilization/cleavage on the previous day's oocytes/embryos; notify the appropriate patient by phone.
   a) Call the patient on the day after laparoscopy to report on fertilization.
   b) Call the patient to report on cleavage prior to embryo transfer (usually two days after laparoscopy). Couples are notified when to be admitted into the hospital for

embryo transfer after cleavage has occurred.

c) Notify Hospital Admissions that the patient is en route. Notify the hospital charge nurse to give diazepam 10 mg p.o. at specified time prior to embryo transfer; inform the operating room of the scheduled transfer time.

d) If no oocytes are fertilized or if cleavage does not occur, couples are so informed and told they can return home and when the next treatment cycle can begin.

5. Meet patients who are scheduled for ultrasound and patients who need Pergonal injections in the ultrasound department. Arrange to meet any post embryo transfer patients who need progesterone injections and any patients who need blood drawn in either the ultrasound department or clinic facilities, as convenient.

6. At a patient's initial ultrasound appointment:
   a) Give the patient's medical history (including number of ovaries, known hydrosalpinges, and limited access to either ovary) to the ultrasonographer.
   b) Give Informed Consent Forms to new patients and answer any questions the patients have.
   c) Obtain a phone number where the patient can be reached during her treatment cycle.
   d) Refer the patients to the IVF-ET program's financial counselor.
   e) Invite the couple to view a 20-minute descriptive videotape of the IVF-ET program.
   f) Review the schedule for the remainder of the treatment cycle with the patient and family.
   g) Re-emphasize to the patient the time and place for the next ultrasound examination.
   h) Interpret the ultrasound results to the patients.
   i) Distribute the daily ultrasound data sheets for any patients who have completed their ultrasound examinations to the IVF-ET team members.

7. Make preparations for scheduled follicular aspirations.
   a) Prepare hCG (2500 or 5000 IU as prescribed) for the patient. Instruct a family member or the patient on how and when to give the injection. (The hCG injection is scheduled for 36 hours prior to follicular aspiration.)
   b) Give preoperative instruction sheet to the patient.
   c) Draw the blood for culture media. (Blood is drawn in special tissue culture tubes and is transported to the embryo laboratory.) Notify the IVF-ET team members of the time and date of surgery.
   d) Give the sperm specimen container to the husband and inform him of the time and place to deliver the specimen.
   e) Request that the patient and her husband abstain from sexual intercourse from this time until the completion of the treatment cycle (positive serum pregnancy test or

onset of menses). Answer any questions the couple might have at this time.

   f) Schedule the follicular aspiration with the operating room and Day Surgery Unit (Monday through Friday surgeries), or schedule for hospital admission the day before surgery (Saturday or Sunday surgeries).

8. See laparoscopy patients postoperatively (after recovery from anesthesia).
   a) Give the patient her follow-up instructions, including how and when she will be informed concerning fertilization and cleavage.
   b) If no oocytes were retrieved, inform the patient when the next treatment cycle is possible and give the phone number to call for further information, questions, or problems.
9. Assist at embryo transfers.
   a) Assist in setting up the room for the embryo transfer.
   b) Show the patient's husband (if he chooses to attend the embryo transfer) where to change into required scrub clothes.
   c) Assist the physician during the embryo transfer procedure by positioning the patient and opening the sterile instruments.
   d) Transport the catheter loaded with the embryos from the laboratory to the physician.
   e) Following the transfer, return the catheter to the laboratory for examination.
   f) Give the patient progesterone 12.5 mg intramuscularly after the transfer catheter has been returned to embryo laboratory and found to be clear.
   g) Give post embryo transfer instructions to the patient and her husband regarding her activities. Give written instructions to the patient including the procedure for progesterone administration by the husband and scheduling and shipping of any follow-up blood samples.
   h) Make arrangement for the patient to have a serum pregnancy test two weeks after the embryo transfer. Request that she call with the results of the test, or at the onset of her next menses.
10. Maintain records for the treatment cycle.
   a) Enter all up-to-date patient data including ultrasound results, laparoscopy findings and fertilization/cleavage information into the computer at the end of day (See chapter 19).
   b) Originate new computer records for patients scheduled to begin a new treatment cycle.
   c) Generate computer status report and post the daily report on the bulletin board (See chapter 19, figure 4).
11. Plan a tentative schedule for the following day.

SUMMARY AND CONCLUSIONS

Successful coordination of a human IVF-ET program requires comprehensive professional knowledge and personal insight to administer an appropriate action plan. The coordinator must insure the smooth, orchestrated functioning of the entire *in vitro* fertilization team, while ensuring that all of the patients' concerns are allayed, that they have been provided all the necessary information, and that all questions are answered.

19

DATA MANAGEMENT IN AN IN VITRO FERTILIZATION AND EMBRYO TRANSFER PROGRAM

Martin M. Quigley

Appropriate collection, storage, correlation, and retrieval of data is critical to the functioning of an *in vitro* fertilization program, whether the program is primarily intended for research or for clinical treatment. There are several inherent reasons why data management is so important to an *in vitro* fertilization program. First, IVF-ET is a unique area in medicine in that it involves close correlation and cooperation between laboratory scientists and clinicians, both of whom are intimately involved in the patients' treatment program. Second, there is a large amount of data generated from each treatment cycle which must be organized in comprehensive patient treatment records. Making this task much more difficult is the fact that the data originates from multiple sources. For example, ultrasonographic follicular measurements are made in the radiology department; serum hormone values come from the radioimmunoassay laboratories; there is clinical input regarding the ovulation induction regimen as well as the observations at laparoscopy; and the embryo laboratory submits data regarding the specific culture media, sperm parameters and preparation as well as oocyte observations and performance. Third, the overall success rate in IVF-ET is still quite low, and it is not possible to predict which factor or factors will be crucial in achieving improvements in this rate. Accordingly, it is desirable that as much data be accumulated and processed as is possible on each treatment cycle to be able to evaluate retrospectively which factors correlate with success or failure.

This chapter is written from the prospective of a physician with no previous training or practical experience in computers, programming, or data processing and management. The large amount of data generated from each treatment cycle and our inability to fully analyze this data led to an odyssey through the microcomputer world leading to a practical system of data management. This system can be adopted and adapted by any group, and does not require programming experience or knowledge, or the addition of a computer specialist to the team. This chapter is by no means intended to be a comprehensive text on computer hardware or software, but will serve to point out the areas of consideration in any IVF-ET data management system, and will describe our solution to these problems.

THE HOW AND WHY OF DATA COLLECTION

Treatment of human infertility by IVF-ET is still in its very early developmental stages and there are substantial differences among the treatment protocols utilized by established groups. With additional groups offering this service, there will be an exponential rise in the individual variations of the "standard" IVF-ET treatment protocol. It will be a disservice to science, and to all of our patients, if all groups involved in IVF-ET do not collect and preserve the data generated during every treatment cycle to share their experience with others in order to examine and compare successess and failures.

Standard medical records techniques represent the minimum system of data management possible and may suffice until records can be computerized. There are several obvious disadvantages to this type of pen, paper, and file folder system. First, the amount of data which can practically be compared and analyzed between patients or between groups of patients is very limited. Second, when the number of treatment cycles completed goes from dozens to hundreds, any type of data analysis becomes impractical. Third, with this system it is difficult to ensure that complete data from each treatment cycle are actually reaching the designated central file. Last, there will be a large expenditure of both time and money when these data are retrospectively computerized.

However, a well conceived and well designed pen, paper, and file folder system should lie at the heart of any computerized system. First, electronic media (i.e., computer disks or tapes) are inherently more fragile and destructible than standard files, and written records should always be maintained as a back-up to the computerized information. In addition, these files can contain more extensive subjective description (say, of the embryos' appearance at transfer) than can be placed in a standard computer field. Second, in most situations it is impractical or impossible to have all the data generating locations, (i.e., the ultrasound department, the radioimmunoassay laboratory, sperm preparation facility, the operating room, and the embryo laboratory) physically "on-line" to a computer system. It it usually more practical to have these locations prepare written reports which are subsequently entered into the computer system at a centralized location on a current basis.

For all practical purposes, the special requirements of an in vitro fertilization program require at least the use of a microcomputer system. With the wisdom of hindsight, it is best that the system be operational before data is actually generated, as it becomes more and more difficult to catch up as time goes on.

DEFINITIONS

For the purposes of this chapter, a microcomputer is a totally self-contained computer (i.e., it is not a terminal connected to a mainframe computer) that is able to handle only one user at a time. The computer contains two types of internal memory, RAM (random access memory) which is transient memory that is used during data processing and any data contained therein is lost when the computer is turned off; and ROM (read only memory) which generally contains only the information needed for internal functioning of the computer system. These computers require an external form of permanent data storage, usually by means of floppy disks (which resemble small flexible phonograph records). Typical examples of this type of computer are the Apple, Radio Shack, and the IBM PC.

A file is defined as the total data stored on a particular subject. (A good analogy would be a file cabinet drawer labeled "In Vitro Fertilization Treatment Cycle Data".) A record is a subdivision of a file and includes all the data with a single unifying feature. The most practical application is to consider all the data generated from a single treatment cycle on one patient to be a record. (A record is analagous to a manilla folder labeled "Mrs. Jones, Treatment #2", filled with data and placed in our file drawer.) A field is a single item of data in the record. An example of a field would be the total number of oocytes recovered at laparoscopy.

REQUIREMENTS OF A COMPUTER SYSTEM

The principle requirement of the in vitro fertilization data storage system, which is not fulfilled by most commercially available data management systems, is the ability to store the large amount of data generated from a single treatment cycle. In other words, there will be a large number of fields in each record. Our current data management system can save over 400 different pieces of information (fields) from every treatment cycle.

There is much more to a data management system than merely collecting and recalling data. The system must have the ability to selectively recall portions of the data from each record, or to examine the relationship between apparently unrelated fields. As an example, you might want to compare the proportion of patients who underwent embryo transfer when there were two follicles aspirated as opposed to three follicles aspirated.

The system chosen must be able to store at least 100, and preferably 200 or more, fields per treatment cycle. It should have the ability to selectively recall data by sorting or selecting with any single or combination of fields. The system should have enough storage capacity so that the entire data file, or at least a year's experience at a time, is "on line" and immediately accessible for processing. As _in vitro_ fertilization is still so new and the treatment protocols are subject to continuing change, the system must have the capacity to alter the file format to accept new and additional data without destroying or losing all the data previously stored. Also very important is the fact that most, if not all, members of the _in vitro_ fertilization team should be able, and in fact expected, to enter and recall data from the system as needed. Accordingly, the system must be sufficiently "user friendly" so that data entry and simple recall can be performed without any knowledge of programming.

DESCRIPTION OF OUR DATA BASE SYSTEM

The following description is not meant to endorse any particular product, and is certainly not meant to imply that there are not other data base systems which can perform the described functions. It is merely intended as an example of a system that fulfills to a greater or lesser degree all of the above requirements.

The heart of our system is a Apple II Plus computer with a video monitor or display screen (CRT). We have modified the standard Apple computer by adding several commercially available plug-in circuit boards. These include one which provides an additional 16K of RAM (Microsoft RAM card), one which allows 80 columns of data to be displayed across the screen instead of 40 (Videx Videoterm), and one which includes a Z80 processor

(Microsoft Soft Card). The Z80 processor allows the use of a computer operating system called CP/M* which is necessary for the operation of most commercially available data base management software which can fulfill the above requirments. In addition, the computer has an attached printer and three disk drives (for permanent storage of the data, to provide additional working space for data processing, and to hold the programs necessary for the data management) (Figure 1).

The computer software (software is the name given to the programs supplied on disks which allow the computer hardware to perform the intended function) is the most important part of the data management system. We have found that there is no commercial software which completely fulfills all of the requirements outlined above. However, the following software has been found to closely fulfill the requirments of our system. We are using a family of software products from MicroPro in San Rafael, California. The key program in the system is their data base management program called DataStar which can accomodate up to 245 fields per record and a file size limited only by the storage capability of the disk drive. This system allows storage of between 225 and 250 typical treatment records on a single 5-1/4 inch floppy disk.

Figures 2 and 3 are the data forms we are currently using for each IVF-ET treatment cycle **. These forms are custom designed using DataStar and can be modified by the user at will.

The second part of the system is a program called SuperSort. This program allows recall of all or part of any record or records in the file by any selected combination of criteria. Records can be selected or excluded based on exmamination of the information in up to 32 fields at a time. For example, SuperSort can select all patient records in which 50 mg of clomiphene were administered, more than three and less than six eggs were recovered, inseminating sperm concentrations were 50,000 per oocyte and a clinical pregnancy resulted. In addition, SuperSort can recall either the entire record or up to 32 individual fields from each record selected.

* The combination of the RamCard, Videx Videoterm, Softcard and CP/M operating system are marketed by Microsoft as the Softcard Premium System.

** We will be happy to provide anyone who wishes to duplicate our data collection system with a copy of these forms on an Apple disk. Obviously, you would then need to have at least the DataStar program and the necessary hardware.

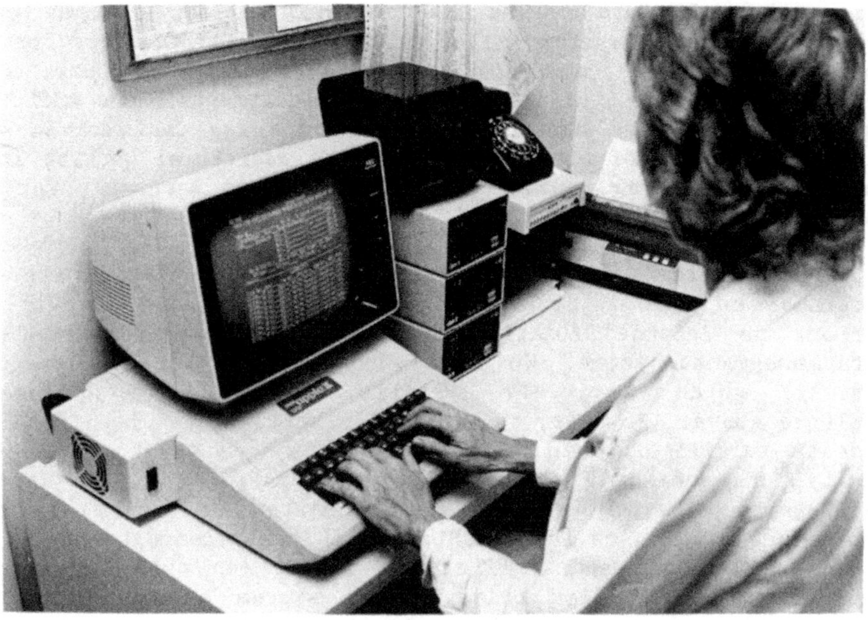

Figure 1

Data base management system in operation.

We have recently incorporated a newly released program called ReportStar (also marketed in a combination of DataStar and ReportStar sold under the name InfoStar). ReportStar has proven useful in three ways. First, Figure 4 is an example of a daily status report on patients in all phases of a treatment cycle. This information is automatically generated each day from sorting the data file in response to a two-word command. Second, ReportStar is a quick, user-friendly system that is capable of generating print-outs (lists) containing any selected fields from all the records in the file. And, third, ReportStar has allowed us to restructure and redesign our data forms (Figures 2 and 3) and then transform all the data stored in the old format into the new format.

The advantage of these selected software programs is the fact that they are already commercially available, and can immediately be used without modification. They also make very efficient use of disk storage space by not requiring space for "empty" fields.

```
***IN VITRO FERTILIZATION-EMBRYO TRANSFER PATIENT TREATMENT RECORD-PART 1***

Name: _______________________ Pat. #: ___ Rx Cycle #: _ Etiology Infert.___
ClomipheneDose:___Days:____PergonalDose(Amp/day):_______________TotAmps:__
LMP:______ Ultrasound:  Day:__ R:______________ L: ______________ Lgst:__mm
                        Day:__ R:______________ L: ______________ Lgst:__mm
                        Day:__ R:______________ L: ______________ Lgst:__mm
                        Day:__ R:______________ L: ______________ Lgst:__mm
                        Day:__ R:______________ L: ______________ Lgst:__mm
   Day 20/16X2 Fol.:__ #Fol. 10-14mm:_ #Fol. 15-19mm:_ #Fol. 20mm+:_
    HCG Dose: _____ HCG Date: ______ HCG Cycle Day: __ Time: ____
Comments:______________________________________________________________
                           <<LAPAROSCOPY>>
Cycle Day:__Date:______Time Asp:____#Fol.Asp.:__ #Eggs Rec:__ #Mat:_ #Imm:_
L1 Dia:__ FF Vol:____Egg(y/n)_ Mat/Imm_ Found(A)spir(N)eedleRinse(F)lush#__
L2 Dia:__ FF Vol:____Egg(y/n)_ Mat/Imm_ Found(A)spir(N)eedleRinse(F)lush#__
L3 Dia:__ FF Vol:____Egg(y/n)_ Mat/Imm_ Found(A)spir(N)eedleRinse(F)lush#__
L4 Dia:__ FF Vol:____Egg(y/n)_ Mat/Imm_ Found(A)spir(N)eedleRinse(F)lush#__
L5 Dia:__ FF Vol:____Egg(y/n)_ Mat/Imm_ Found(A)spir(N)eedleRinse(F)lush#__
L6 Dia:__ FF Vol:____Egg(y/n)_ Mat/Imm_ Found(A)spir(N)eedleRinse(F)lush#__
L7 Dia:__ FF Vol:____Egg(y/n)_ Mat/Imm_ Found(A)spir(N)eedleRinse(F)lush#__
R1 Dia:__ FF Vol:____Egg(y/n)_ Mat/Imm_ Found(A)spir(N)eedleRinse(F)lush#__
R2 Dia:__ FF Vol:____Egg(y/n)_ Mat/Imm_ Found(A)spir(N)eedleRinse(F)lush#__
R3 Dia:__ FF Vol:____Egg(y/n)_ Mat/Imm_ Found(A)spir(N)eedleRinse(F)lush#__
R4 Dia:__ FF Vol:____Egg(y/n)_ Mat/Imm_ Found(A)spir(N)eedleRinse(F)lush#__
R5 Dia:__ FF Vol:____Egg(y/n)_ Mat/Imm_ Found(A)spir(N)eedleRinse(F)lush#__
R6 Dia:__ FF Vol:____Egg(y/n)_ Mat/Imm_ Found(A)spir(N)eedleRinse(F)lush#__
R7 Dia:__ FF Vol:____Egg(y/n)_ Mat/Imm_ Found(A)spir(N)eedleRinse(F)lush#__
Comments:______________________________________________________________

     Medium(Specify/Water/Gas Phase): ________________________________
     Semen #1 (Pre-wash): Vol: ___ml Conc: ____ mil  Motilty: __% Prog:____
     Vol.Washed: ___ ml  Post-Conc: ____ mil Post-Motil: __% Post-Prog:____
     Semen #2 (Pre-wash): Vol: ___ml Conc: ____ mil  Motilty: __% Prog:____
     Vol.Washed: ___ ml  Post-Conc: ____ mil Post-Motil: __% Post-Prog:____

            (INSERT "D" IN "FERT" COLUMN FOR DISPERMIC FERTILIZATION)
Egg#01:Fol____Mat/Imm_EggIncbHrs____Sp#_______SpIncbHrs____Fert_Clev_Trans_
Egg#02:Fol____Mat/Imm_EggIncbHrs____Sp#_______SpIncbHrs____Fert_Clev_Trans_
Egg#03:Fol____Mat/Imm_EggIncbHrs____Sp#_______SpIncbHrs____Fert_Clev_Trans_
Egg#04:Fol____Mat/Imm_EggIncbHrs____Sp#_______SpIncbHrs____Fert_Clev_Trans_
Egg#05:Fol____Mat/Imm_EggIncbHrs____Sp#_______SpIncbHrs____Fert_Clev_Trans_
Egg#06:Fol____Mat/Imm_EggIncbHrs____Sp#_______SpIncbHrs____Fert_Clev_Trans_
Egg#07:Fol____Mat/Imm_EggIncbHrs____Sp#_______SpIncbHrs____Fert_Clev_Trans_
Egg#08:Fol____Mat/Imm_EggIncbHrs____Sp#_______SpIncbHrs____Fert_Clev_Trans_
Egg#09:Fol____Mat/Imm_EggIncbHrs____Sp#_______SpIncbHrs____Fert_Clev_Trans_
Egg#10:Fol____Mat/Imm_EggIncbHrs____Sp#_______SpIncbHrs____Fert_Clev_Trans_

Egg #01:Hr/Obs1:______________________Hr/TranObs/Gr:___________________
Egg #02:Hr/Obs1:______________________Hr/TranObs/Gr:___________________
Egg #03:Hr/Obs1:______________________Hr/TranObs/Gr:___________________
Egg #04:Hr/Obs1:______________________Hr/TranObs/Gr:___________________
Egg #05:Hr/Obs1:______________________Hr/TranObs/Gr:___________________
Egg #06:Hr/Obs1:______________________Hr/TranObs/Gr:___________________
Egg #07:Hr/Obs1:______________________Hr/TranObs/Gr:___________________
Egg #08:Hr/Obs1:______________________Hr/TranObs/Gr:___________________
Egg #09:Hr/Obs1:______________________Hr/TranObs/Gr:___________________
Egg #10:Hr/Obs1:______________________Hr/TranObs/Gr:___________________

Trans hrs.:____ Cath Used:____________________ #Attempts/Bleed/Cramp:_____
No.EmbryosTrans:_ Progesterone(Dose/Days):_______________Next Menses:______
Outcome:_ Lap Dr.:_________ Trans Dr.:_________ Group:____________________
Comments:_______________________________________________________________
         _______________________________________________________________
```

Figure 2

Blank treatment record, part I - clinical observations.

```
***IN VITRO FERTILIZATION-EMBRYO TRANSFER PATIENT TREATMENT RECORD-PART 2***
                          <<HORMONE DATA>>

Name: _______________________________ Pat. #: ___  Rx Cycle #: _ LMP:______
Clomiphene Dose:___ Days:____Pergonal(Amps/Days):_______________Tot.Amps:__
HCG Date:______HCG Cycle day:__ HCG Dose:_____LapDate:______ LapCycleDay:__
Day for 20mm/16mmX2 Follicles:__  #Fol.10-14mm:_ #Fol.15-19mm:_ #Fol.20+mm_
# Fol.Asp:__ # Eggs Rec:__# Mat Eggs:_ # Imm Eggs:_ # Emb Trans:_ Outcome:_
Comments:__________________________________________________________________

                       <<PRE-HCG HORMONES>>
                       (LMP is Cycle Day 1)
Cycle Day:__Time:____LH:____mIU/ml FSH:___mIU/ml E2:______Pg/ml P:____Ng/ml
Cycle Day:__Time:____LH:____mIU/ml FSH:___mIU/ml E2:______Pg/ml P:____Ng/ml
Cycle Day:__Time:____LH:____mIU/ml FSH:___mIU/ml E2:______Pg/ml P:____Ng/ml
Cycle Day:__Time:____LH:____mIU/ml FSH:___mIU/ml E2:______Pg/ml P:____Ng/ml
Cycle Day:__Time:____LH:____mIU/ml FSH:___mIU/ml E2:______Pg/ml P:____Ng/ml
Cycle Day:__Time:____LH:____mIU/ml FSH:___mIU/ml E2:______Pg/ml P:____Ng/ml
Cycle Day:__Time:____LH:____mIU/ml FSH:___mIU/ml E2:______Pg/ml P:____Ng/ml
Cycle Day:__Time:____LH:____mIU/ml FSH:___mIU/ml E2:______Pg/ml P:____Ng/ml
Cycle Day:__Time:____LH:____mIU/ml FSH:___mIU/ml E2:______Pg/ml P:____Ng/ml
Cycle Day:__Time:____LH:____mIU/ml FSH:___mIU/ml E2:______Pg/ml P:____Ng/ml
Cycle Day:__Time:____LH:____mIU/ml FSH:___mIU/ml E2:______Pg/ml P:____Ng/ml
Cycle Day:__Time:____LH:____mIU/ml FSH:___mIU/ml E2:______Pg/ml P:____Ng/ml
Cycle Day:__Time:____LH:____mIU/ml FSH:___mIU/ml E2:______Pg/ml P:____Ng/ml
Cycle Day:__Time:____LH:____mIU/ml FSH:___mIU/ml E2:______Pg/ml P:____Ng/ml

                       <<POST-HCG HORMONES>>
                       (Day of HCG is Day 0)
Cycle Day:+__ Time:____   E2: ______Pg/ml   P: ____Ng/ml   B-HCG _____mIU/ml
Cycle Day:+__ Time:____   E2: ______Pg/ml   P: ____Ng/ml   B-HCG _____mIU/ml
Cycle Day:+__ Time:____   E2: ______Pg/ml   P: ____Ng/ml   B-HCG _____mIU/ml
Cycle Day:+__ Time:____   E2: ______Pg/ml   P: ____Ng/ml   B-HCG _____mIU/ml
Cycle Day:+__ Time:____   E2: ______Pg/ml   P: ____Ng/ml   B-HCG _____mIU/ml
Cycle Day:+__ Time:____   E2: ______Pg/ml   P: ____Ng/ml   B-HCG _____mIU/ml
Cycle Day:+__ Time:____   E2: ______Pg/ml   P: ____Ng/ml   B-HCG _____mIU/ml
Cycle Day:+__ Time:____   E2: ______Pg/ml   P: ____Ng/ml   B-HCG _____mIU/ml
Cycle Day:+__ Time:____   E2: ______Pg/ml   P: ____Ng/ml   B-HCG _____mIU/ml
Cycle Day:+__ Time:____   E2: ______Pg/ml   P: ____Ng/ml   B-HCG _____mIU/ml

                    <<FOLLICULAR FLUID STEROIDS>>
Follicle:__ E2:________ P:________ T:________ A:________ Other:____________
Follicle:__ E2:________ P:________ T:________ A:________ Other:____________
Follicle:__ E2:________ P:________ T:________ A:________ Other:____________
Follicle:__ E2:________ P:________ T:________ A:________ Other:____________
Follicle:__ E2:________ P:________ T:________ A:________ Other:____________
Follicle:__ E2:________ P:________ T:________ A:________ Other:____________
Comments:__________________________________________________________________
         __________________________________________________________________
         __________________________________________________________________
```

Figure 3

Blank treatment record, part II - hormone values.

IVF TREATMENT CYCLE DAILY REPORT
8/ 5/83

PATIENTS SCHEDULED FOR TREATMENT

PATIENT NAME	PAT.NO	RX	LMP	CLOM	PERGONAL
TEST PATIENT 1	999	1	840000	30	10/1-2-3
TEST PATIENT 6	999	6	840000	30	10/1-2-3

Number of Patients Scheduled for Treatment: 2

PATIENTS UNDERGOING FOLLICULAR MONITORING

TEST PATIENT 2 Pat.No:999 Rx.No:2 LMP:840000 Clom:30 Perg:10/1-2-3
Cycle Day: 10 Largest Follicle: 13

TEST PATIENT 7 Pat:No:999 Rx.No:7 LMP:840000 Clom:30 Perg:10/1-2-3
Cycle Day: 10 Largest Follicle: 16
Cycle Day: 11 Largest Follicle: 17
Cycle Day: 12 Largest Follicle: 19

Number of Patients Undergoing Ultrasound Monitoring: 2

PATIENTS SCHEDULED FOR LAPAROSCOPY

TEST PATIENT 3 Pat.No:999 RxNo:3 LMP:840000 Clom:30 Perg:10/1-2-3
HCG:Date:840012 Day:12 Time:2200 #FOL 10-14:2 #FOL 15-19:1 #FOL>=20mm:1
Right Follicles: 13 Left Follicles: 14 17 20
Laparoscopy Date: 840014 Laparoscopy Cycle Day: 14 Laparoscopy Time: 1000

TEST PATIENT 8 Pat.No:999 RxNo:8 LMP:840000 Clom:30 Perg:10/1-2-3
HCG:Date:840013 Day:13 Time:2100 #FOL 10-14:0 #FOL 15-19:2 #FOL>=20mm:1
Right Follicles:18 19 21 Left Follicles:
Laparoscopy Date: 840015 Laparoscopy Cycle Day: 15 Laparoscopy Time: 900

Number of Patients Scheduled for Laparoscopy: 2

PATIENTS POST-LAPAROSCOPY

TEST PATIENT 4 Pat.No:999 RxNo:4 LMP:840000 Clom:30 Perg:10/1-2-3
Lap date:840015 #Fol Asp: 09 #Egg Rec: 03 #Mat Eggs: 2 #Imm Eggs: 1

TEST PATIENT 9 Pat.No:999 RxNo:9 LMP:840000 Clom:30 Perg:10/1-2-3
Lap date:840015 #Fol Asp: 8 #Egg Rec: 5 #Mat Eggs: 3 #Imm Eggs: 2

Number of Patients Post Laparoscopy/Awaiting Transfer: 2

PATIENTS POST-TRANSFER/AWAITING PREGNANCY TEST

TEST PATIENT 5 Pat.No:999 RxNo:5 LMP:840000 Clom:30 Perg:10/1-2-3
Lap Date:840015 Transfer Date:840017 #Embryos Trans:1 Preg Test Sched:8/25/83

TEST PATIENT 10 Pat.No:999 RxNo:0 LMP:840000 Clom:30 Perg:10/1-2-3
Lap Date:840014 Transfer Date:840016 #Embryos Trans:1 Preg Test Sched:9/1/83

Number of Patients Post-Transfer/Awaiting Pregnancy Test: 2

Figure 4

Example of daily treatment cycle status report.

NAME ____________________

PATIENT # ________ TREATMENT # ____________________

ETIOLOGY OF INFERTILITY ____________

(enter up to three, e.g. 1 2 4)

1)	tubal	5)	cervical
2)	oligospermia	6)	immunologic
3)	unexplained	7)	other, female (specify in "comments")
4)	endometriosis	8)	other, male (specify in "comments")

Clomiphene (dose per day) ________ (cycle days) ________

Pergonal (amps per day) ________ (cycle days) ________

LMP ____________

(Enter #8 (treatment in progress) into Outcome Field and enter group number into Group Field)

Comments: ____________________

Figure 5

Clinical information data collection form.

They are available for a large variety of micro- and mini-computer systems and do not require a programmer or programming knowledge for implementation, maintenance, or modification.

Examples of the forms we use for the initial data collection and from which the data is entered into the computer are shown in Figures 5 through 14. Figure 5 contains the clinical information, including the patient identifiers, details of the planned ovulation induction regimen, the couple's infertility diagnoses as well as the date of the menstrual period initiating this cycle. When this information is received a new record is created in the computer file. The top half of Figure 6 is completed on each day that an ultrasound examination is performed. The bottom section of this form is completed when the decision has been made to administer hCG for final oocyte maturation. Figure 7 lists the observations made at laparoscopy. Figure 8 is prepared by the

NAME ______________________________

PATIENT # __________ TREATMENT # __________ LMP __________

CYCLE DAY __________ DATE __________

Right __________ Left __________ Largest __________ mm

(e.g. Right 12, 10 Left 16, 13 Largest 16 mm

Comments: ______________________________

____

____

(If more than five ultrasound examinations, enter only the last five.)

COMPLETE ON DAY PATIENT IS READY FOR hCG:

Total ampules of Pergonal given __________
Cycle day for 20 mm (clomiphene) or 16 mm X 2 (Pergonal) ______

Number follicles 10 to 14 mm on that day ______

Number follicles 15 to 19 mm on that day ______

Number follicles 20+ mm on that day ______

hCG dose __________ IU

hCG date __________

hCG cycle day __________

hCG time __________

Comments: ______________________________

____

____

Figure 6

Follicular ultrasound and hCG administration data collection form.

NAME ____________________

PATIENT # ________ TREATMENT # ________ LMP ________

CYCLE DAY ________ DATE ________ TIME 1st ASP ________

TOTAL FOLLICLES ASPIRATED ______ TOTAL OOCYTES RECOVERED ______

NUMBER MATURE OOCYTES RECOVERED ______ NO. IMMATURE OOCYTES RECOVERED ______

L1: Dia. __mm Fol. Fluid Vol. __ml Egg ____ Mature/Immature ____
Found: * (A)spirate (N)eedle rinse (F)lush # ____
Comment ____________________

L2: Dia. __mm Fol. Fluid Vol. __ml Egg ____ Mature/Immature ____
Found: * (A)spirate (N)eedle rinse (F)lush # ____
Comment ____________________

L3: Dia. __mm Fol. Fluid Vol. __ml Egg ____ Mature/Immature ____
Found: * (A)spirate (N)eedle rinse (F)lush # ____
Comment ____________________

L4: Dia. __mm Fol. Fluid Vol. __ml Egg ____ Mature/Immature ____
Found: * (A)spirate (N)eedle rinse (F)lush # ____
Comment ____________________

L5: Dia. __mm Fol. Fluid Vol. __ml Egg ____ Mature/Immature ____
Found: * (A)spirate (N)eedle rinse (F)lush # ____
Comment ____________________

L6: Dia. __mm Fol. Fluid Vol. __ml Egg ____ Mature/Immature ____
Found: * (A)spirate (N)eedle rinse (F)lush # ____
Comment ____________________

L7: Dia. __mm Fol. Fluid Vol. __ml Egg ____ Mature/Immature ____
Found: * (A)spirate (N)eedle rinse (F)lush # ____
Comment ____________________

R1: Dia. __mm Fol. Fluid Vol. __ml Egg ____ Mature/Immature ____
Found: * (A)spirate (N)eedle rinse (F)lush # ____
Comment ____________________

R2: Dia. __mm Fol. Fluid Vol. __ml Egg ____ Mature/Immature ____
Found: * (A)spirate (N)eedle rinse (F)lush # ____
Comment ____________________

R3: Dia. __mm Fol. Fluid Vol. __ml Egg ____ Mature/Immature ____
Found: * (A)spirate (N)eedle rinse (F)lush # ____
Comment ____________________

R4: Dia. __mm Fol. Fluid Vol. __ml Egg ____ Mature/Immature ____
Found: * (A)spirate (N)eedle rinse (F)lush # ____
Comment ____________________

R5: Dia. __mm Fol. Fluid Vol. __ml Egg ____ Mature/Immature ____
Found: * (A)spirate (N)eedle rinse (F)lush # ____
Comment ____________________

R6: Dia. __mm Fol. Fluid Vol. __ml Egg ____ Mature/Immature ____
Found: * (A)spirate (N)eedle rinse (F)lush # ____
Comment ____________________

R7: Dia. __mm Fol. Fluid Vol. __ml Egg ____ Mature/Immature ____
Found: * (A)spirate (N)eedle rinse (F)lush # ____
Comment ____________________

* Enter "A", "N", "F" - if found in flush, enter number, e.g., "F2"

Figure 7
Laparoscopy observations data collection form.

NAME ______________________________
PATIENT # __________ TREATMENT # __________ LMP __________

MEDIUM __________ WATER USED __________ GAS PHASE __________

SEMEN ANALYSIS #1

(Pre-wash):
Volume _____ml Concentration _____mil Motility _____% Progression _____
(post-washed):
Vol.washed _____ml Concentration _____mil Motility _____% Progression _____

SEMEN ANALYSIS #2

(Pre-wash):
Volume _____ml Concentration _____mil Motility _____% Progression _____
(postwashed):
Vol.washed _____ml Concentration _____mil Motility _____% Progression _____

OOCYTE #1: Follicle _____ Mature/Immature _____ Egg preincubated ____ hours
Motile sperm inseminated __________ Sperm preincubated ____hours
OOCYTE #2: Follicle _____ Mature/Immature _____ Egg preincubated ____ hours
Motile sperm inseminated __________ Sperm preincubated ____ hours
OOCYTE #3: Follicle _____ Mature/Immature _____ Egg preincubated ____ hours
Motile sperm inseminated __________ Sperm preincubated ____ hours
OOCYTE #4: Follicle _____ Mature/Immature _____ Egg preincubated ____ hours
Motile sperm inseminated __________ Sperm preincubated ____ hours
OOCYTE #5: Follicle _____ Mature/Immature _____ Egg preincubated ____ hours
Motile sperm inseminated __________ Sperm preincubated ____ hours
OOCYTE #6: Follicle _____ Mature/Immature _____ Egg preincubated ____ hours
Motile sperm inseminated __________ Sperm preincubated ____ hours
OOCYTE #7: Follicle _____ Mature/Immature _____ Egg preincubated ____ hours
Motile sperm inseminated __________ Sperm preincubated ____ hours
OOCYTE #8: Follicle _____ Mature/Immature _____ Egg preincubated ____ hours
Motile sperm inseminated __________ Sperm preincubated ____ hours
OOCYTE #9: Follicle _____ Mature/Immature _____ Egg preincubated ____ hours
Motile sperm inseminated __________ Sperm preincubated ____ hours
OOCYTE #10: Follicle _____ Mature/Immature _____ Egg preincubated ____ hours
Motile sperm inseminated __________ Sperm preincubated ____ hours

Figure 8

Media, semen washing and insemination data collection form.

NAME ______________________________

PATIENT # __________ TREATMENT # __________ LMP __________

OOCYTE #1 FOLLICLE __________ FERTILIZED (Y/N) __________

OBSERVATION #1: HOURS POST INSEMINATION __________

OBSERVATION ______________________________

OOCYTE #2 FOLLICLE __________ FERTILIZED (Y/N) __________

OBSERVATION #1: HOURS POST INSEMINATION __________

OBSERVATION ______________________________

OOCYTE #3 FOLLICLE __________ FERTILIZED (Y/N) __________

OBSERVATION #1: HOURS POST INSEMINATION __________

OBSERVATION ______________________________

OOCYTE #4 FOLLICLE __________ FERTILIZED (Y/N) __________

OBSERVATION #1: HOURS POST INSEMINATION __________

OBSERVATION ______________________________

OOCYTE #5 FOLLICLE __________ FERTILIZED (Y/N) __________

OBSERVATION #1: HOURS POST INSEMINATION __________

OBSERVATION ______________________________

OOCYTE #6 FOLLICLE __________ FERTILIZED (Y/N) __________

OBSERVATION #1: HOURS POST INSEMINATION __________

OBSERVATION ______________________________

OOCYTE #7 FOLLICLE __________ FERTILIZED (Y/N) __________

OBSERVATION #1: HOURS POST INSEMINATION __________

OBSERVATION ______________________________

OOCYTE #8 FOLLICLE __________ FERTILIZED (Y/N) __________

OBSERVATION #1: HOURS POST INSEMINATION __________

OBSERVATION ______________________________

OOCYTE #9 FOLLICLE __________ FERTILIZED (Y/N) __________

OBSERVATION #1: HOURS POST INSEMINATION __________

OBSERVATION ______________________________

OOCYTE #10 FOLLICLE __________ FERTILIZED (Y/N) __________

OBSERVATION #1: HOURS POST INSEMINATION __________

OBSERVATION ______________________________

Figure 9.

Oocyte observations from day after laparoscopy data collection form.

NAME ____

PATIENT # __________ TREATMENT # _______ LMP_________

OOCYTE #1 FOLLICLE _____ CLEAVED (Y/N) _____ TRANSFERRED (Y/N) _______
TRANSFER OBSERVATION: HOURS POST INSEMINATION ______________
OBSERVATION ______________________________ GRADE _______

OOCYTE #2 FOLLICLE _____ CLEAVED _____ TRANSFERRED _______
TRANSFER OBSERVATION: HOURS POST INSEMINATION ______________
OBSERVATION ______________________________ GRADE _______

OOCYTE #3 FOLLICLE _____ CLEAVED _____ TRANSFERRED _______
TRANSFER OBSERVATION: HOURS POST INSEMINATION ______________
OBSERVATION ______________________________ GRADE _______

OOCYTE #4 FOLLICLE _____ CLEAVED _____ TRANSFERRED _______
TRANSFER OBSERVATION: HOURS POST INSEMINATION ______________
OBSERVATION ______________________________ GRADE _______

OOCYTE #5 FOLLICLE _____ CLEAVED _____ TRANSFERRED _______
TRANSFER OBSERVATION: HOURS POST INSEMINATION ______________
OBSERVATION ______________________________ GRADE _______

OOCYTE #6 FOLLICLE _____ CLEAVED _____ TRANSFERRED _______
TRANSFER OBSERVATION: HOURS POST INSEMINATION ______________
OBSERVATION ______________________________ GRADE _______

OOCYTE #7 FOLLICLE _____ CLEAVED _____ TRANSFERRED _______
TRANSFER OBSERVATION: HOURS POST INSEMINATION ______________
OBSERVATION ______________________________ GRADE _______

OOCYTE #8 FOLLICLE _____ CLEAVED _____ TRANSFERRED _______
TRANSFER OBSERVATION: HOURS POST INSEMINATION ______________
OBSERVATION ______________________________ GRADE _______

OOCYTE #9 FOLLICLE _____ CLEAVED _____ TRANSFERRED _______
TRANSFER OBSERVATION: HOURS POST INSEMINATION ______________
OBSERVATION ______________________________ GRADE _______

OOCYTE #10 FOLLICLE _____ CLEAVED _____ TRANSFERRED _______
TRANSFER OBSERVATION: HOURS POST INSEMINATION ______________
OBSERVATION ______________________________ GRADE _______

Transfer hours (post first insemination) ________ Catheter used ________
Number attempts _____* Bleeding (Y/N) ______ Cramping (Y/N) ________
Comments ____
Number embryos transferred ____________
Progesterone administered: dose/day ________ days of cycle __________**
Laparoscopy physician ____________ Transfer physician ______________
* An attempt is each time the embryo is loaded into a catheter
** Day of cycle - day of hCG administration is day 0, day of transfer is usually +4.

Post transfer: enter 9 into outcome field
Serum pregnancy test due ________________

Figure 10.
Oocyte observations from day of embryo transfer data collection form.

NAME ______________________________

PATIENT # __________ TREATMENT # __________ LMP __________

Next menses ______________

Outcome (code) ____________

Comments: ______________________________

____

____

Outcome code:

0 - Laparoscopy not done

1 - No egg recovered

2 - No transfer

3 - No pregnancy

4 - Elevated hCG only

5 - Clinical pregnancy, aborted

6 - Clinical pregnancy, in progress

7 - Term delivery

8 - Treatment in progress

9 - Post transfer awaiting pregnancy test

Serum pregnancy test due ________________

Figure 11.

Treatment cycle outcome data collection form.

embryo laboratory and includes the details of the culture media preparation, the semen analysis and washing results, and the incubation times and sperm concentrations at insemination. Figure 9 contains the oocyte observations made on the day following insemination.

The oocyte observations from the day of transfer as well as the transfer information (time, number of embryos transferred, catheter used, etc.) are listed in Figure 10. Figure 11 contains information pertaining to the clinical outcome of the cycle. Figures 12, 13, and 14 are for the results of the various hormone radioimmunoassays performed.

NAME: ____________________

PATIENT #: __________ CYCLE # __________

LMP: __________ hCG INJECTION DATE __________ CYCLE DAY __________

DATE	CYCLE DAY	TIME	SAMPLE IN?	RESULTS		
				LH (mIU/ml)	FSH (mIU/ml)	β-hCG (mIU/ml)
	5					
	6					
	7					
	9					
	10					
	11					
	12					
	13					
	14					
	15					
	16					
	+ 7					
	+10					
	+12					
	+14					

Figure 12

LH, FSH, and β-hCG radioimmunoassay result reporting form.

NAME: ______________________

PATIENT #: __________ CYCLE # __________

LMP: __________ hCG INJECTION DATE __________ CYCLE DAY __________

DATE	CYCLE DAY	TIME	SAMPLE IN?	E_2 RESULTS (pg/ml)
	5			
	6			
	7			
	8			
	9			
	10			
	11			
	12			
	13			
	14			
	15			
	16			
	+ 1			
	+ 2			
	+ 3			
	+ 4			
	+ 5			
	+ 7			
	+10			
	+12			

Figure 13

Estradiol radioimmunoassay result reporting form.

NAME: ______________________

PATIENT #: __________ CYCLE # __________

LMP: __________ hCG INJECTION DATE __________ CYCLE DAY ________

DATE	CYCLE DAY	TIME	SAMPLE IN?	P_4 RESULTS (ng/ml)
	- 1			
	0			
	+ 1			
	+ 2			
	+ 3			
	+ 4			
	+ 5			
	+ 7			
	+10			
	+12			

Figure 14

Progesterone radioimmunoassay result reporting form.

The information from each of these forms is entered into the record on a daily basis so the computer file is continuously up-to-date with respect to the ongoing treatments.

SUMMARY AND CONCLUSIONS:

Hopefully, in the coming years the success rate following IVF-ET will be substantially improved and the factor or factors critical in successful treatments will be better known. At that time there will be much less need for as extensive a data collection system as is currently required. However, until that time is reached, it is vitally important both for the acquisition of knowledge and the most successful treatment of our patients that we make every effort to learn as much as possible from every in vitro fertilization attempt. The amount of data generated by each treatment cycle essentially requires that this data be computerized if any attempt at correlation and analysis of results is to be made.

20

ETHICAL CONSIDERATIONS IN *IN VITRO* FERTILIZATION AND EMBRYO TRANSFER

Lori B. Andrews

Since the initial proposal of human *in vitro* fertilization, attacks and counterattacks regarding the ethics of the procedure have been so frequent and so heated that it is difficult to believe that both sides are talking about the same enterprise. Proponents of the technique stress its benefit to couples who would otherwise remain childless. Opponents concentrate on the dangers to society of future applications of the process: experimentation, interspecies fertilization, cloning and eugenics. Both groups claim to represent the child. The proponents speak of his right to be born, desperately wanted, into a loving family. The opponents urge his protection as the unconsenting victim of a manipulation whose dangers are not yet fully recognized.

The clinician establishing an *in vitro* fertilization program should be aware of the varying public and professional perceptions of what constitutes ethical practice in this field. In an area as emotionally charged as this one, there is a need to separate out each of the concerns involved and reflect over how likely it is that a harm could occur and how it could be prevented. This can best be done by analyzing the various viewpoints on the status of the embryo, the concerns raised by *in vitro* fertilization as an infertility treatment and the potential benefits and dangers of application of the procedure in other scientific endeavors.

Before undertaking such an analysis, it is necessary to consider the role of medical ethics in clinical practice. The Royal College of Obstetricians and Gynaecologists (RCOG) Ethics

Committee on In Vitro Fertilisation and Embryo Replacement or Transfer[1] found useful a definition expounded by Dunstan, Dunstan and Welbourne: "Medical ethics are obligations of a moral nature which govern the practice of medicine....They embody the standards by which each practitioner should inform his conscience, his capacity for moral reasoning and so govern himself in his practice.... It is the responsibility of the profession to develop its ethics to accommodate new demands and circumstances not encountered before...."[2] In developing standards that apply to in vitro fertilization, various ethical concerns must be kept in mind - fairness, voluntariness, protection of society and the parties involved, and maintenance of values we hold dear regarding the procreative process. Yet each of these concerns may have different meanings for different individuals.

THE FORUM IN WHICH ETHICAL ISSUES HAVE BEEN SCRUTINIZED

During the past decade, ethical concerns have affected policy considerations regarding whether in vitro fertilization should be undertaken at all and, if so, whether it should be federally funded. In 1972, an editorial in the Journal of the American Medical Association called for a moratorium on IVF research.[3] A 1975 federal law provided for the creation of an Ethics Advisory Board (EAB) within the Department of Health, Education, and Welfare, to review proposals for federal funding of in vitro fertilization research. In 1977, the Board analyzed a NIH grant application from Dr. Pierre Soupart of Vanderbilt University, who proposed to examine the composition of oocytes fertilized in vitro.

The Ethics Advisory Board had before it the task of studying in vitro fertilization, analyzing all the arguments pro and con, and making suggestions for a government policy on in vitro fertilization. The Secretary of HEW (at the time, Joseph Califano) did not want the Board to limit its consideration to Soupart's proposal. Rather, the Board was charged with a massive fact-finding mission about the scientific, ethical, legal, and social issues raised by in vitro fertilization.

The 15-member Board, which included physicians, medical ethicists, three lawyers, a psychiatrist, and three civic leaders, worked from May 1978 to May 1979 gathering information and preparing their report. They held hearings across the nation, taking testimony from medical and scientific experts, theologians, infertility patients, concerned individuals, professional organizations and various special interest groups. The conclusions of their report, touching on the full spectrum of ethical issues raised by in vitro fertilization are the closest thing we have to a national policy on the matter.[4] These conclusions, and the recommendations of a similar endeavor by the Royal College of Obstetricians and Gynaecologists Committee on In Vitro Fertilisation and Embryo Replacement or Transfer,[1] are discussed throughout this chapter.

STATUS OF THE EMBRYO - WHEN DOES PROTECTABLE LIFE BEGIN?

The issue on which there is most disagreement in the area of *in vitro* fertilization is that of the status of the embryo. A *plethora* of viewpoints exists regarding when life actually begins.

The well-known Roman Catholic viewpoint is that life begins at conception. A biological basis for that viewpoint is expressed by Krimmel and Foley: "Viewed from the perspective of an adult organism, the zygote represents the first time there is a specific form of life present and a specific identity attributable to the life."[5] The hereditary blueprint is in place; an individualized identity is secure.

Another commentator places the beginning of life at implantation.[6] That event has had significance in other inquiries as well. The regulations regarding federally funded research with pregnant women or with fetuses define both pregnancy and fetal life as beginning with implantation.[7]

Yet at these early stages, the embryo does not possess many of the traits we regard as human. "There is no feeling nor thought of which we know," wrote Heymann and Barzelay. "There is no memory or fear. What most of us mean by life, what most of us care about when we think of protecting life, is not true of the 12 or 16 cells present on the third or fourth day after pregnancy nor is it present for some time thereafter."[8]

Further along the continuum, Curran puts personhood at two to three weeks after implantation.[9] Another possible turning point might be the seventh or eighth week after conception, at which time the embryo is responsive to stimuli.[10] Similarly, some commentators use the ability to feel pain as the marker for when an embryo should be recognized as a person. Horan points out the flaw in that approach: we don't consider someone who is comatose or sedated to be a non-person and ready subject for experimentation.[11]

Grobstein feels the relevant inquiry is whether the embryo has "some degree of sentience or even an active volition."[10] He asserts that the emergence of a rudiment of self occurs no earlier than the second trimester and is therefore quite unlikely to be present at the point when the embryo is *in vitro*.

Quickening, the point at which the pregnant woman feels the motions of the fetus as a separate being, or viability, the point at which the fetus can live independently of the woman, are also candidates for the time at which the fetus becomes a person. But birth or developments after birth have also been suggested as the operative events. For example, important developments occur in the brain for the first two years after birth that contribute to the child's ability to be independent.[12]

The question of when the product of human conception becomes a person thus has numerous answers. Theologians differ in their responses, as do scientists. No amount of research or soul searching will produce an answer that is acceptable to all.

Often, the debate on the issue gets stalled in semantics. For those who refer to the embryo as a mere "collection of tissues," there is Tiefel's reply that we are all just a collection of tissues.[13]

Since the attempt to pinpoint the beginning of personhood has not yielded a consistent response, some of the groups considering the ethics of *in vitro* fertilization have chosen a different focus. The RCOG Committee, for example, has said "The proper moral question, then, is not 'When does life begin?' but, 'At what point in the development of the embryo do we attribute to it the protection due to a human being?'"[1]

The federal Ethics Advisory Board answered this question in the following manner: "After much analysis and discussion regarding both scientific data and the moral status of the embryo, the Board is in agreement that the human embryo is entitled to profound respect; but this respect does not necessarily encompass the full legal and moral rights attributed to persons."[4] The determination of the precise moral rights of the embryo requires an analysis of the purposes to which the embryo is being put and by whom.

ETHICAL CONCERNS REGARDING *IN VITRO* FERTILIZATION WITH HUSBAND'S SPERM AND WIFE'S OOCYTE AS TREATMENT FOR INFERTILITY

Just as there is a chorus of opinions on when life begins, there has been a wide range of views on the ethics of the *in vitro* fertilization process itself. Even its most conservative application - to provide an infertile married couple with a genetically related child - has been branded as unethical by some commentators. Ramsey,[14] Kass,[15] Tiefel[16] and others have eloquently expressed their qualms about the procedure while Edwards,[17] Francoeur,[18] Fletcher[19] and others have responded equally articulately with support for the morality of *in vitro* fertilization.

An initial set of attacks on the morality of *in vitro* fertilization are primarily resource allocation arguments, focusing on how medical funds might otherwise be spent or how maintaining the couple's infertility might further other social goals by reducing overpopulation or enhancing the adoption of "special needs" children. This line of attack suggests that *in vitro* fertilization should not be undertaken because there are more pressing medical or social problems on which attention should be focused. Hellegers and McCormick frame the issue as follows: "With limited resources should our country be pouring money into life-creating technologies when basic health needs go unmet?....We are not arguing against medical progress, for a great deal of useful knowledge is potentially available through *in vitro* research. We are simply concerned that Americans spell out carefully what progress means before they endorse it."[20]

Although the existence of alternative pressing problems might serve as a basis for judgments regarding governmental funding of *in vitro* fertilization, it certainly is not sufficient to ban the procedure. If a hierarchy of necessity existed for every medical procedure, wouldn't plastic surgery have to be banned before *in vitro* fertilization?

In the early days of research on fertilization of human ova *in vitro* the procedure viewed by some as inappropriate since the world faced problems of overpopulation. Edwards and Steptoe take issue with the claim that the "cure" for overpopulation lies in denying treatment to infertile couples. "Adopting this suggestion," they point out, "would lead to changes in the doctor-patient relationship and could demand that an unfortunate minority be penalized for the sake of the majority."[21] Additionally, Watson points out that research regarding *in vitro* fertilization may ease the population problem by leading to the development of better contraceptives.[22]

Another view of ethics that penalizes infertile couples suggests that *in vitro* fertilization should not be undertaken since there are homeless children infertile couples could adopt. But there seems to be little ethical about thrusting children who are strangers upon couples who want the chance to create biological children of their own. After all, the constitutional right to privacy gives great weight to the personal choice of couples regarding how to constitute their family. In addition, many of the children available for adoption are "special needs" children who are physically or mentally handicapped.[23] It takes a special couple to care for such children and it may not be in the children's best interest to be adopted by the infertile couples who would prefer in vitro fertilization.

A second line of attack on in vitro fertilization charges that the procedure is unethical because infertility is not a disease and treating infertility through in vitro fertilization is nontherapeutic and artificial. Kass argues that infertility is not a disease within the usual meaning of the word since it "is not life theatening or crippling, nor does it lead to detectable bodily damage."[15] But Lappé counters that, "When we speak of justification for medical practice, we are talking simply about a universal obligation to relieve suffering. And childlessness is a particularly acute form of such suffering."[24]

"The physical health of the parents does not demand that their infertility be cured," concede Edwards and Sharpe. "Yet the desire to have children must be among the most basic of human instincts, and denying it can lead to considerable psychological and social difficulties."[17]

In vitro fertilization has been criticized as nontherapeutic since, unlike tubal surgery or a varicocelectomy, the process does not aid the underlying cause of the infertility.[15] But Edwards points out that many medical treatments - such as insulin for a diabetic and spectacles for those with poor eyesight - rely on the same principle: "the clinical condition itself remains, but treatment modifies its expression."[17]

A related attack criticizes the technique as being unnatural. Anderson explains the argument as follows, "IVF separates the physical dimensions of intercourse from the emotional and spiritual ones. Procreation becomes reproduction (in the mechanical sense) and turns the marriage bed into a chemistry set."[25] This view overlooks the fact that infertile couples do not prefer the artifice of in vitro fertilization over the naturalness of traditional reproduction; rather, the latter has been denied to them. In that respect, their request parallels the request of any other patient who seeks medical aid. "Actually, every request of a physician to diagnose and treat disease is a request to manipulate nature," states Howard Jones. "If it is ethically acceptable to seek medical care for a reproductive disorder, it is ethically acceptable to seek care which requires in vitro fertilization."[26]

Kilbrandon notes that in vitro fertilization "is analogous to a caesarean birth: simply an artificial means of organizing an ordinary birth."[27] In addition, the amount of time that the embryo spends outside the natural environment of its mother's womb is a mere fraction of the pregnancy. Premature babies are maintained in an artificial environment, an incubator, for up to 20 weeks, much longer than the few days an IVF embryo is in its artificial environment, the petri dish.[28]

Of course, the major concern about the seeming unnaturalness of in vitro fertilization is that it represents an unparalleled opportunity for man to apply technology to his own shaping. Should in vitro fertilization be discouraged as "playing God?" Francoeur responds: "these moral positions assume that only God can make a tree or a man. They ignore the fact that God has shared with us His creative power so that we may contribute to the ongoing task of creating man and nature."[29]

The claims that in vitro fertilization is somehow suspect because it changes nature without effecting a cure for a medically-demonstrated ill do not provide us with a useful framework for contemplating the morality of the procedure. After all, man's lot on earth has been to change nature. And even if in vitro fertilization appears to be a departure from a traditional medical approach, there is no reason to think that childbearing is ethical only if undertaken for medical reasons. (In fact, the converse may be true - a couple would probably be viewed as morally suspect if the reason they had a child was a medical one, such as to cure the woman's endometriosis,[30] rather than because of the love and nurturing they could offer that child.)

The third, and most compelling, set of concerns about in vitro fertilization focuses on the potential harm to the child created by the procedure. Tiefel urges that "It makes good moral sense never to beget offspring when would-be parents cannot reasonably ensure a future child a fair chance of health."[16] Ramsey argued in 1972 that in vitro fertilization "constitutes unethical experimentation on possible future human beings, and therefore is subject to absolute moral prohibition."[14] He felt that no animal trial could reveal all the possible defects that the IVF procedure might cause (since, for example, research on monkeys would not reveal whether the procedure would induce mental retardation).[14] Since it could not be said with certainty that IVF children would be healthy, Ramsey concluded that the procedure should never be undertaken.

But whatever the morality of the first attempt at human in vitro fertilization, experience with the procedure to date has not shown an increase in abnormalities when compared to normal births.[1] Thus, predictions about physical harm have not been borne out.

Opponents of in vitro fertilization also point to potential harm to children through stigmatization or notoriety. However, as the ranks of the "test tube" babies grow, there is a diminishing chance that they will suffer ill effects from society's knowledge of their unique origins. To prevent such problems, couples can and do maintain confidentiality about their use of the procedure. Even if the word might get out, publicity itself is no reason to ban a medical practice. As we have seen with the artificial heart, notoriety with respect to new medical procedures goes beyond the area of infertility treatment - yet generally is not considered a reason to ban medical developments.

In vitro fertilization in married couples using their own gametes has also been attacked on the grounds that it is destructive of the family. "On the contrary," counters Grobstein, "the immediate purpose is to create a family, an objective exactly opposite to the concern expressed."[10] Besides, as Reilly points out, "given the myriad other pressures operating upon the marriage institution, the threat of I.V.F. appears miniscule."[31] Edwards expresses a similar idea: "how the notion of the family, which has survived abortion, divorce, sexual freedom, and rejection of the parents by children, is to be preserved by withholding treatment from the infertile is not clear...."[17]

ETHICAL CONCERNS REGARDING IN VITRO FERTILIZATION USING DONOR GAMETE(S) OR A SURROGATE CARRIER

For those troubled about how in vitro fertilization will affect our notion of family, an additional schism is added when a third party enters the procreative process. If the woman is anovulatory, has missing or inaccessible ovaries or carries a genetic defect that she does not wish to pass on, another woman may be recruited to donate an oocyte. If the man in the couple is azoospermic or carries a genetic defect, a sperm donor may be used. Even in situations where the couple provide the gametes, they may wish to have the in vitro fertilized embryo transferred to another woman for the period of gestation - either for medical reasons or as a personal preference on the part of the genetic mother not to be pregnant.

A precedent has already been established for third party involvement in the reproductive process with artificial insemination by donor. Insemination of the donor sperm into the petri dish rather than the woman's reproductive tract introduces no additional ethical dilemmas.

Although biologically analogous, the donation of an oocyte raises more concerns than does the provision of sperm. The oocyte donor faces greater physical risks than does the sperm donor. She may need to undergo hormone treatment; a laparoscopy will generally be necessary to recover the eggs. However, physical danger alone does not make the use of a donor unethical. (After all, kidney donors face even greater physical risks.) To protect the well-being of the donor, though, the risks involved should be carefully explained to her in advance. Coercion should not be used or condoned. For example, it would be unfair to use the coercive tactic of limiting entry into an *in vitro* fertilization program to women who were willing to donate some of their oocytes. Likewise, if the infertile woman brings a relative or donor with her to provide an oocyte, the physician involved should attempt to learn whether unfair coercion has been used to get the donor to participate. At a minimum, the potential donor should be interviewed separately. If it is clear that she does not really want to participate, the physician should help her extricate herself from the situation. This is similar to the situation of a coerced kidney donor; in the transplant situation, the physician will talk to the donor alone and, if the donor does not want to go through with it but yet does not wish to offend the relative who needs the organ, the physician will tell the relative that the proposed donor is not suitable.[32]

It seems ethically appropriate to try to recruit female donors who are undergoing abdominal surgery for other reasons so that the additional risk of providing an oocyte would not be great. This would include women who are undergoing tubal ligation or hysterectomy and women enrolled in an *in vitro* fertilization program, provided that they are not coerced. For example, in the *in vitro* fertilization program directed by Alan Trounson, John Leeton and Carl Wood at the Queen Victoria Medical Centre in Melbourne, Australia, only three embryos are transferred back into a patient (in order to avoid the danger of a multiple pregnancy). If more than three oocytes are removed, the couple can have the excess ones fertilized and either donate them or freeze them. The alternatives are carefully explained to couples when they contact the program. Since the clinic has a two year waiting list, there is ample time to reach a considered decision.[33]

The professional undertaking an *in vitro* fertilization program should protect against potential physical or psychological harm to the donor. The RCOG Report advocates non-directive counselling of the potential donor. It also recommends that, as is the case with sperm donation, anonymity of the oocyte donor be preserved and the donor not be told whether or not her oocyte actually produced a pregnancy. When the Trounson group performs *in vitro* fertilization with a donated oocyte, the donor and recipient are cared for in two different hospitals to preserve their anonymity "thus preventing the possibility of interaction or argument between the genetic and rearing parents."[33]

Additional ethical issues are raised by the use of a surrogate carrier, a woman who agrees to gestate the IVF embryo of a couple and then turn the child over to the couple after the birth. A couple may wish to use this technique if the woman has a medical or physical problem that prevents her from carrying a pregnancy (such as severe diabetes or hypertension or a uterine malformation). Or the woman may wish to use a surrogate carrier for convenience (for example, if the genetic mother is an actress who does not want to interrupt her career).

An initial issue is whether it is ethical to use a surrogate carrier when the genetic mother has no physical problem that would prevent her from carrying the child. Revillard comments that "the application of embryo transfer should be subservient to therapeutic considerations: any other motivation - coquetry, ambition or pursuit of a career where aesthetics are essential - should exclude such action."[34] Rassaby argues that "I do not belive that we are entitled to argue (as some have argued) that the need of the woman who physically cannot give birth is an actual one whereas the need of the busy female executive or model is more perceived than actual. To the latter, the need may be just as great as to the former."[35] But the issue is not between actual and false needs, rather it is between qualitatively different types of needs. The use of a surrogate carrier by a healthy woman may lead us to question a woman's commitment to parenthood. If she can't be bothered for nine months nurturing the child internally, how will she find the time in the next 18 years to attend to the child's needs?

Even in instances where use of a carrier is medically indicated for the genetic mother, there is concern for its effect on the surrogate. Might a poor woman be coerced into serving as a carrier just because she needs the money?[15] Rassaby says that "it seems rather counterproductive to deny her this option. Given a choice between poverty and exploitation, many people may prefer the latter."[35] Karp and Donahue[36] add that "it seems inconsistent to categorically deny such women this kind of livelihood while we permit and even encourage people to earn money by such dangerous means as coal mining, or racing little cars around a track at 200 miles per hour".

Before use of a surrogate carrier is permitted, the issue of a possible coercion of the woman warrants a thorough examination. Coercion may occur either as a compelling economic incentive or as a case of undue influence. Both types have already surfaced in the transplant situation. A graphic example of economic coercion took place when a rich Italian man bought one testicle from a poor Italian,[32] apparently so that the rich man could increase his sexual prowess.

Undue influence can occur when the party suggesting the procedure has an independent source of power over the potential donor - such as when a prisoner is offered a reduced sentence for donating an organ or a certain quantity of blood.[32] In the surrogate situation, undue influence might be exercised by a relative, an employer, or a court.

In addition to the potential harm from possible coercion, some ethicists argue that surrogacy may cause harm to the carrier since she cannot predict at the time she agrees to gestate another couple's embryo how she will feel once the child is born. "She cannot possibly predict before the baby is born what her attitude will be towards the child which she has been carrying for nine months," wrote the RCOG Committee. "A change in her attitude and intentions would create emotional stress in herself if she gives up the child or to the potential parents if she does not."[1]

Protection of the couple from harassment by the donor or surrogate is also a consideration. Some organ donors have persecuted or blackmailed recipients;[32] biological mothers have intruded into the life of the couples adopting their children.[37] The RCOG Committee was also concerned about the risky legal position of the surrogate arrangement, since the woman who gives birth is considered its legal mother. Thus, the couple's right to parenthood would not be sufficiently protected, despite their genetic link to the child. Because of these unresolved social, psychological and legal issues, the RCOG Committee considers it unethical to implant IVF embryos into surrogate mothers.[1]

Another criticism leveled against donor or surrogate participation in *in vitro* fertilization is that it will "commercialize" childbearing. Sperm donors are paid for their contribution and surrogate mothers have commanded fees from $5,000 to $20,000. Anderson argues that use of a surrogate "dehumanizes the aspect of prenatal care for the infant and opens up a realm of commercialization of fetal rights".[25] Yet spending money in furtherance of childbearing does not of itself seem unethical. After all, even without donor involvement, infertile couples spend substantial sums to investigate their condition and treat it with drugs and surgery. And no one has yet tried to argue that payment for a Caesarean section or neonatal care will "commercialize" childbearing.

Rassaby dismisses the argument that children will be "devalued" because they were bought and sold. "In most cases, the services of a surrogate will only be sought after all other viable alternatives have been exhausted," he points out. "Far from being devalued, this child is likely to be especially loved."[35]

It is probably not the fee itself that is troublesome so much as the potential attitude it fosters on the part of the donor or carrier. Should society approve of people who "create" children, but then have no moral responsibility for them? This is an issue that needs attention and the place to begin would be with sperm donors for traditional artificial insemination. How do they feel years later about the experience? How do they treat the children they raise within their own marriages? It would seem wrong to condemn one type of donation (womb rental) and not the others (oocyte or sperm donation). As a principle, they would seem to stand or fall together.

ETHICAL CONCERNS REGARDING EMBRYO FREEZING

The potential now exists for an embryo created with a couple's gametes (or with donor gametes) to be frozen for future implantation into a woman's uterus.[38] This would allow a couple to have embryos implanted in a subsequent unstimulated cycle of the woman which might offer a greater chance of pregnancy than implantation in the cycle in which the superovulation and the laparoscopy was undertaken. Or it could make it possible for couples to have several embryos fertilized _in vitro_ at the same time and to space the pregnancies of their children without the need for subsequent laparoscopies. It could also foster the wider availability of embryo donation, since it would no longer be necessary to choose a donor and recipient who had matched menstrual cycles.

For those who believe that life begins at conception, embryo freezing poses insurmountable ethical problems. While the appropriate freezing technique is being perfected, some embryos will be destroyed by the process. Once the process is perfected embryos will be condemned to a sentence of suspended animation.

In rebuttal to the claim that freezing embryos is unethical, Trounson and Conti assert that there may be situations in which it is unethical _not_ to freeze embryos. They point out that "there may be an obligation on in-vitro fertilisation clinics to develop freezing so that in circumstances where embryos cannot be transplanted - because of illness or unexpected difficulty - or where excess embryos develop they are not disposed of or used for other purposes".[39]

In any discussion of the ethics of embryo freezing, however, potential harm to the fetus must be considered. Biggers reports that while there is no evidence that freezing itself is mutagenic, the background radiation may increase the mutation rate.[40] However, short term freezing should not present these difficulties.

A problem more likely to arise is what to do with excess frozen embryos. Before freezing of a particular embryo is attempted, provisions should be made for what will be done with the embryo if the couple divorces, one or both gamete donors dies or the couple lose interest in the embryo. Tiefel argues that "prolonged freezing may rob a thawed and growing life of its genetic progenitors, of its roots and support".[16]

The RCOG Committee, deliberating about the issue of embryo freezing concluded that it "would be wise at first to limit the storage time to that required for a foreseeable and specific purpose, e.g., a second pregnancy for the same couple".[1] The Committee felt that such a limitation was warranted on social rather than scientific grounds "to avoid unpredictable legal hazards."

The RCOG Report also concluded that once a successful pregnancy has been achieved, the remaining frozen embryos produced by the couple's gametes should not be donated to another infertile couple. This recommendation is an attempt to limit the creation of siblings unknown to one another. The report, however, suggests that spare embryos could be used for certain research purposes (but not beyond the stage of early neural development, 17 days after conception).

ETHICAL CONCERNS REGARDING IN VITRO FERTILIZATION IN SITUATIONS OTHER THAN INFERTILITY TREATMENT

There are many research uses to which an embryo conceived through <u>in vitro</u> fertilization might be put. When Pierre Soupart of Vanderbilt University submitted an IVF proposal to the National Institutes of Health, he wanted to study such embryos to determine the incidence of chromosomal abnormality. Embryos conceived <u>in vitro</u> could provide valuable information that might lead to advances in infertility treatment and in contraception development. They could also be used to test the effects of medicine or suspected environmental toxins. They might even be useful for therapeutic purposes. Edwards, for example, suggests that cells from early embryos might be used for bone marrow transplants to children.[1] If <u>ex utero</u> development becomes possible for extensive periods beyond the implantation stage, the IVF conceptus might be used to provide replacement organs for existing human beings.

One recurring criticism of in vitro fertilization is that it will lead to the creation of an experimental class of human beings created only for laboratory uses. And, indeed, the prospect of creating a sibling, twin, or child to provide spare body parts for an individual does sound like a science fiction story run amuck.

The ethical dilemmas in this area arise from the fact that, no matter what one's answer is to the question of when life begins, one cannot help but recognize the special nature of an embryo. An embryo, with its unique genetic blueprint, is not like other body tissue. Consequently, any research on it must be designed with a profound respect for the embryo. When the Ethics Advisory Board considered the issue of IVF research, it found that "concerns regarding the moral status of the embryo and the potential long-range consequences of this research were among the most difficult that confronted the Board."[4] After extensive analysis, the Board concluded that such research is "acceptable from an ethical standpoint," if the following guidelines are met: the research meets other regulations governing work with human subjects,[41] the research is designed primarily to establish the safety and efficacy of embryo transfer and to obtain important scientific information toward that end not reasonably attainable by other means, informed consent of the gamete donors has been received, no embryo is sustained beyond 14 days after fertilization, and the public is advised if there is evidence that in vitro fertilization leads to greater risks of abnormal offspring than does natural procreation.

The conclusions of the Ethics Advisory Board regarding IVF research are similar to those reached by other august bodies. The Judicial Council of the American Medical Association adopted guidelines for in vitro fertilization research that acknowledge its value to further knowledge of "how genetic defects arise and are transmitted and how they might be prevented or treated." The guidelines prohibit research on an embryo that will be implanted in a woman and state that in vitro fertilization research should comply with the AMA's fetal research guidelines.

The British Medical Research Council [42] found research involving in vitro fertilization between human gametes to be ethically acceptable on the condition that it is scientifically sound, informed consent of the donors is obtained, and the embryos are not cultured in vitro beyond the implantation stage and are not stored for unspecified research use, there is no intent to transfer to the uterus any embryo resulting from or used in such experiments, and the aim of the research is clearly defined and directly relevant to clinical problems. The Council opined that human embryos resulting from clinical in vitro fertilization treatment programs that are no longer required for that purpose may be used for research with the informed consent of both donors. The Medical Research Council of Australia also issued guidelines recommending that research not continue beyond the stage at which implantation would normally occur.[43]

Beyond research with human gametes, some scientists may attempt to use the in vitro fertilization procedure to cross species. Joseph Fletcher describes two potential uses for human-animal creations - providing organs for transplants or doing dangerous or demeaning jobs.[19]

Kass is especially concerned that researchers will try to merge ape and man by fertilizing an ape oocyte with human sperm.[44] Anderson points out that "One important implication of the sanctity of human life is human beings are distinct from animals because we are created in the image of God (Gen 1:27, 5:1-2)".[25] This may counsel against using the in vitro fertilization technology in an attempt to merge animal and man. Edwards also finds such a possibility questionable ethically "for the human component would be condemned to a situation unworthy of it".[17]

But the difficult moral issue of interspecies fertilization was not born with the IVF procedure. Already, a Chinese surgeon has used artificial insemination in an attempt to fertilize a chimpanzee with human sperm in order to create a subhuman field worker.[30]

The creation of such a creature - whether through in vitro fertilization or otherwise - would have profoundly disturbing effects on society. Some argue that the attempt alone is unethical; others believe that even in vitro fertilization for infertile couples should be banned to prevent the possibility of interspecies fertilization in vitro. In considering this issue, the British Medical Research Council has adopted a middle position, favoring studies on interspecies fertilization, so long as the embryo is not allowed to develop beyond the early cleavage stage.[42] Yet Walters points out that "The moral status of human-animal hybrids, even at this early stage of development, is a matter that will require further philosophical and ethical exploration".[45]

Watson criticizes in vitro fertilization as a first step toward cloning.[46] But cloning is not an inevitable by-product of fertilizing the gametes of a childless married couple in vitro. As Edwards points out "Cloning depends on embryo transfer, but the converse is not true."[17] Watson himself admits that cloning need not necessarily occur as a result of in vitro fertilization research, but he believes that some medical professionals undertaking IVF would ultimately get involved in cloning. "Some people may sincerely believe the world desperately needs many copies of really exceptional people if we are to fight our way out of the ever-increasing computer-mediated complexity that makes our individual brains so frequently inadequate," he states.[46]

Yet even if the cloning were determined to be ethically unacceptable, it could be banned without a need to stop the entire in vitro fertilization process. Serious ethical concerns are raised by cloning since it deprives an individual of the right to a unique identity. If a couple raises a clone of a famous violinist, it is unlikely that they would let him pursue his interests in sports or mathematics. Edwards and Sharpe note "There would be a strong impulse to treat cloned children as laboratory subjects to be analysed repeatedly during their lifetime".[17] The Medical Research Council of Australia has specifically found cloning ethically unacceptable.[43]

Finally, several critics have opposed the procedure of in vitro fertilization on the grounds that it may facilitate eugenics. Leon Kass opposed in vitro fertilization for infertile couples, in part because he considers it "a great step toward the full laboratory control of human reproduction."[15]

In the United States from approximately 1900 to the 1930's, the American Eugenics Movement advocated the improvement of mankind by encouraging proliferation among people presumed to have desirable genes and by discouraging childbearing among those people presumed to have undesirable genes.[47] As part of that movement, 30 states tried to legislate standards of "worthiness" for childbearing by passing laws to sterilize people who were thought to be alcoholic, feeble-minded or to have criminal tendencies. A 1927 U.S. Supreme Court case upheld the sterilization of a mentally retarded woman so that she would not give birth to a similarly afflicted child.[48] But now in vitro fertilization followed by embryo transfer to a second woman provides the possibility that eugenics could be practiced not by sterilization, but by forcing a woman to carry and raise a child of "superior" donors.

The late Nobel Prize winner Hermann J. Muller foresaw such possibilities when artificial insemination by donor was introduced. "Foster pregnancy, which is already possible, will become socially acceptable and even socially obligatory," he asserted. "It will seem wrong to breed children who mirror parents' peculiarities and weaknesses. In the future, children will be produced by the union of ovum and sperm, both derived from persons of proved worth, possibly long deceased, and who exemplify the ideals of the foster-parents."[49] Similarly, Dobzansky has advocated "What we want is not simply natural selection, but selection, natural and artificial, directed toward humanly desirable goals".[50]

But the ethical issues raised by such approaches are particularly troublesome. A National Academy of Sciences Committee has posed some of the social problems raised by eugenics: "Selection is a harsh process. To make speedy progress, reproduction should be limited primarily to those who possess genotypes for the desired traits. But who will decide what is desirable? How much genotypic and phenotypic variability would be optimal in the human society? Who would dare to prohibit procreation to a majority of men and women, limiting this activity only to an elite group? And to whom would society entrust such decisions?"[51]

Even if a societal consensus could be reached about what characteristics people should be bred to have, aggressive eugenics could actually harm rather than improve the gene pool by diminishing genetic variety and possibly proliferating unwanted recessive genes of donors chosen for other traits.[52]

PUBLIC PARTICIPATION IN THE DEBATE OVER THE ETHICS OF _IN VITRO_ FERTILIZATION

In 1980, the federal Ethics Advisory Board, charged with the task of scrutinizing _in vitro_ fertilization, ceased to exist. Yet it is clear that as _in vitro_ fertilization becomes more widespread and it becomes scientifically feasible to clone or socially feasible to undertake eugenics, additional consideration of evolving ethical issues will be necessary. Already, one federal legislator has suggested the creation of a Commission on Human Genetic Engineering. But attention to the ethics of _in vitro_ fertilization should not be confined to elite governmental bodies.

It is clear that the issues surrounding reproductive technology are, as Watson has said, "a matter far too important to be left in the hands of the scientific and medical communities".[46] Edwards has pointed out that "What is to be feared is that if the biologists do not invent a method of taking counsel of mankind, society will thrust its advice on biologists and other scientists and probably in a manner or form seriously hampering to science."

The first step toward taking the public's counsel has been accomplished by pollsters. A month after the first IVF birth, in August 1978, a Harris poll of around 1,500 American women found that 85% felt in vitro fertilization should be an option for infertile women. Overall, 58% of the women said they would themselves consider using in vitro fertilization. Among younger women, age 18 to 39, the number was even higher (61%).

A similar Gallup poll of both men and women, also taken in August 1978, found that 60% favored the availability of the procedure to anyone who needed and wanted it. Gallup found that "an extraordinary 93% had heard or read about the baby." Forty-two percent could fully and correctly explain in vitro fertilization.

Given the widespread level of knowledge and understanding of in vitro fertilization, it is possible to explore the ethical issues with society at large. "It will be important for infertility programs to engage meaningful involvement of their communities in the evolution of whatever policy they adopt for regulating reproductive technologies," explains Kenneth Ryan. "There appear to be no simple right or wrong answers to the broad social questions. They seem to be inherently context bound. In our pluralistic society that honors individual liberty and privacy above all else, we have to be prepared for diversity and change. It will be difficult to hold on to cherished traditions unless they can be widely embraced and validated for our time".[53]

FOOTNOTES

1. Royal College of Obstetricians and Gynaecologists, 1983, "Report of the RCOG Ethics Committee on In Vitro Fertilisation and Embryo Replacement or Transfer, Chameleon Press, London.
2. Dunstan, A.S., Dunstan, G.R., Welbourne, R.B., 1981, "Dictionary of Medical Ethics," Darton, Longman & Todd, London.
3. Editorial, 1972, Genetic engineering in man: Ethical considerations, J. Amer. Med. Assoc., 220:721.
4. Department of Health, Education, and Welfare, Office of the Secretary: Protection of Human Subjects; HEW Support of Human In Vitro Fertilization and Embryo Transfer: Report of the Ethics Advisory Board, 1979, Federal Register, 44:35034.
5. Krimmel, H.T., Foley, M.J., 1977, Abortion: An inspection into the nature of human life and potential consequences of legalizing its destruction, Univ. of Cincinnati Law Review, 46:725.

6. Carney, T., 1980, Instant evolution: We'd better get good at it, cited in Lorio, K.V., In vitro fertilization and embryo transfer: Fertile areas for litigation, Southwestern Law J., 35:973.
7. 45 C.F.R.§ 46, 203(b) and (c), 1982.
8. Heymann, P.B., Barzelay, D.E., 1973, The forest and the trees: Roe v. Wade and its critics, Boston Univ. Law Review, 53:765.
9. Curran, C.E. In vitro fertilization and embryo transfer: From a perspective of moral theology, a paper prepared for the federal Ethics Advisory Board.
10. Grobstein, C., 1981, "From Chance to Purpose: An Appraisal of of External Human Fertilization", Addison-Wesley, Reading, Massachusetts.
11. Horan, D.J., 1976-77, Fetal experimentation and federal regulation, Villanova Law Review 22:325.
12. Grobstein, C., 1981, citing J. M. Tanner, 1978, "Fetus Into Man", Harvard Univ. Press, Cambridge, Massachusetts.
13. Tiefel, H.O., 1974, The cost of fetal research: Ethical considerations, New Eng. J. of Med., 294:85.
14. Ramsey, P., 1972, Shall we "reproduce"? I. The medical ethics of in vitro fertilization, J. Amer. Med. Assoc., 220:1346, and Shall we "reproduce"? II. Rejoinders and future forecast, J. Amer. Med. Assoc., 220:1346;1480.
15. Kass, L.R., 1979, "Making babies" revisited, Public Interest, 54:32; 1971, Babies by means of in vitro fertilization: Unethical experiments on the unborn?, New Eng. J. of Med., 285:1174; 1972, Making babies - The new biology and the "old" morality, Public Interest, 26:18.
16. Tiefel, H.O. 1982, Human in vitro fertilization, J. Amer. Med. Assoc, 247:3235.
17. Edwards, R., 1974, Fertilization of human eggs in vitro: Morals, ethics and the law, Quarterly Review of Biol., 49:3; Edwards, R.G., Sharpe, D.J., 1971, Social values and research in human embryology, Nature, 231:87.
18. Francoeur, R.T., 1970, "Utopian Motherhood: New Trends in Human Reproduction," Doubleday, Garden City, New York.
19. Fletcher, 1974, "The Ethics of Genetic Control: Ending Reproductive Roulette," Anchor Press, Doubleday, Garden City, New York.
20. Hellegers, A.E., and McCormick, R.A., 1978, Unanswered questions on test tube life, America, 139:74
21. Edwards, R.G., and Steptoe, P.C., 1973, Biological aspects of embryo transfer, in CIBA Foundation Symposium "Law and Ethics of A.I.D. and Embryo Transfer," Associated Scientific Publishers, Amsterdam.
22. Watson, J.D., 1971, Excerpts from potential consequences of experimentation with human eggs, Congressional Record, 117:7674.

23. Plumez, J.H., 1982, "Successful Adoption," Harmony Books, New York.
24. Lappé, M., 1972, Risk taking for the unborn, Hastings Center Report, 2 (1):1.
25. Anderson, J.K., 1982, "Genetic Engineering," Zondervan, Grand Rapids, Michigan.
26. Jones, H., 1982, The ethics of in vitro fertilization - 1982, Fertil. Steril., 37:146.
27. Stone, O.M., 1973, English law in relation to A.I.D. and embryo transfer, in CIBA Foundation Symposium "Law and Ethics of A.I.D. and Embryo Transfer," Associated Scientific Publishers, Amsterdam.
28. Marlow, J.L., (interview), 1978, British birth poses many problems to society, U.S. News & World Report, 24:(August 7).
29. Francoeur, R.T., 1972, We can - we must; reflections on the technological imperative, Theological Studies, 33:428.
30. Andrews, L.B., 1984, "New Conceptions," St. Martin's Press, New York, New York.
31. Reilly, P., 1976, In vitro - A legal perspective, in "Genetics and the Law," A. Milunsky and G.J. Annas, eds., Plenum Press, New York, New York.
32. Scott, R., 1981, "The Body as Property," Viking Press, New York, New York.
33. Trounson, A., Leeton, J., Bensanko, M., Wood, C., and Conti, A., 1983, Pregnancy established in an infertile patient after transfer of a donated embryo fertilised in vitro, Brit.Med. J., 286:835.
34. Revillard, M., 1973, Legal aspects of artificial insemination and embryo transfer in French domestic law and private international law, in CIBA Foundation Symposium, "Law and Ethics of A.I.D. and Embryo Transfer," Associated Scientific Publishers, Amsterdam.
35. Rassaby, A., 1982, Surrogate motherhood: The position and problem of substitutes, in "Test Tube Babies," W. A. W. Walters and Peter Singer, eds., Oxford University Press, Melbourne.
36. Karp, L., Donahue, R., 1976, Preimplantational ectogenesis: Science and speculation concerning in vitro fertilization and related procedures, Western Journal of Medicine, 124:295.
37. Meezan, W., Katz, S., Russo, E.M., 1978, "Adoptions Without Agencies: A Study of Independent Adoptions," Child Welfare League of America, Inc., New York, New York.
38. Branigin, W., 1983, "Frozen Embryos Trigger Debate by Australians," Washington Post, page 1, column 5, May 17.
39. Trounson, A., Conti, A., 1982, Research in human in-vitro fertilisation and embryo transfer, Brit. Med. J., 285:224.
40. Biggers, J.D., 1981, In vitro fertilization and embryo transfer in human beings, New Eng. J. of Med., 304:336.

41. 45 C.F.R., 1982, § 46.101 et. seq.
42. Editorial, 1982, Research related to human fertilization and embryology, Brit. Med. J., 285:1480.
43. Levine,C., 1983, In Britain and Australia, new in vitro guidelines, Hastings Center Report, 13 (2):2.
44. Presentation at Biology and Ethics Roundtable Discussion at the University of Chicago, February 16, 1983.
45. Walters, L., 1979, A review of the ethical literature, Hastings Center Report, 9 (4):23.
46. Watson, J., 1971, Moving toward clonal man - Is this what we want?, Cong. Rec - Senate, 117:1275.
47. Fiddler, M. B., 1978, Social and ethical dimensions of population control and attempts to modify the gene pool: An overview of genetics, in "Workshop/Symposium on Frontiers in Genetics Research," University of Illinois, Chicago.
48. Buck v. Bell 274 U.S. 200 (1927).
49. Daly, C.B., 1962, "Morals, Law and Life," Clonmore and Reynolds, Dublin.
50. Dobzhansky, T., 1961, Man and natural selection, American Scientist, 49:285.
51. Handler, P., 1970, in "Biology and the Future of Man," P. Handler, ed., Oxford University Press, New York.
52. Kindegran, C.P., 1973, State power over human fertility and individual liberty, Hastings Law Journal, 23:1401.
53. Ryan, Kenneth J., 1983, "Ethical Issues in Reproductive Technology," presented at the 39th Annual Meeting of the American Fertility Society, San Francisco, California.

APPENDIX A

DETAILS OF LABORATORY PROCEDURES

IVF Glassware Washing Procedure

1. All glassware is rinsed in reverse osmosis (R/O) water and soaked in a 2% solution of 7 X detergent in R/O water for at least 24 hours.
2. Wash all glassware in fresh 7 X. Scrub with a brush if necessary. Transfer 7 X and glassware to a stainless steel pot and bring to a boil. Let simmer for 30 minutes. (Caution: Do not let water level drop below top of glassware.)

   Handle Glassware Only with Gloves for the Rest of the Procedure

3. Before the glassware cools, rinse well in deionized water.
4. Soak for 24 hours in R/O water
5. Rinse with distilled-R/O water.
6. Soak in distilled-R/O water for 24 hours.
7. Rinse with distilled milli-Q (Millipore) purified water.
8. Soak for 24 hours in distilled-milli-Q water..
9. Dry in oven.

IVF Pasteur Pipette Washing Procedure

Using a Pipette Washer:

1. Aspirate one jar of a 2% solution of 7 X detergent in R/O water.
2. Aspirate two jars of R/O water.
3. Aspirate one jar of distilled-R/O water.
4. Dry in oven.
5. Package appropriately and sterilize with ethylene oxide.

IVF Teflon Tubing Washing Procedure

(Aspirating needles, transfer catheters)

1. Soak for 24 hours in a 2% solution of 7 X detergent in R/O water.
2. Flush several times with 2% 7 X solution.
3. Flush several times with R/O water.
4. Flush several times with distilled-R/O water.
5. Air dry.
6. Package appropriately and sterilize with ethylene oxide.

5x Glass Redistilled Water

The distilled water used for media production is made by sequentially distilling house R/O water five times in a commercially available glass distillation apparatus (Fisher 09-107) and using each collection flask (Fisher 10-067P) as the next distillization pot to avoid contamination. The final water is transferred to storage bottles (1 liter glass) and stored at 4° C until use.

MATERIALS AND SUPPLIES

This list is not meant as an endorsement for any of the companies mentioned.

Chemicals

Description	Company	Catalog No.
Ham's F-10 (powdered)	GIBCO [1]	430-1200
Calcium lactate $1.5H_2O$	Calbiochem [2]	4272
Penicillin G	Sigma [3]	PEN-NA
Sodium bicarbonate	Fisher [4]	S233
Sodium heparin	Sigma	H-3125
Streptomycin sulfate	Sigma	S-6501

Major Equipment

Description	Company	
Video equipment	Hitachi color camera JVC video recorder and color monitor	HV9017
Laminar flow hood (horizontal)	Baker [5]	EG3252 or EG6252

Incubator, 3 gas	Forma [6]	3315
Dissecting scope	Wild*	M8

* We use a Nikon diascopic base and illuminator

Plasticware; sterile, disposable

Description Number	Company	Catalog
0.22 um filter	Amicon 7	022255
0.45 um filter	Amicon	3042255
5 ml pipette	Falcon 8	7543
10 ml pipette	Falcon	7551
50 ml flask	Falcon	3013
250 ml flask	Falcon	3024
15 ml conical centrifuge tube	Falcon	2095
16 x 125 mm culture tube	Falcon	3033
12 x 75 mm culture tube	Falcon	2003
35 x 10 mm petri dish	Falcon	3001
60 x 15 mm petri dish	Falcon	1007
60 x 15 mm organ culture dish with center well	Falcon	3037

1. Grand Island Biological Company, Grand Island, NY.
2. Calbiochem-Behring, Division of American Hoechst Corporation, San Diego, CA.
3. Sigma Chemical Company, St. Louis, MO.
4. Fisher Scientific Company, Pittsburgh, PA.
5. Baker Company, Inc., Sanford Airport, Sanford, ME.
6. Forma Scientific, Division of Mallinckrodt, Inc., Marietta, OH.
7. Amicon Corporation, Danvers, MA.
8. Falcon, a trademark of Becton, Dickinson and Company, Oxnard, CA.

APPENDIX B

IN VITRO FERTILIZATON AND EMBRYO TRANSFER INFORMED CONSENT

I have been unable to become pregnant due to blocked or absent Fallopian tubes which cannot be corrected surgically (or attempted surgical correction has been unsuccessful or I have some other reason for infertility which is not treatable with any other currently available method). I have consented to attempt to become pregnant using *in vitro* fertilization and embryo transfer ("test-tube baby"). I understand that the following is an outline of the steps required in this procedure: 1) Determine by standard infertility tests (including laparoscopy) that I am a suitable candidate for the procedure. 2) The use of "fertility drugs" (clomiphene, hCG and/or Pergonal) to produce ovulation at a predictable time. 3) Ultrasound examinations to assist in predicting the time of expected ovulation. 4) Undergoing laparoscopy ("belly-button surgery" or "band-aid surgery") about 1 to 4 hours before I am expected to ovulate and insertion of a needle into my ovary to obtain the egg. 5) Obtaining of one or two sperm specimens from my husband by masturbation and laboratory treatment of the sperm to prepare them for fertilization. 6) Mixing the egg and the sperm together to allow fertilization to occur. 7) After fertilization transferring the egg into a different media for growth. 8) After several cell divisions, if the embryo is developing normally, transferring the embryo into my uterus by means of a small tube inserted through my cervix. 9) Obtaining blood samples up to 20 times during the treatment cycle to measure hormone levels.

I understand that I may be hospitalized for up to three days for the above procedure to be accomplished. I also understand that any of the following may occur which would prevent the establishment of a pregnancy. 1) The time of ovulation may be misjudged, may be unable to be predicted, may occur prior to laparoscopy, or ovulation may not occur in the monitored cycle, thus precluding any attempt at obtaining an egg. 2) Pelvic adhesions may prevent access to the ovary with the follicles. 3) Ovulation may have occurred by the time laparoscopy is performed. 4) Medical emergencies may make an operating room and/or anesthesia unavailable. 5) Attempted obtaining of an egg may be unsuccessful. 6) The egg may not be normal. 7) My husband may be unable to obtain a semen specimen. 8) Fertilization may not occur. 9) Cleavage or cell division of the fertilized egg may not occur. 10) The embryo may not develop normally. 11) Implantation may not occur. 12) A laboratory accident may result in loss or damage to the fertilized egg or embryo.

If pregnancy is successfully established, miscarriage, ectopic pregnancy, stillbirth and/or congenital abnormalities (birth defects) may occur. There is no indication that the occurrence of these are increased or decreased by this procedure.

I understand that insurance coverage for any or all of the above procedures may not be available and that I will be personally responsible for the expenses of this treatment. The expenses will consist of hospital charges, laboratory charges and physician professional fees.

From presently available information I understand that the chances that I will become pregnant by this procedure are between 10 and 20%.

I understand that the following are some of the risks and discomforts associated with the procedure. 1) Blood drawing - mild discomfort and a little risk of developing a bruise at the needle site. 2) Laparoscopy - possibility of bleeding or infection; moderate discomfort after the procedure; possible damage to intestines or other abdominal organs, especially likely if I have had other pelvic surgery. 3) The risks associated with anesthesia. 4) Reimplantation - minimal discomfort, minimal risks of developing infection. 5) Ultrasound examinations - no known risks, minimal discomfort.

If the procedure is successful I understand that I will achieve a pregnancy as well as aid in the development of a technique which may help many couples with similar problems to mine.

I understand that there is no currently available alternative procedure to allow me to become pregnant.

I have had the opportunity to ask any questions I might have about my participation. Future questions will be answered by Dr. Martin Quigley, 713/792-5360.

My participation is purely voluntary. I understand that I may withdraw my consent at any time. My present or future care will not be affected by my decision.

I have been assured that all information about me obtained during this study will be handled confidentially and that neither my identity nor specific medical details will be revealed by the investigators without my consent. Specific medical details may be revealed in professional publications as long as my identity is concealed. It has been recommended that I refrain from granting interviews or having any contact with the news media. All information provided to the media by the investigators will be controlled by the Public Affairs Office of The University of Texas Health Science Center at Houston in coordination with the Office of Public Affairs at Hermann Hospital.

I have been informed that should I suffer any physical injury as a result of participation in this reserch activity all of the necessary medical facilities are available for treatment. I understand, however, that I cannot expect to receive any payment for hospital expenses or any financial compensation for such an injury.

I have read this form and acknowledge receipt of a copy of this form.

____________________ ____________________
Date Wife

____________________ ____________________
Date Husband

____
Witness

---

*This research study has been reviewed by the Committee for the Protection of Human Subjects at The University of Texas Health Science Center at Houston, (713)792-5048.

CONTRIBUTORS

Lori B. Andrews, J.D.
American Bar Foundation, Chicago, Illinois

Pedro J. Beauchamp, M.D.
Department of Obstetrics, Gynecology, and Reproductive Sciences, Medical School, The University of Texas Health Science Center, Houston, Texas

Jeffrey Boldt, Ph.D.
Department of Obstetrics, Gynecology, and Reproductive Sciences, Medical School, The University of Texas Health Science Center, Houston, Texas

William Byrd, Ph.D.
Department of Obstetrics, Gynecology, and Reproductive Sciences, Medical School, The University of Texas Health Science Center, Houston, Texas

Stanley R. Glasser, Ph.D.
Department of Cell Biology, Baylor College of Medicine, Houston, Texas

Bernard Gonik, M.D.
Department of Obstetrics, Gynecology, and Reproductive Sciences, Medical School, The University of Texas Health Science Center, Houston, Texas

Julane Hotchkiss, Ph.D.
Department of Physiology, Graduate School of Biomedical Sciences, The University of Texas Health Science Center, Houston, Texas

Nabil F. Maklad, M.D. Ph.D.
Department of Radiology, Medical School, The University of Texas Health Science Center, Houston, Texas

Sylvia Pace-Owens, R.N.-C.
Department of Obstetrics, Gynecology, and Reproductive Sciences, Medical School, The University of Texas Health Science Center, Houston, Texas

Martin M. Quigley, M.D.
Department of Obstetrics, Gynecology, and Reproductive Sciences, Medical School, The University of Texas Health Science Center, Houston, Texas

Griff T. Ross, M.D., Ph.D.
Department of Obstetrics, Gynecology, and Reproductive Sciences, Medical School, The University of Texas Health Science Center, Houston, Texas

Cecilia L. Schmidt, M.D.
Department of Obstetrics, Gynecology, and Reproductive Sciences, Medical School, The University of Texas Health Science Center, Houston, Texas

Joseph E. Sokoloski, B.S.
Department of Obstetrics and Gynecology, School of Medicine, The University of Mississippi Medical Center, Jackson, Mississippi

Paul D. Webb, Ph.D.
Department of Immunology, The University of Liverpool, Liverpool, United Kingdom

Don P. Wolf, Ph.D.
Department of Obstetrics, Gynecology, and Reproductive Sciences, Medical School, The University of Texas Health Science Center, Houston, Texas

INDEX

Batch number: 10855257

Printed by Printforce, the Netherlands